Textbook of Sports Medicine

Textbook of Sports Medicine

Edited by
Finley Edwards

Larsen & Keller
www.larsen-keller.com

Textbook of Sports Medicine
Edited by Finley Edwards
ISBN: 978-1-63549-010-7 (Hardback)

© 2017 Larsen & Keller

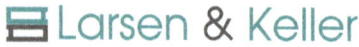

▤ Larsen & Keller

Published by Larsen and Keller Education,
5 Penn Plaza,
19th Floor,
New York, NY 10001, USA

Cataloging-in-Publication Data

Textbook of sports medicine / edited by Finley Edwards.
      p. cm.
Includes bibliographical references and index.
ISBN 978-1-63549-010-7
1. Sports medicine--Textbooks. I. Edwards, Finley.
RC1210 .T49 2017
617.1027--dc23

The publisher's policy is to use permanent paper from mills that operate a sustainable forestry policy. Furthermore, the publisher ensures that the text paper and cover boards used have met acceptable environmental accreditation standards.

Printed and bound in the United States of America.

For more information regarding Larsen and Keller Education and its products, please visit the publisher's website www.larsen-keller.com

Table of Contents

Preface   **VII**

Chapter 1 **Introduction to Sports Medicine**   **1**

Chapter 2 **Popular Sports and Injuries Related to Them**   **6**
    i. Boxer's Fracture   6
    ii. Little League Elbow   9
    iii. Footballer's Ankle   10
    iv. Injuries in Netball   11
    v. Golfer's Elbow   20
    vi. Volleyball Injuries   22
    vii. Swimming Injuries   25
    viii. Tennis Injuries   27
    ix. Musculoskeletal Injury   30
    x. Skin Infections and Wrestling   31
    xi. Sports-Related Traumatic Brain Injury   34
    xii. Sports Injury   45
    xiii. Infectious Disease (Athletes)   54

Chapter 3 **Various Sports Injuries**   **61**
    i. Tennis Elbow   61
    ii. Shin Splints   69
    iii. Achilles Tendon Rupture   72
    iv. Athletic Heart Syndrome   78
    v. Patellar Tendinitis   83
    vi. Commotio Cordis   85
    vii. Patellar Dislocation   88
    viii. Climbing Injuries   94
    ix. Saddle Sore   96
    x. Fencing Response   97
    xi. Female Athlete Triad   99
    xii. Exertional Rhabdomyolysis   104
    xiii. Major Trauma   109
    xiv. Strain (Injury)   119
    xv. Surfer's Ear   120

Chapter 4 **Health Issues in Sports**   **124**
    i. Health Issues in Athletics   124
    ii. Health Issues in Youth Sports   127

Chapter 5   **Physical Exercise: An Overview**   **132**
     i. Physical Exercise   132
     ii. Physical Fitness   217

Chapter 6   **Risk Reduction in Sports Injuries**   **229**
     i. Altitude Training   229
     ii. Conconi Test   235
     iii. Fascia Training   235
     iv. Sports Hypnosis   238
     v. Overtraining   240
     vi. Exercise Hypertension   246
     vii. Athletic Training   246
     viii. Cross-Training   253
     ix. Athletic Trainer   254

Chapter 7   **Treatment and Therapies of Sports Injuries**   **259**
     i. Physical Therapy   259
     ii. Ice Bath   270
     iii. Dry Needling   279
     iv. Tommy John Surgery   286
     v. Aquatic Therapy   289
     vi. Sports Chiropractic   291
     vii. Ulnar Collateral Ligament Reconstruction   293
     viii. Sports Hypnosis   296
     ix. Hypopressive Exercise   297

Chapter 8   **Interdisciplinary Fields of Sports Medicine**   **302**
     i. Sport Psychology   302
     ii. Physical Medicine and Rehabilitation   314
     iii. Sports Science   316
     iv. Orthopaedic Sports Medicine   318
     v. Sports Nutrition   319

Permissions

Index

Preface

Athletic activities and sports can often result in serious injuries. Sports medicine in the modern day is an individual branch of study under medicine which only focuses on injuries related to sports and exercises. This book provides a comprehensive overview of this field along with discussing some of the most popular sports injuries, their diagnosis and treatment as well. It will also glance upon some methods to reduce the risk of injuries in sports and health issues related to it. The aim of this textbook is to serve as a valuable source of reference for anyone interested in this field.

A short introduction to every chapter is written below to provide an overview of the content of the book:

Chapter 1 - Sports medicine has emerged as an independent field of study in the past few decades. This all encompassing chapter provides a brief overview of sports medicine and its fundamental areas which will be further elaborated in the other chapters of this book; **Chapter 2 -** There are a number of popular sports which have specific injuries related to them such as boxer's fracture, footballer's ankle, golfer's elbow, etc. The aim of this chapter is to shed light on such injuries, their causes, diagnostic methodologies and prevention. This chapter will help the readers in understanding these injuries in detail; **Chapter 3 -** This chapter is the further classification of injuries that are listed in chapter two. The following topics will provide the reader an elaborate understanding of the other major types of injuries that are prevalent in sports like tennis elbow, shin splints and saddle sore to name a few. The chapter will offer new perspectives and insights into the field; **Chapter 4 -** Health and sports are closely associated. The major health issues in sports are elaborated in the following chapter. It also presents a detailed account on health issues in athletics and youth sports. It will help readers gain a broader perspective on sports medicine; **Chapter 5 -** Physical exercise is an integral part of sports medicine. This chapter will not only provide an overview of physical exercise but it will also comprehensively discuss about the various types of physical exercises like aerobic exercise, strength training, bodyweight exercise and weight training, etc; **Chapter 6 -** Risk reduction is also a significant aspect of sports medicine. The major risk management strategies related to sports injuries are discussed in this chapter. This chapter is a compilation of various measures to avoid and abort risks of sports injuries. Methods like altitude training, athletic training, conconi test, sports hypnosis amongst others are described to provide an overview on the different practices to reduce risks in sports injuries. It also glances at some reasons that increase the risk of injury in sports such as overtraining, etc; **Chapter 7 -** Preventive measures related to sports are a critical component for understanding sports medicine comprehensively. This chapter unfolds a plethora of preventive measures that are essential in order to deal with injuries and trauma related to sports. The following chapter serves as a source to understand the major preventive techniques like ice bath, dry needling and physical therapy to treat sports related injuries; **Chapter 8** - Sports medicine is an interdisciplinary field of study. It spreads to other fields like sports science, sports psychology, physical medicine and rehabilitation to name a few. This chapter will provide an overview of the various significant fields related to it.

Finally, I would like to thank my fellow researchers who gave constructive feedback and my family members who supported me at every step.

Editor

Introduction to Sports Medicine

Sports medicine has emerged as an independent field of study in the past few decades. This all encompassing chapter provides a brief overview of sports medicine and its fundamental areas which will be further elaborated in the other chapters of this book.

Sports medicine
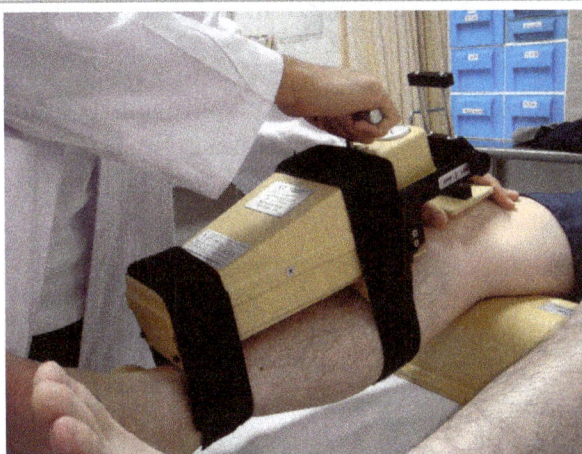
Orthopaedics is a large part of sports medicine, and knee injuries a common theme. Here a subject is having the anterior-posterior laxity of his knee tested..

Sports medicine, also known as sport and exercise medicine (SEM), is a branch of medicine that deals with physical fitness and the treatment and prevention of injuries related to sports and exercise. Although most sports teams have employed team physicians for many years, it is only since the late 20th century that sports medicine has emerged as a distinct field of health care.

Scope

Sport and exercise medicine doctors are specialist physicians who have completed medical school, appropriate residency training and then specialize further in sports medicine or 'sports and exercise medicine' (the preferred term). Specialization in sports medicine may be a doctor's first specialty (as in Australia, Netherlands, Norway, Italy). It may also be a sub-specialty or second specialisation following a specialisation such as physiatry or orthopedic surgery. The various approaches reflect the medical culture in different countries.

Specializing in the treatment of athletes and other physically active individuals, sports and exercise medicine physicians have extensive education in musculoskeletal medicine. SEM doctors treat injuries such as muscle, ligament, tendon and bone problems, but may also treat chronic illnesses that can affect physical performance, such as asthma and diabetes. SEM doctors also advise on managing and preventing injuries.

Specialists in SEM diagnose and treat any medical conditions which regular exercisers or sports persons encounter. The majority of a SEM physicians' time is therefore spent treating musculoskeletal injuries, however other conditions include sports cardiology issues, unexplained underperformance syndrome, exercise-induced asthma, screening for cardiac abnormalities and diabetes in sports. In addition team physicians working in elite sports often play a role in performance medicine, whereby an athletes' physiology is monitored, and aberrations corrected, in order to achieve peak physical performance.

SEM consultants also deliver clinical physical activity interventions, negating the burden of disease directly attributable to physical inactivity and the compelling evidence for the effectiveness of exercise in the primary, secondary and tertiary prevention of disease.

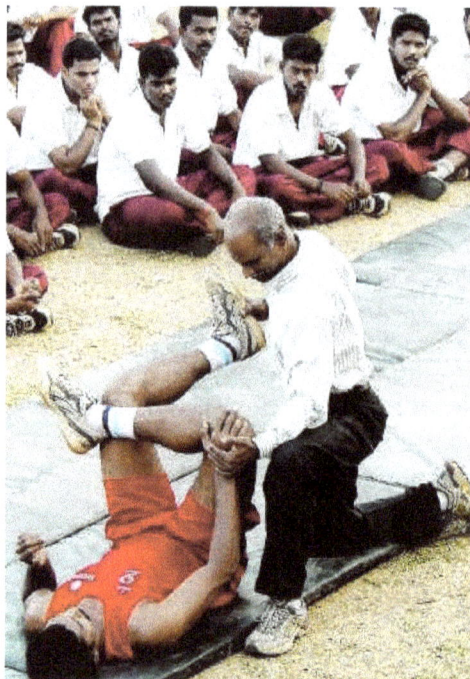

Exercise Medicine

The Foresight Report issued by the Government Office for Science, 17 October 2007, highlighted the unsustainable health and economic costs of a nation that continues to be largely sedentary. It forecasts that the incremental costs of this inactivity will be $10 billion per year by 2050 and the wider costs to society and businesses $49.9billion. Physical inactivity inevitably leads to ill-health and it forecasts the cost of paying for this impact will be unsustainable in the future. No existing group of medical specialists is equipped with the skills and training to deal with this challenge.

The concept of Exercise as Health tool or Exercise is Medicine™ is becoming increasingly important. SEM physicians are able to evaluate medical patients co-morbidities, perform exercise testing and provide an exercise prescription, together with a motivational programme and exercise classes.

Public Health

SEM physicians are frequently involved in promoting the therapeutic benefits of physical activity, exe rcise and sport for the individuals and communities. SEM Physicians in the UK spend a period of their training in public health, and advise public health physicians on matters relating to physical activity promotion. An example of published work includes the Royal College of Physicians publications.

Common Sports Injuries

Concussion – caused by severe head injury where the brain moves violently within the skull so that brain cells all fire at once, much like a seizure

Muscle cramps – a sudden tight, intense pain caused by a muscle locked in spasm. Muscle cramps are also recognized as an involuntary and forcibly contracted muscle that does not relax

ACL sprains – The anterior cruciate ligament (ACL) is a ligament involved in knee stabilization. An ACL rupture can occur when the foot is planted and the knee twists to change direction.

ACL tears – The anterior cruciate ligament; one of four major knee ligament necessary for comfortable knee movement, tears, causing major pain and causes the knee to "give out". The knee ACL can tear for a number of reasons.

Ankle sprain – The ligaments that hold the ankle bones in place can easily be overstretched.

Shin splints – The tissue that attaches the muscles of your lower leg to the shin bone may be pulling away from the bone, or it may be inflamed from overuse.

Muscle strains – tears in muscle that cause pain and or loss of function

History

In recent years Western society has increasingly recognized the dangers of physical inactivity, and significant efforts have been made within the public health community to encourage the nation to become more physically active. To reflect this paradigm shift BASM has renamed itself BASEM (British Association of Sport and Exercise Medicine) and the speciality itself has rebranded from Sports Medicine to Sport & Exercise Medicine. Since 2007 several deaneries across the UK have established training programmes in SEM, and recurrent funding for 50 National Training Numbers (NTN's) is available.

Organizations

- American College of Sports Medicine (ACSM) Founded in 1954, the American College of Sports Medicine is the largest and most prominent sports medicine and exercise science organization in the world. ACSM has more than 45,000 International, National and Regional Chapter members.

- American Orthopaedic Society for Sports Medicine (AOSSM) The American Orthopaedic Society for Sports Medicine is a world leader in sports medicine education, research, communication, and fellowship. Founded in 1972, AOSSM is an international organization of orthopaedic surgeons and other allied health professionals dedicated to sports medicine. Essentially every professional and collegiate team has a team physician who is a member of the AOSSM.

- American Medical Society for Sports Medicine (AMSSM) Founded in 1991, AMSSM is a multi-disciplinary organization of physicians whose members are dedicated to education, research, collaboration and fellowship within the field of Sports Medicine. It now comprises over 2100 Sports Medicine Physicians whose goal is to provide a link between the rapidly expanding core of knowledge related to sports medicine and its application to patients in a clinical setting.

- National Athletic Trainers' Association(NATA) Founded in 1950, the mission of the National Athletic Trainers Association is to enhance the quality of health care provided by certified athletic trainers and to advance the athletic training profession.

- Canadian Athletic Therapists' Association(CATA) Founded in 1965. The Canadian Athletic Therapists Association (CATA) is an organization devoted to the comprehensive health care of an individual at any level of physical ability by Certified Athletic Therapists.

- American Medical Association(AMA) The American Medical Association recognized Athletic Training(AT) as an allied health profession in 1990.

- International Society of Arthroscopy, Knee Surgery and Sports Medicine (ISAKOS) The ISAKOS - International Society of Arthroscopy, Knee Surgery and Orthopaedic Sports Medicine is an international society with over 4,000 surgeons members, dedicated to advancing of education, research and patient care in arthroscopy, knee surgery and orthopaedic sports medicine around the world.

- International Association for Dance Medicine and Science (IADMS) The International Association for Dance Medicine & Science was formed in 1990 by an international group of dance medicine practitioners, dance educators, dance scientists, and dancers. Membership is drawn equally from the medical and dance professions, and has grown from an initial 48 members in 1991 to over 900 members at present world-wide, representing 35 countries.

Popular Sports and Injuries Related to Them

There are a number of popular sports which have specific injuries related to them such as boxer's fracture, footballer's ankle, golfer's elbow, etc. The aim of this chapter is to shed light on such injuries, their causes, diagnostic methodologies and prevention. This chapter will help the readers in understanding these injuries in detail.

Boxer's Fracture

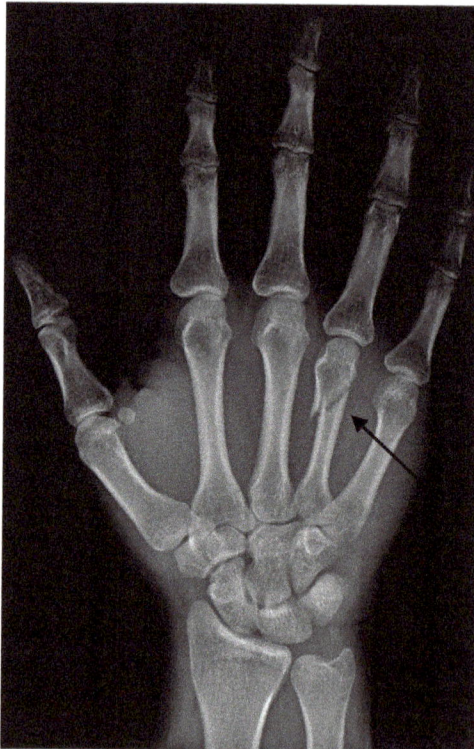

DP (PA) right hand x-ray showing fracture at the neck of fourth metacarpal bone

Boxer's Fracture is a colloquial term for a fracture of one of the metacarpal bones of the hand. Classically, the fracture occurs transversely across the neck of the bone, after the patient strikes an object with a closed fist. Alternate terms include scrapper's fracture or bar room fracture.

As these are colloquial terms, texts and medical dictionaries do not universally agree on precise meanings. Various authorities state that a "Boxer's fracture" means a break in specifically the second metacarpal bone or third metacarpal bone, with "Bar Room fracture" being specific to the fourth metacarpal bone or fifth metacarpal bone. Though some writers assert that Boxer's fracture and Bar Room fracture are distinct terms representing injuries to different bones, this distinction seems to have been lost over time and most medical professionals now describe any metacarpal fracture as a "Boxer's Fracture".

Signs and Symptoms

The symptoms are pain and tenderness in the specific location of the hand, which corresponds to the metacarpal bone around the knuckle. When a fracture occurs, there may be a snapping or popping sensation. There will be swelling of the hand along with discoloration or bruising in the affected area. Abrasions or lacerations of the hand are also likely to occur. The respective finger may be misaligned, and movement of that finger may be limited and painful.

Causes

Metacarpal fractures are usually caused by the impact of a clenched fist with a hard, immovable object, such as a skull or a wall, using improper punching technique. When a punch impacts with improper form, the force occurs at an angle towards the palm, creating a dorsal bend in the bone, ultimately causing the fracture when the bone is bent too far.

When a boxer punches with proper form, the knuckles of the second and third metacarpal align linearly with the articulating radius, followed linearly by the humerus. Due to the linear articulation of bones, the force is able to travel freely across these joints and bones and be dissipated without injury. Therefore, fractures of the second or third metacarpals are rare, with fractures of the 4th and 5th metacarpals comprising the vast majority of metacarpal fractures.

Diagnosis

Diagnosis by a doctor's examination is the most common, often confirmed by x-rays. X-ray is used to display the fracture and the angulations of the fracture. A CT scan may be done in very rare cases to provide a more detailed picture.

Prevention

Boxers and other combat athletes routinely use hand wraps and boxing gloves to help stabilize the hand, greatly reducing pain and risk of injury during impact. Proper punching form is the most important factor to prevent this type of fracture.

Treatment

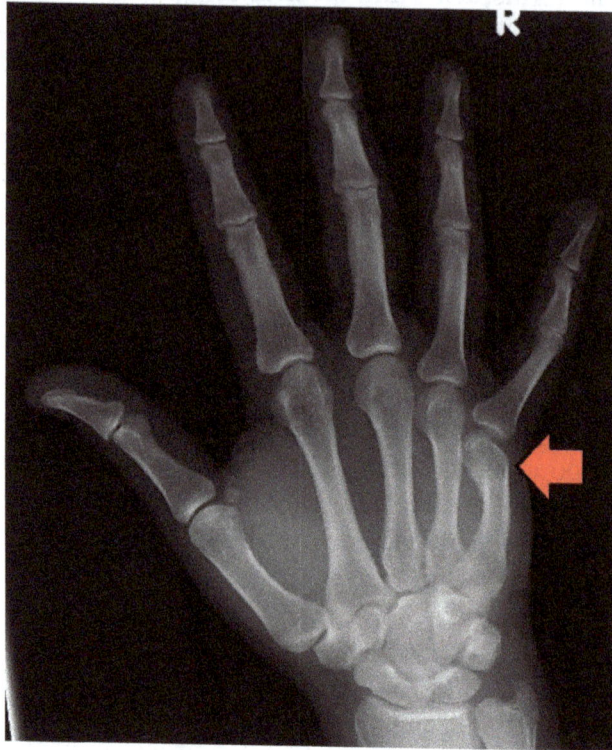

A healed fracture of the base of the 5th metacarpal

Once injured, the subject will feel both the swelling and associated pain in the hand. Ice is applied to relieve pain and swelling. Any open wounds are cleansed to avoid infection. The injured hand must remain immobilized, to avoid moving the broken end of the bone, which can cause damage to the muscles, blood vessels, tendons, ligaments and nerves.

Conservative treatment is to apply a splint to immobilize the affected part of the hand and allow healing. If the broken parts of the bone are misaligned by more than 70 degrees, or if the physician is unable to reduce (realign) the fragments by manipulation, surgery may be required to place pins or plates in the bone to hold the pieces in place.

Prognosis for these fractures is generally good, with total healing time not exceeding 12 weeks. The first two weeks will show significantly reduced overall swelling, with improvement in clenching ability showing up first. Ability to extend the fingers in all directions appears to improve more slowly. Hard casts are rarely required, and soft casts or splints can be removed for brief periods of time to allow for cleaning and drying the skin underneath the splint. Pain from this injury is generally very mild and rarely requires medications beyond over the counter drugs such as ibuprofen or acetaminophen. Muscle atrophy of 5 to 15 percent may be expected, with a rehabilitation period of approximately 4 months given adequate therapy. In the mildest of cases, full rehabilitation status can be achieved within 3 to 4 months.

Epidemiology

Hand and wrist injuries are reported to account for fifteen to twenty percent of emergency room injuries, and metacarpal fractures represent a significant number of those injuries. Hand injuries of this sort are most prevalent among fifteen- to thirty-five-year-old males, and the fifth metacarpal is the one most commonly affected.

Males are nearly fifty percent more likely to sustain fracture from a punch mechanism than females. Male punch injuries are correlated predominantly with social deprivation, while female punch injuries show correlation with psychiatric disorders.

Approximately 3.7 male hand injuries, per 1000, per year, and 1.3 female hand injuries, per 1000, per year, have been reported. Common mechanisms of injury are gender specific. Although the fiscal cost is not available, it can be asserted that the cost is reasonably significant per individual, depending on the cost of emergency care, immobilization, surgery, follow up doctors' visits, etc. in addition to the fiscal impact from loss of and/or limited work abilities.

Little League Elbow

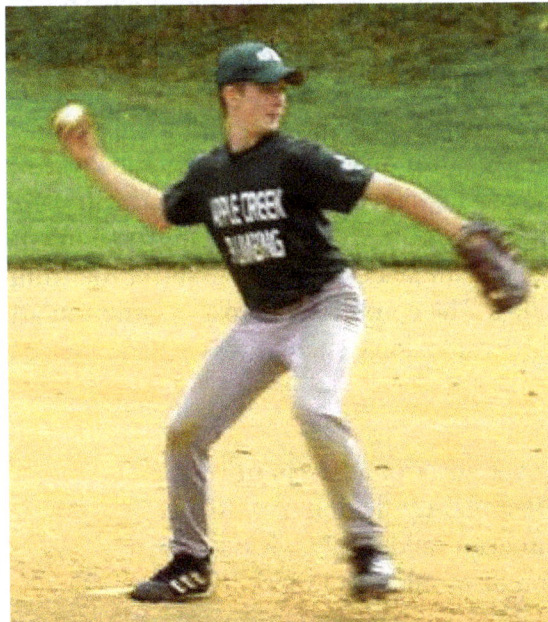

Repetitive overhead throwing motions, like those in baseball, can lead to this medical condition.

Little League elbow is a condition that is caused by repetitive throwing motions, especially in children who play sports that involve an overhand throw. "Little Leaguer's elbow" was first coined by Brogdon and Crow in an eponymous 1960 article in the American Journal of Radiology.

The name of the condition is derived from the game of baseball; it is most often seen in young pitchers under the age of sixteen. The pitching motion causes a valgus stress to be placed on the elbow joint which can cause damage to the structures of the elbow, resulting in an avulsion of the medial epiphyseal plate (growth plate).

The first diagnosis of the injury in 1960 set off a firestorm of controversy regarding how much youth baseball players can and should be asked to pitch. The ailment even appeared in the comic strip *Peanuts* in 1963 when Charlie Brown received a diagnosis. In 2007, in order to protect against overuse injuries, Little League Baseball began limiting the number of pitches a player could throw per day.

Adult pitchers do not experience the same injury because they do not have an open growth plate in the elbow. Instead, in adult athletes a more common injury is to the ulnar collateral ligament of the elbow, an injury that often requires Tommy John surgery in order for the athlete to resume high-level competitive throwing.

Footballer's Ankle

Footballer's Ankle is a pinching or impingement of the ligaments or tendons of the ankle between the bones, particularly the talus and tibia. This results in pain, inflammation and swelling.

Causes

A common cause of anterior impingement is a bone spur on anklebone (talus) or the shinbone (tibia). Repeated kicking actions can cause the anklebone to hit the bottom of the shinbone, which can lead to a lump of bone (or bone spur) developing. This bone spur may then begin to impact on the soft tissue at the front of the ankle, causing inflammation and swelling. The condition is most common in athletes who repeatedly bend the ankle upward (dorsiflexion), such as footballers, hence the name.

Symptoms

- pain and tenderness over anterior ankle joint
- pain on dorsiflexion and plantar flexion
- band of pain across anterior ankle when kicking a ball
- palpable bony lump on distal tibia or superior talus

Treatment

- soft tissue techniques to stretch muscles crossing the ankle to relieve tension
- mobilisation of ankle joint
- steroid injection to reduce inflammation
- surgery to remove bony spurs

Injuries in Netball

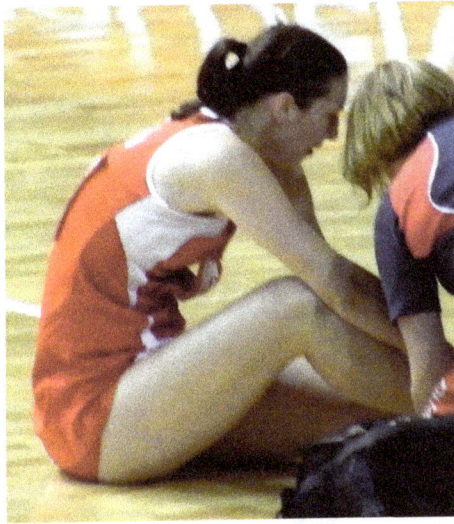

Rachel Dunn from Australia v England - Netball Test - Adelaide, October 2008 with an ankle injury.

Netball is a sport that has one of the largest female participation rates within the commonwealth, most popular in the United Kingdom, Australia and New Zealand, with more than 20 million athletes participating in the sport. Netball is a ball sport played by two teams of seven players in which goals are scored by shooting the ball through a netted ring. Netball relies heavily on muscular endurance and bursts of rapid acceleration to "break free" from an opponent as well as, sudden and rapid change of directions in combination with jumping to receive a pass, intercept a ball or rebound. The sudden stop-start motion of the game is what often leads to serious injuries in participants. Higher grade players, in both senior and junior competitions, are more susceptible to injuries than lower grade players, due to the high intensity and rapid pace of the game. An injury is most commonly defined as one that has occurred while participating in sport and which led to one of the following consequences: a reduction in the amount or level of sports activity; need for medical advice or treatment; and/or adverse economic or social effects for the athlete.

Common Soft Tissue Injuries in Netball

A soft tissue injury is the damage of muscles, ligaments or tendons in the body. The most common soft tissue injuries in netball occur to the ankles, knees and hands. The main cause of these injuries is due to incorrect landing. Other factors influencing injury include; tripping, collisions with other players, being struck by the ball, over-exertion and fatigue.

Ankles

In netball the ankle joint is most susceptible to injury and accounts for 31% of the injuries sustained in the sport. A sprained ankle is a tear or complete rupture of a ligament. The most commonly injured ligament is the Anterior Talofibular Ligament. This ligament is on the outside of the ankle and injury occurs when the sole of the foot rolls inwards. A minor sprain may only need a week to recover, however severe ankle sprains can result in a player being out for 6–10 weeks.

Knees

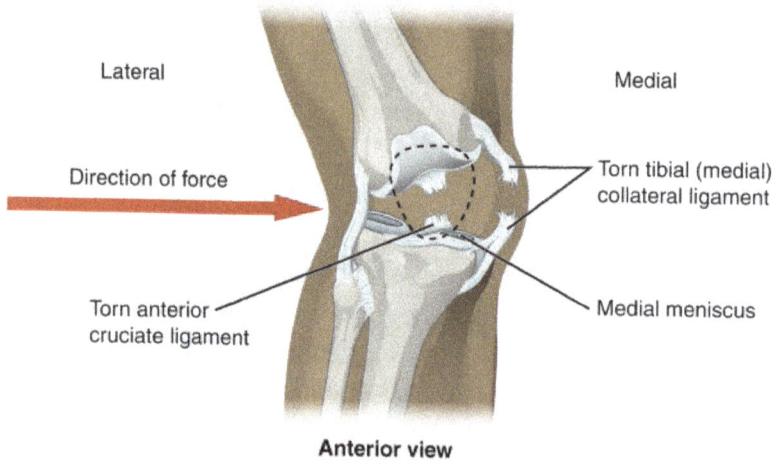

Anterior view

Ruptured Anterior Cruciate Ligament(ACL)

Knee injuries are the second most common injury in netball and are the most serious in regards to cost and disability. Studies show that majority of knee injuries are new injuries, and those who sustain a knee injury often withdraw from participation in netball. The most common knee injuries are meniscal and major ligament sprains/ruptures. The most commonly injured ligament is the Anterior Cruciate Ligament(ACL). The ACL allows a twisting motion at the knee. Common symptoms of an ACL rupture include a "popping" sound at the time of the injury, severe pain, swelling and a feeling of instability. ACL injuries are difficult to effectively diagnose without the assistance of Medical Resonance Imaging (MRI). A ruptured ACL will require knee reconstruction surgery that will result in the athlete being out of the game for 9–12 months.

Hands/Other

Hand injuries usually involve joint ligamentous sprains and fractures. Children most commonly injure hands, in particular their fingers. "Other" types of injuries in netball vary including; lower leg strain, quadriceps haematoma, rotator cuff shoulder problems, an elbow joint dislocation, a radial fracture, and back problems.

Treatment

As soon as an injury occurs game time must be held until the player has been properly assessed and removed from the court if need be. It is essential that players seek immediate help from a qualified first aid provider or health practitioner. Any netball injury should be treated by using the P.R.I.C.E.S., D.R.S.A.B.C., T.O.T.A.P.S. AND R.I.C.E.R. regimes:

P - Protect

R - Rest

I - Ice

C - Compression

E - Elevation

S - Stabilise

D - Danger

R - Response

S - Send for help

A - Airway

B - Breathing

C - Circulation

T - Talk

O - Observe

T - Touch

A - Active movement

P - Passive movement

S - Skills test

R - Rest

I - Ice

C - Compression

E - Elevation

R - Referral

If an injury occurs ensure that all netball players receive adequate treatment and full rehabilitation before returning to play. Serious ankle and knee ligament ruptures will require reconstructive surgery. It is essential to follow all recovery and rehabilitation programs fully to prevent any injury from re occurring.

Netball Injury Prevention

Good Preparation

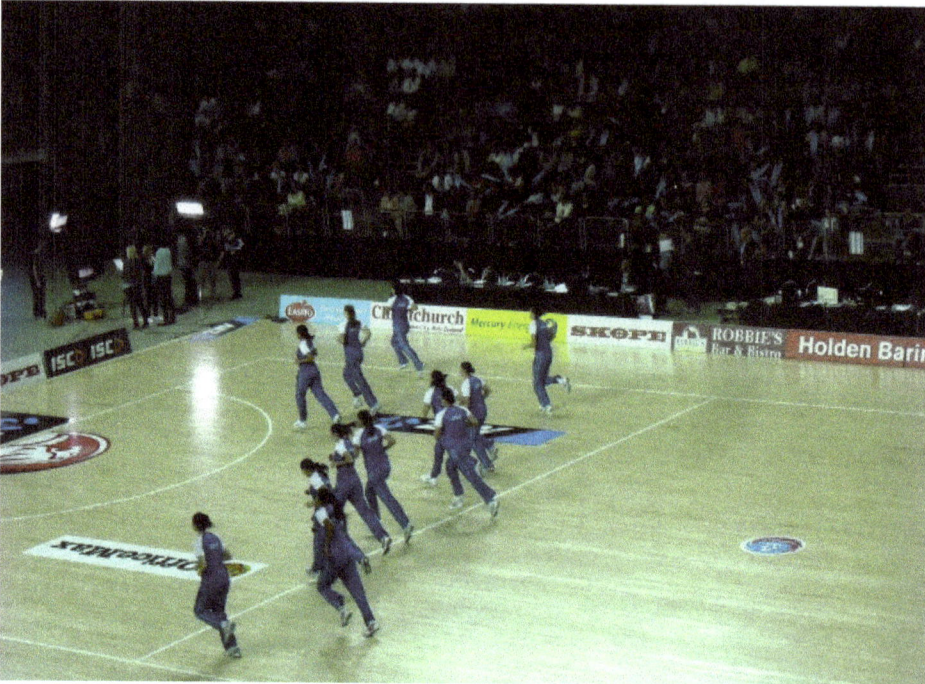

Northern Mystics warming up for their match against the Canterbury Tactix.

In order to prevent netball injuries, essential pre-season training is required before commencing the playing season. The distance travelled by elite players over a game ranges from 7 km (shooters/ defenders) to 8.8 km (centre court players). A game does not only consist of basic running; players are required to accelerate in rapid bursts for the majority of the game. In pre-season training players must undertake fitness programs that focus on power, strength, agility and flexibility, especially of muscles around the ankles and feet. It is important that fitness testing is conducted prior to competition to ensure readiness to play the game.

Good Technique

Training should consist of netball specific exercises that focus on enhancing body balance, landing control, change of direction and catching passes. It is essential for coaches to undergo regular educational updates to make sure the information they have about correct training drills is current. It is very important that children are properly taught the fundamentals of netball before they participate in game situations. Any incorrect techniques should be corrected at a young age before they become a bad habit.

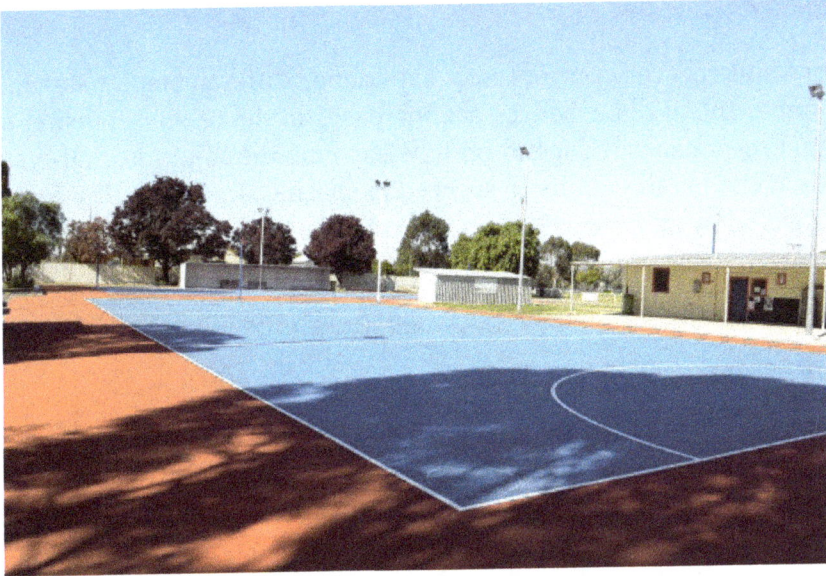

A hard but smooth netball court surface.

Warm Up

A warm-up should never be overlooked in netball as it plays a vital and effective role in preventing injury. A warm-up is essential before physical activity to; prepare the body for vigorous exercise, reduce the risk of injury, reduce muscle stiffness and mentally prepare the athlete. Any warm-up should consist of running, dynamic movements and dynamic stretches. It should last for a minimum of ten minutes.

Equipment/Clothing

In netball it is essential that the goal posts are firmly fixed to the ground and have a padded post protector around them. All courts should be a firm, smooth surfaces with no loose gravel or hazards. The most important uniform item for any netball player is the shoes. It is highly recommended that players wear netball specific shoes, as they are tailored to the demands of the game and provide the correct level of support and cushioning. It is also recommended that players should wear braces or strap their ankles to provide extra support and decrease the risk of a major injury occurring.

Psychological Effects of Having a Major Injury

For many netball players a serious injury can be a traumatic life event that results in physical and psychological ramifications. The main psychological effects include the initial emotional response of experiencing an injury, the psychological factors that influence the recovery process, and the psychological impact of an injury on the athletes future performance. It is important to remember that not all injured athletes will experience the same cognitive and emotional responses.

Emotional Responses

During injury and recovery players may experience different mood states. The most commonly found mood disturbances are increases in depression, tension and anger. The emotional response will depend on how extreme the injury is. Self-efficacy is defined as one's belief in ones ability to succeed in specific situations. Physical self-efficacy is often affected by an injury. Players will often enter an extremely negative state of mind immediately after an injury, however; during recovery they often become exceedingly positive.

Self-Motivation

Most often players will be highly motivated to get back to playing netball as soon as possible. However it is important to remember that injured athletes will have good and bad days. During rehabilitation an athletes motivation and enthusiasm for treatment may decrease if they are experiencing setbacks or a period of little or no improvement. It is important for athletes to have a good support network to keep them positive and focused during these harder times.

Confidence

Physical recovery is critical, however, psychological rehabilitation is the most important part of recovery. Even though a player may be physically ready to return to netball, they may not be psychologically ready to play. Various doubts, fears and anxieties may surface when thinking about returning to netball. The athlete may fear they are going to be a different player, they will not meet their coach or teammates expectations or that their physical fitness will not return to pre-injury state. This will result in the athlete putting a huge amount of pressure on themselves. This anxiety and tension can lead to the following outcomes: reinjury; injury to another body part; lowered confidence resulting in a temporary or permanent performance decrement; general depression; and fear of further injury, which can sap motivation and the desire to return to competition.

Dealing with Psychological Effects

The most successful psychological techniques that aid injury recovery are; good interpersonal communication skills, positive reinforcement, setting realistic goals, knowing methods for positive self-thoughts, coach support, and keeping the athlete involved with the team.

Returning to Pre-Injury Levels & Goal Setting

Determining a successful return to netball from injury for most athletes is the ability to train and compete at pre-injury levels and standards. Measuring this includes things such as; reaching past endurance fitness test levels (beep tests); the ability to perform and complete sport-specific training exercises; and maintaining performance. Achieving these goals at training will best prepare an athlete for what they will experience during competition standards.

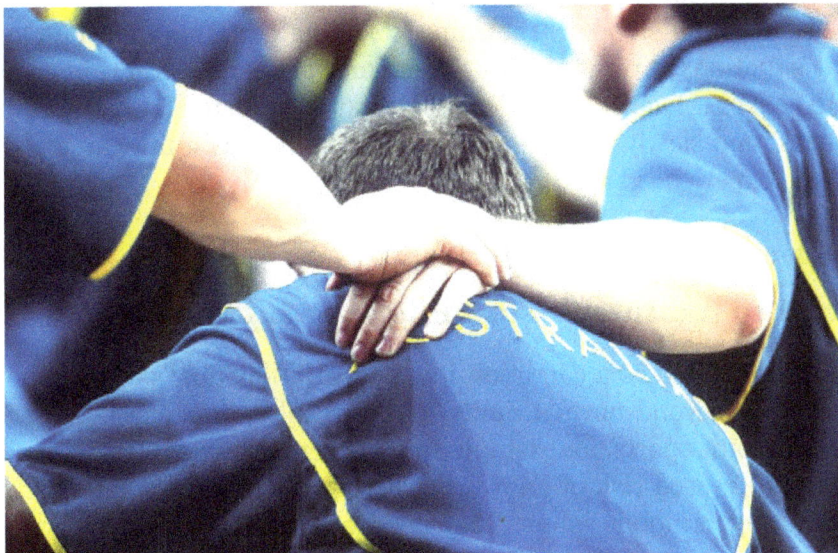

Strong support is needed from teammates, coaches, friends and family.

It is important for the athlete to set realistic goals that they are able to achieve. They must understand that these goals may need to be long term, as not everything can be achieved over night. It is important that goals are flexible because when injured the rehab progress is often unpredictable.

Active Participation in Rehabilitation

Athletes that are engaged in their rehabilitation program are likely to cope with their injury more successfully. Physiotherapists state that athletes who show interest in their rehabilitation by; communicating well, asking questions, listening well to advice, and providing feedback, are more likely to have a positive psychological response to their injury.

Strong Support Systems

It is very important to have social support during the injury, rehabilitation and sports returning phase. This may include coaches, trainers, friends and family. The support of these people is essential for times when the athlete may need positive encouragement around them. The athlete should talk to someone they feel most comfortable with and who is going to listen and support them.

Sports Psychologist

It can be beneficial for an injured player to work with a sports psychologist. Coach and family can be helpful, however there may be times when they are too close to the situation and where an outside point of view is needed to help.

Take It Slow

It is important to remember that there is no rush to get back to netball. Athletes should feel prepared and confident before returning to competition. It is important to take part in game play situations at training. The athlete may also want to start in a lower grade then usual to help ease back into the game. They should aim to play one quarter in their first game back, and slowly build from there aiming to play a full game as they have progressed and experienced success.

Controversies

Hypermobility and Injuries in Junior Netball Players

Hypermobility is defined as a condition in which an individual's synovial joints have a range of motion beyond normal limits. Hypermobile joints can be a performance enhancement in some sports, for example spin bowlers in cricket. However some studies suggest the increased risk of joint dislocations, sprains and joint hyperextension in athletes with hypermobile joints. They believe that recognising hyper mobility in young female athletes may reduce the risk of injuries occurring. On the contrary, others suggest that hyper mobility is not associated with an increased incidence of injuries in junior netball players.

Serious/Career Threatening Injuries in Elite Netball Players

- 2005

In October 2005, Australian captain Liz Ellis, suffered a career-threatening knee injury after tearing her ACL in a match against New Zealand. This injury ruled her out of the chance to play at the 2006 Melbourne Commonwealth games. Ellis said that she had to reignite her passion and love for the game that had been her life. Ellis states that "It was soul-destroying to watch my team walk out without me and realise, hey, they can play without me".

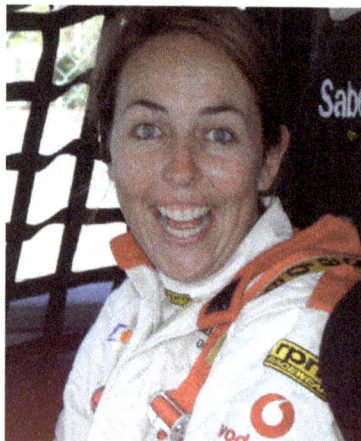

Australian netball player Liz Ellis

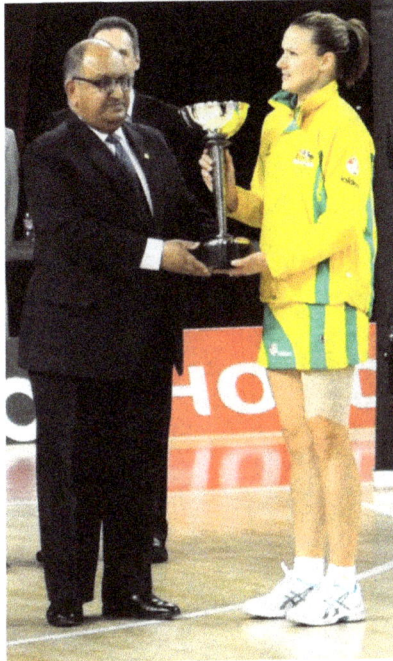

Constellation Cup Presentation 2010

She worked extremely hard on her rehabilitation, her knee repaired and her passion was restored. Ellis produced some of the best netball of her career in the two years that followed. She ended her 18-year career in her 122nd test with Australia winning the world championship 42-38. She overcame all critics and odds after coming back from her knee injury.

- 2012

West Coast Fever captain, Ashleigh Brazill, ruptured the meniscus in her left knee late in the 2012 ANZ championship season. Brazill had been selected to represent Australia in the Constellation Cup, but unfortunately had to withdrawal from the team. Brazil worked to build the strength back in her knee and went on to resume playing in the following 2013 season.

- 2014

In October 2014, KIA Magics inspirational captain, Casey Kopua suffered a knee injury during the Test of the Constellation Cup Series between Australian and New Zealand. Kopua ruptured the patella tendon in her left knee and had knee surgery to repair the tendon that would result in her missing up to 6 months of netball.

- 2015

In April 2015, Melbourne Vixens mid courter, Madi Robinson ruptured the anterior cruciate ligament in her right knee. Robinson missed out on the 2015 Netball World Cup. She is on track to return to play in the 2016 season.

Golfer's Elbow

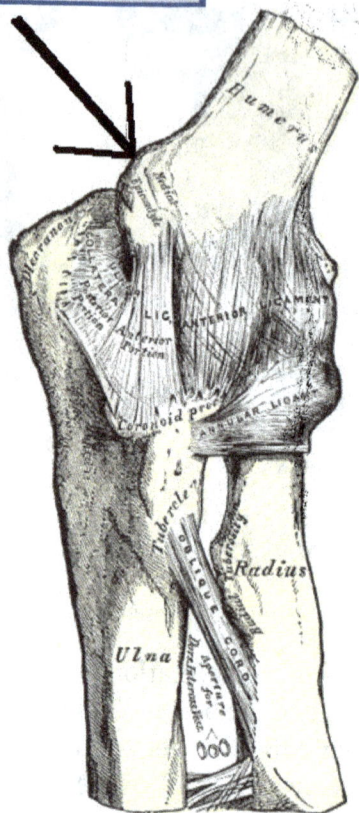

Left elbow-joint, showing anterior and ulnar collateral ligaments.
(Medial epicondyle labeled at center top.)

Golfer's elbow, or *medial epicondylitis*, is tendinosis of the medial epicondyle of the elbow. It is in some ways similar to tennis elbow.

The anterior forearm contains several muscles that are involved with flexing the digits of the hand, and flexing and pronating the wrist. The tendons of these muscles come together in a common tendinous sheath, which originates from the medial epicondyle of the humerus at the elbow joint. In response to minor injury, or sometimes for no obvious reason at all, this point of insertion becomes inflamed.

Causes

The condition is called *Golfer's Elbow* because in making a golf swing this tendon is stressed, especially if a non-overlapping (baseball style) grip is used; many people, however, who develop the condition have never handled a golf club. It is also sometimes called *Pitcher's Elbow* due to the same tendon being stressed by the throwing of objects such as a baseball, but this usage is much less frequent. Other names are *Climber's Elbow* and *Little League Elbow*: all of the flexors of the fingers and the pronators of the forearm insert at the medial epicondyle of the humerus to include: pronator teres, flexor carpi radialis, flexor carpi ulnaris, flexor digitorum superficialis, and palmaris longus; making this the most common elbow injury for rock climbers, whose sport is very grip intensive. The pain is normally caused due to stress on the tendon as a result of the large amount of grip exerted by the digits and torsion of the wrist which is caused by the use and action of the cluster of muscles on the condyle of the ulna.

Epicondylitis is much more common on the lateral side of the elbow (tennis elbow), rather than the medial side. In most cases, its onset is gradual and symptoms often persist for weeks before patients seek care. In golfer's elbow, pain at the medial epicondyle is aggravated by resisted wrist flexion and pronation, which is used to aid diagnosis. On the other hand, tennis elbow is indicated by the presence of lateral epicondylar pain precipitated by resisted wrist extension. Although the condition is poorly understood at a cellular and molecular level, there are hypotheses that point to apoptosis and autophagic cell death as causes of chronic lateral epicondylitis. The cell death may decrease the muscle density and cause a snowball effect in muscle weakness - this susceptibility can compromise a muscle's ability to maintain its integrity. So athletes, like pitchers, must work on preventing this cell death via flexibility training and other preventive measures.

Treatment

Non-specific palliative treatments include:

- Non-steroidal anti-inflammatory drugs (NSAIDs): ibuprofen, naproxen or aspirin
- Heat or ice
- A counter-force brace or "elbow strap" to reduce strain at the elbow epicondyle, to limit pain provocation and to protect against further damage.

Before anesthetics and steroids are used, conservative treatment with an occupational therapist may be attempted. Before therapy can commence, treatment such as the common rest, ice, compression and elevation (R.I.C.E.) will typically be used. This will help to decrease the pain and inflammation; rest will alleviate discomfort because golfer's elbow is an overuse injury. The patient can use a tennis elbow splint for compression. A pad can be placed anteromedially on the proximal forearm. The splint is made in 30–45 degrees of elbow flexion. A daytime elbow pad also may be useful, by limiting additional trauma to the nerve.

Therapy will include a variety of exercises for muscle/tendon reconditioning, starting with stretching and gradual strengthening of the flexor-pronator muscles. Strengthening will slowly begin with isometrics and progresses to eccentric exercises helping to extend the range of motion back to where it once was. After the strengthening exercises, it is common for the patient to ice the area.

Simple analgesic medication has a place, as does more specific treatment with oral anti-inflammatory medications (NSAIDs). These will help control pain and any inflammation. A more invasive treatment is the injection into and around the inflamed and tender area of a long-acting glucocorticoid (steroid) agent. After causing an initial exacerbation of symptoms lasting 24 to 48 hours, this may produce a resolution of the condition in some five to seven days.

The ulnar nerve runs in the groove between the medial humeral epicondyle and the olecranon process of the ulna. It is most important that this nerve should not be damaged accidentally in the process of injecting a golfer's elbow.

If all else fails, epicondylar debridement (a surgery) may be effective. The ulnar nerve may also be decompressed surgically.

The overall prognosis is good. Few patients will need to progress to steroid injection and even fewer, less than 10%, will need surgical intervention.

Volleyball Injuries

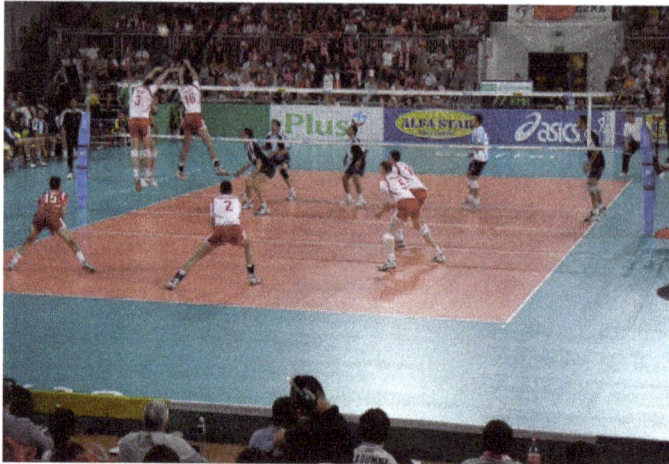

An image of a volleyball match between Poland and Argentina

Volleyball is a game played between two opposing sides, with six players on each team, where the players use mainly their hands to hit the ball over a net and try to make the ball land on the opposing team's side of the court. Volleyball is played by over 800 million people world wide, making it one of the most popular sports in the world. Volleyball has some risks involved with it because there are some injuries which occur to players that are quite common; these include ankle injuries, shoulder injuries, foot injuries and knee injuries.

Ankle Sprains

The Majority of sprained ankles in volleyball occur when a player is at the net, either blocking or Spiking. The reason why ankle sprains occur at the net is because both block-ing and spiking involve jumping and possibly of landing on an opponents foot causing the injury. Approximately 50 percent of all sprained ankles in volleyball occur when a blocker lands on the attacking players foot, while about 25 percent occur when a blocker lands on their own teammates foot following a block with multiple blockers involved.

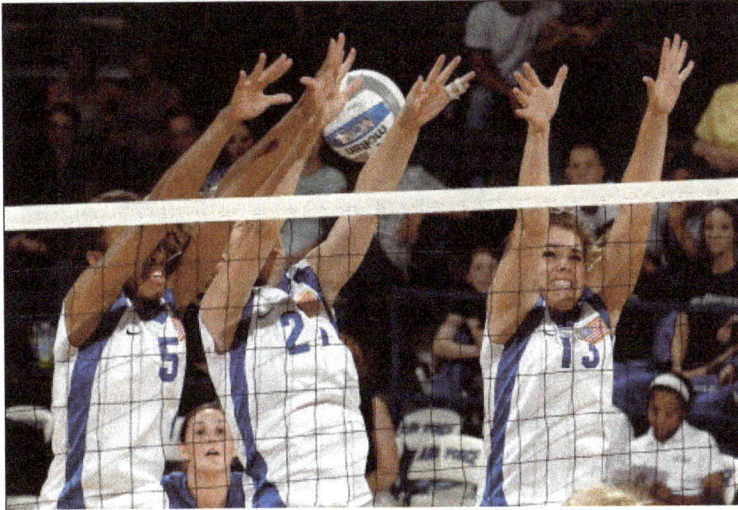

Three teammates who are attempting to block a ball have a greater risk of landing on each other's feet and spraining their ankle.

One possible situation that has the possibility to cause a player to sprain their ankle is when the ball is set to tight or close to the net. As the ball is to close to the net the player who is attempting to spike the ball has to jump closer to the net meaning that they have a higher possibility of landing on or over the center line on the court. By doing this both the blockers and attacker are at an increased risk of spraining their ankle. There are some simple ways in which ankle sprains can be prevented, which include rule changes, technical training and strapping or bracing the ankle.

Shoulder Injuries

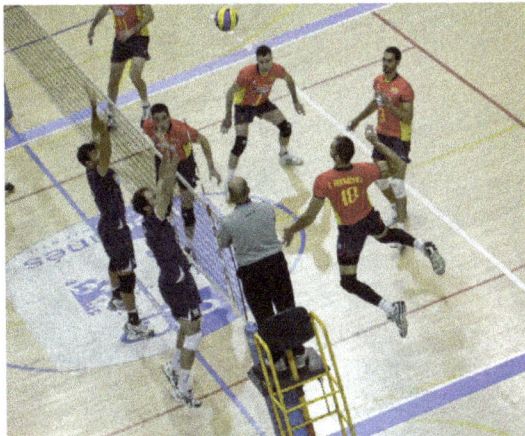

Spiking in volleyball places the shoulder under stress and can result in injury to the shoulder.

There is currently a high number of shoulder injuries in volleyball and it is still unknown to how this number can be managed. Shoulder injuries are great in number because the shoulder is constantly placed under stress during the spiking movements and can often result in injuries to the shoulder. The stress is caused by the rotating of the arm around the shoulder joint at a high velocity. There are however multiple spiking techniques, including traditional and alternative techniques, that have different risks to the shoulder. The alternative spiking method is said to be a possible prevention to some injuries that occur in the shoulder and also enhance an athletes performance.

Jumper's Knee

Jumper's knee is injury term used in volleyball circles that describes the mechanism of the injury known as patella tendinopathy, patella tendinosis or patella tendonitis. Jumper's knee is defined as a syndrome of tendon pain, localized tenderness and swelling that is detrimental to an athletes performance. in the initial phase of the Jumper's knee injury the tendons with the knee are usually inflamed. If Jumper's knee becomes a chronic injury ,which usually occurs as age increases, the tendons show an increasing degree of degeneration and little to no inflation present. As the etiology and pathology of Jumper's knee is not know the treatment varies and is largely based on a trial and error basis.

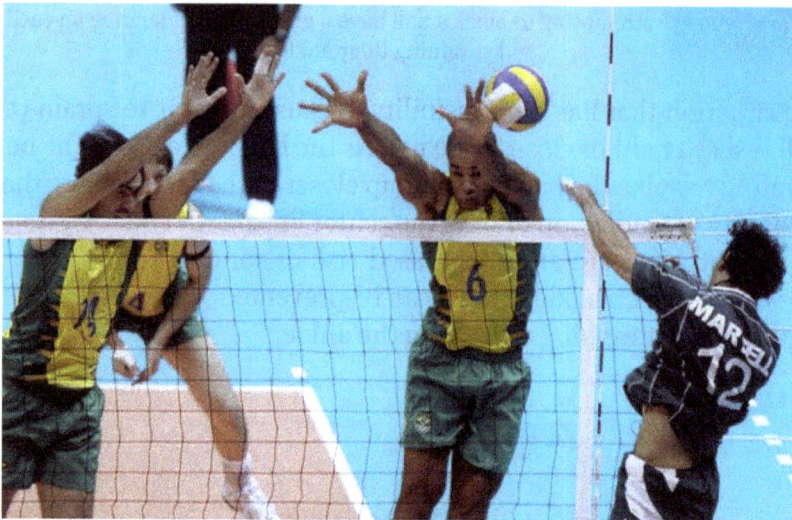

Both blocking and spiking involve jumping and have the possibility to cause Jumper's knee.

Jumpers knee is said to occur after frequent actions involving quick accelerations and declarations, eccentric activities and quick cutting actions. As spiking involves jumping, in which a quick acceleration occurs when jumping and quick deceleration when landing, this action is a possible cause of Jumper's knee. Also blocking is a possible cause of Jumper's knee because it to involves jumping and landing quickly. However, Jumper's knee is less common among athletes who compete in beach volleyball rather than those who play indoor volleyball. This is because beach volleyball is played on sand which reduces the impact of landing on the knee.

Swimming Injuries

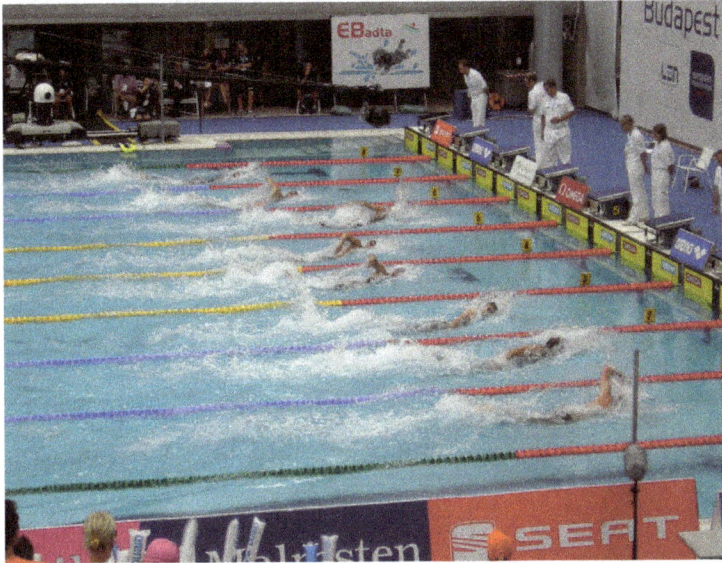

The most common type of injury individuals associate with swimming is pain felt within or around the shoulders, most commonly known as swimmer's shoulder. However while this type of injury may be the most well known injury there are also a few other common injuries associated with swimming. These include knee problems also known as Breastroker's knee and lower back pain also known as Butterfly swimmer's back.

Swimmer's Shoulder

Swimmers shoulder is the name given to a broad range of shoulder injuries that occur in swimmers and results in pain felt within the shoulder and in areas surrounding the shoulder, including down the arm and up the neck. Pain associated with swimmers shoulder often starts as an irritating niggle when swim training and can persist to intense pain while swim training and also a constant pain while resting.

While there are a number of contributing factor leading to the development of swimmers shoulder, it is believed that the two main causes of swimmers shoulder are overuse and the biomechanics of the stroke also known as stroke technique.

The first cause of swimmers shoulder is overuse. Overuse of the shoulder muscles and surrounding muscles can lead to fatigue of the muscles. Due to the muscles being fatigued they are in a weakened state and with continuous use will therefore work less effectively when swimming and will result in the swimmer having to work the shoulder muscles twice as hard by taking double the amount of strokes they would usually take in order to cover the same distance. This would ultimately result in more fatigue and inflammation of the muscles. Unilateral breathing may also cause swimmers shoulder due to the fact that the opposite shoulder to the breathing arm has to work harder to support balanced position and forward movement while the head is turned. Some training equipment such as paddles and kick boards can also put stress on the shoulder and surrounding muscles and cause fatigue and inflammation.

The second cause of swimmer shoulder is the biomechanics of the stroke also known as stroke technique. Incorrect stroke technique for example the swimmers hand entering the water across the mid-line of the swimmers body then proceeding to stroke back or the swimmers hand entering the water palm out thumb down and any other type of incorrect technique when done repetitively can cause pain, fatigue and inflammation of the shoulder and surrounding muscles.

Treatment Methods

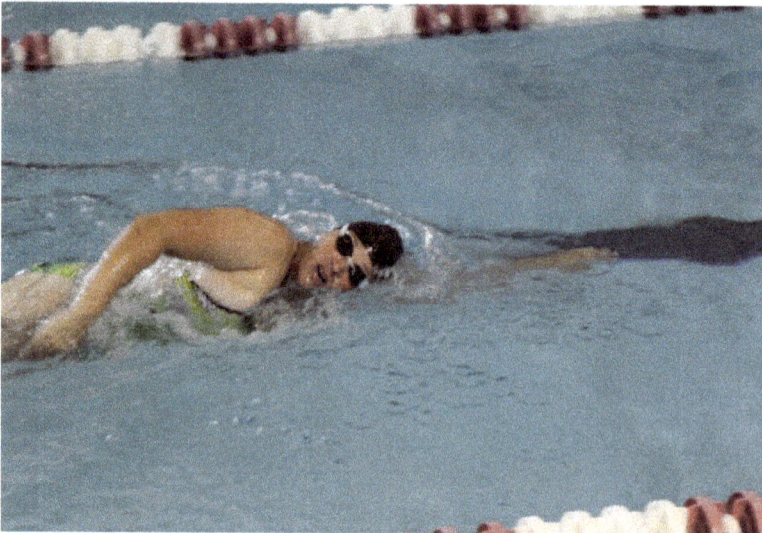

Some treatment methods include; warming up slowly prior to training, avoiding strokes & positions that cause pain (butterfly/freestyle), fixing any bad technique that could be causing the pain, adjusting the distance and frequency of training to avoid further overuse of the muscles, discontinue the use of paddles, increase kick sets to allow the shoulder to rest however limit the use of kickboards and avoid pulling sets. Increase the use of fins to assist with maintaining a good body position and to avoid drag, avoid dry land upper body weight training, ice the shoulder daily, consider the use of anti-inflammatory creams and medicines and seek the advice of a medical professional.

Breastroker's Knee

Breastroker's knee is the name given to pain felt within and around the knee that is experienced by swimmers. It is named this due to the fact it is most commonly only breastrokers that experience pain within the knee and around the knee. Most swimmer will have no problems with their knees however 'the majority (86%) of breaststroke swimmers will have experienced knee pain at one point in their career and 47.2% of them will have had this problem at least one time every week.'

There are several factors that increase the swimmers chances of developing knee pain and inflammation of the knee muscles such as, the increasing age of the swimmer, the length of the competitive career, the length of the event, inadequate warm-up, strength imbalance of hip abductors/adductors and flexibility imbalance of hip abductors/adductors.

Prevention and Treatment

In order to prevent the development of knee pain and inflammation of the knee muscles it is recommended that swimmers use a well-designed strength and stretching program, warm-up adequately, use correct breastroke kick technique, gradually build up the distance of breastroke swimming and have a balanced training program that focuses on not only breastroke and also has training sessions that allows for adequate recovery of the knee muscles to prevent fatigue of the muscles causing overuse, inflammation and pain.

Treatment of breastroker's knee includes resting the knee muscles, icing daily, elevating the limb, strengthening and stretching, support e.g. strapping or knee braces, seeking medical advice which can lead to physiotherapy, cortisone injections and in few cases surgery.

Tennis Injuries

Muscle strain is one of the most common injuries in tennis. When an isolated large-energy appears during the muscle contraction and at the same time body weight apply huge amount of pressure to the lengthened muscle which can result in the occurrence of muscle strain. Inflammation and bleeding are triggered when muscle strain occur which resulted in redness, pain and swelling. Overuse is also common in tennis players from all level. Muscle, cartilage, nerves, bursae, ligaments and tendons may be damaged from overuse. The repetitive use of a particular muscle without time for repair and recover in the most common case among the injury.

Types of Injuries

Lateral Epicondylitis

Lateral epicondylitis is an overuse injury that frequently occur in tennis. It is also known as tennis elbow. This injury categorise as tendon injury where it occur in the forearm muscle called the extensor carpic radialis brevis (ECRB). The injury is regularly developed in the recreational players. Experienced players are less likely to develop lateral epicondylitis than the inexperienced players due to poorer technique. Tennis elbow or lateral epicondylalgia is a common injury that occurs in 40-50% of tennis players.

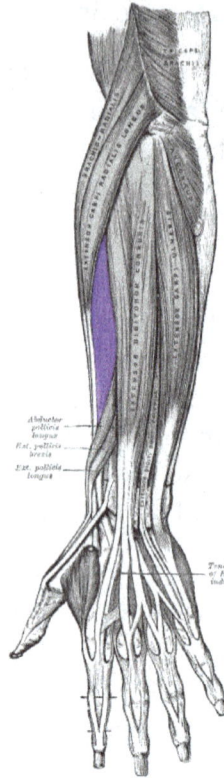

Coloured in purple: the Extensor Carpi Radialis Brevis muscle

It is more prominent at the lower levels of play and usually comes from any incorrect use of the wrist or grip on the forehand or one-handed backhand strokes. Players at higher levels often have more relaxed grips and have a larger racquet extension out to the ball after they make contact, where professionals have less emphasis on the arm and more on the use of every part of the body in order exert the natural power behind the ball, lower level players don't get the training to discover how to use their whole body for a tennis stroke and are often reduced to using their arms in order to exert all of the power therefore putting heavy strain on the arm. Holding the grip tightly will put more tension on the arm therefore when going for a swing the muscles will be absorbing all of the shock from the initial contact of the ball. Symptoms of tennis elbow include the slow pain which occurs around the elbow. Simple tasks such as shaking hands or moving the wrist with force, like lifting weights or doing push ups, will worsen the pain. Tennis Elbow has actually shown that inflammatory tendons are only part of the early stages or acute stages with a treatment of anti-inflammatory or steroids being appropriate uses for this symptom. Most players respond well to simple rest, but other means of treatment include physical therapy, strength training, and electrical stimulation. Some players make alterations to their racquet such as increasing grip size which will ultimately prevent any unwanted movement of the wrist when extending out and finishing the tennis stroke.

ommon types of injury in tennis. Shoulder injury caused by
...oulder when serving and striking the ball. The injury also rele-
... cuffs pathology, toscapular dyskinesis or glenohumeral internal rota-
...it which leads to internal impingement and/or labral pathology. There is 24%
... the high-level tennis players aged 12–19 suffered from shoulder pain and rise up to
50% for middle-aged players.

Back

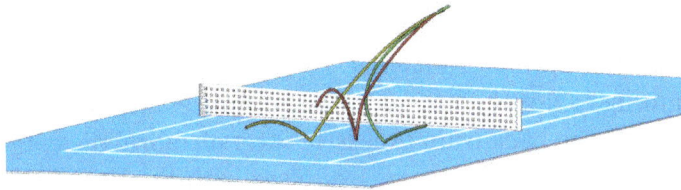

There are 3 different type of tennis serves. Yellow represent: Flat serve Red represent:
Topspin serve Green represent: Slice serve

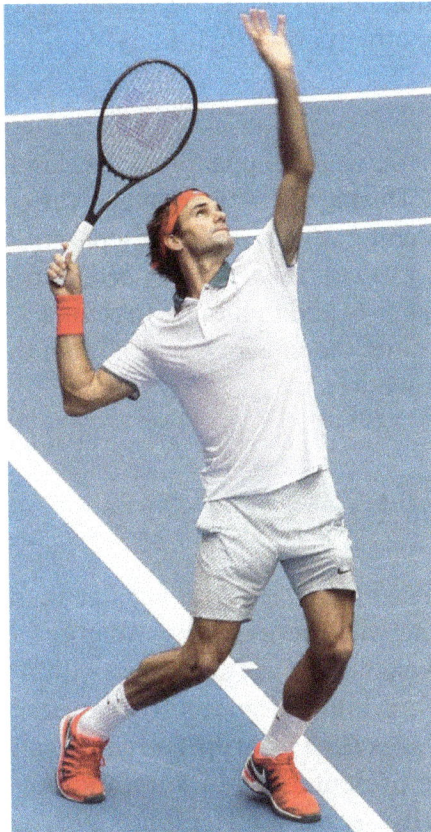

Roger Federer at Australian Open in 2014. Throughout his career back injury always been the problem
for him.

It is common for tennis players in all level of play have experienced back injury th[?] out their career. In fact, more than 85% of the active athletes clarified that they [?] experienced back pain. According to 148 professional tennis player in one particu[?] study, back pain forcing 39% of players to withdraw from the tournament. Furthermore, 29% of the player said they experienced chronic back pain. Lower back pain is the most common injury amongst tennis players with instances of postural abnormalities and general overuse which may occur during the back rotation and extension of the serve. In order to relieve pain in the lower back people are often told to rest it, but not for more than two days because of its potential damage to the bones, connecting tissue, and cardiovascular system. Once the back pain has dispersed stretching is recommended in order to prevent the stiffness from the initial pain, with examples being the squatting position or spinal extensions. In order to prevent future lower back injuries strength training to the abdominal muscles is necessary because with a stronger abdomen it will protect the back from excessive intervertebral disk strain. The straight crunch, the Oblique crunch, and balance exercises with the gym ball are some of the workouts for abdominal strengthening, but the exercises should be done with caution because if done incorrectly the strain on the back will be amplified. After the injury is dealt with, players of any level return to the court, the higher level players will often go through a thorough stretching period before any matches so they can assure that they won't hurt their back or any other part of their body.

Blister

Blister can be described as a patch that appears on the skin filled with a clear fluid and sometimes filled with blood. During physical activities, the continuous force of friction, cutting, squeezing and scratching which cause the separation of the epidermal cell layer, as a result the blister is formed. Blister (foot) occurs frequently among marathon runners, walk racers, backpackers and in hiking. In tennis, blister development site often occur on the hand or around the fingers because often time the skin is consistently rubbing against the tennis racquet.

Musculoskeletal Injury

Musculoskeletal injury refers to damage of muscular or skeletal systems, which is usually due to a strenuous activity. In one study, roughly 25% of approximately 6300 adults received a musculoskeletal injury of some sort within 12 months—of which 83% were activity-related. MI spans into a large variety of medical specialties including orthopedic surgery (with diseases such as arthritis requiring surgery), sports medicine, emergency medicine (acute presentations of joint and muscular pain) and rheumatology (in rheumatological diseases that affect joints such as rheumatoid arthritis). In many cases, during the healing period after a musculoskeletal injury, a period in which the healing area will be completely immobile, a cast-induced muscle atrophy can occur.

Routine sessions of physiotherapy after the cast is removed can help return strength in limp muscles or tendons. Alternately, there exist different methods of electrical stimulation of the immobile muscles which can be induced by a device placed underneath a cast, helping prevent atrophies.

Skin Infections and Wrestling

Skin infections and wrestling is the role of skin infections in wrestling. This is an important topic in wrestling since breaks in the skin are easily invaded by bacteria or fungi and wrestling involves constant physical contact that can cause transmission of viral, bacterial, and fungal pathogens. These infections can also be spread through indirect contact, for example, from the skin flora of an infected individual to a wrestling mat, to another wrestler. According to the National Collegiate Athletic Association's (NCAA) Injury Surveillance System, ten percent of all time-loss injuries in wrestling are due to skin infections.

Common Forms of Infection

Bacterial infections, or pathogens, make up the largest category of include Furuncles, Carbuncles, Folliculitis, Impetigo, Cellulitis or Erysipelas, and Staphylococcal disease. These range in severity, but most are quickly identified by irritated and blotchy patches of skin. Bacterial infections, of all skin infections, are typically the easiest to treat, using a prescribed anti-bacterial lotion or crème.

Molluscum Contagiosum is caused a DNA poxvirus called the molluscum contagiosum virus. For adults, molluscum infections are often sexually transmitted, but in wrestling, it is spread either through direct contact or through contact with shared items such as gear or towels. Molluscum Contagiosum can be identified by pink bulbous growths that contain the virus. These typically grow to be 1–5 millimeters in diameter, and last from 6 to 12 months without treatment and without leaving scars. Some growths may remain for up to 4 years. Treatment for Molluscun Contagiosum must be designated by a healthcare professional because they can be dangerous. Usually for treatment liquid nitrogen can be used to freeze the molluscum off but other methods include other creams that burn the warts off, or oral medications.

The herpes simplex virus comes in two different strains, though only one is spread among wrestlers. Type 1 (HSV-1) can be transmitted through contact with an infected individual, and usually associated with sores on the lips, mouth, and face. HSV-1 can also cause infection of the eye, or even infection of the lining of the brain, known as meningoencephalitis. The lesions will heal on their own in 7 to 10 days, unless the infected individual has a condition that weakens the immune system. Once an infection occurs, the virus will spread to nerve cells, where it remains for the rest of the person's life. Occasionally, the virus will suddenly display recurring symptoms, or flares. There is no complete treatment for Herpes Simplex 1 but there is prescription medication to help ease and relieve the symptoms of the virus. Antiviral oral medication and topic medication can be prescribed to relieve the pain and soreness of the herpes virus.

Verrucae are small skin lesions which can be found on the bottom surface of the foot. They vary in length, from one centimeter in diameter upwards. Verrucae are caused by the human papilloma virus, which is common in all environments but does often attack the skin. The color of the lesion is usually paler then the normal tone of the skin, and is surrounded by a thick layer of calloused skin. Depending on the development of the Verrucae, the surface may show signs of blood vessels, which feed the infection.

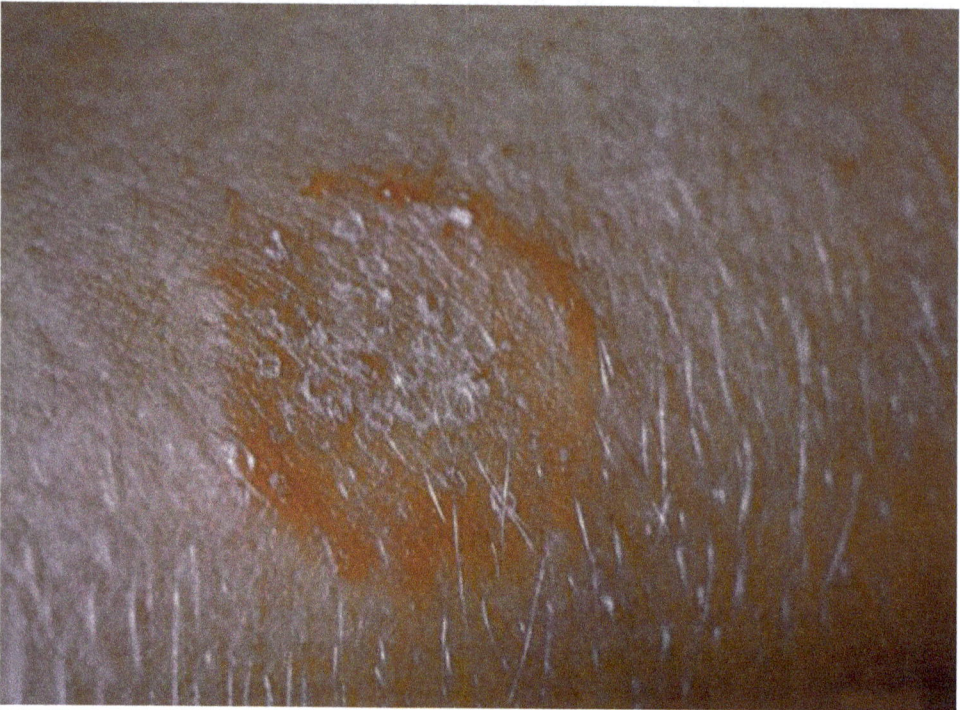

Advanced Tinea Corporis

Tinea infections, more commonly known as Ringworm, are the most common skin infections transmitted through wrestling. It is caused by parasitic fungi that survive on keratin, an organic material that is found in skin, hair, and nails. There are several varieties of Tinea, which are classified depending on their location. Tinea corporis is found on the body, tinea cruris (jock itch) on the groin, tinea capitis on the scalp, and tinea pedis (athlete's foot) on the foot. Although they are not harmful, they are highly contagious and difficult to treat. The symptoms of ringworm include patches of skin that are red, swollen, and irritated, forming the shape of a ring. Ringworm will last between two and four weeks with treatment. Tinea infections can be combatted orally or topically with numerous amount of different medications. Some topical treatments include Mentax 1%, Lamisil 1%, Naftin 1% and Spectazole and these creams should be applied two times a day until the infection is gone. Oral treaments for Tinea include Lamisil, Sporanox, and Diflucan.

Rules

At the start of each wrestling meet, trained referees examine the skin of all wrestlers before any participation. During this examination, male wrestlers are to wear shorts; female wrestlers are only permitted to wear shorts and a sports bra. Open wounds and infectious skin conditions that cannot be adequately protected are considered grounds for disqualification from both practice and competition. This essentially means that the skin condition has been deemed as non-infectious and adequately medicated, covered with a tight wrapping and proper ointment. In addition, the wrestler must have developed no new lesions in the 72 hours before the examination. Wrestlers who are undergoing treatment for a communicable skin disease at the time of the meet or tournament shall provide written documentation to that effect from a physician. This documentation should include the wrestler's diagnosis, culture results (if possible), date and time therapy began, and the exact names of medication for treatment. These measures aren't always successful, and the infection is sometimes spread regardless.

Prevention

According to the NCAA Wrestling Rules and Interpretations, used by all high schools in the United States: "Infection control measures, or measures that seek to prevent the spread of disease, should be utilized to reduce the risks of disease transmission. Efforts should be made to improve wrestler hygiene practices, to utilize recommended procedures for cleaning and disinfection of surfaces, and to handle blood and other bodily fluids appropriately. Suggested measures include: promotion of hand hygiene practices; educating athletes not to pick, squeeze, or scratch skin lesions; encouraging athletes to shower after activity; educating athletes not to share protective gear, towels, razors or water bottles; ensuring recommended procedures for cleaning and disinfection of wrestling mats, all athletic equipment, locker rooms, and whirlpool tubs are closely followed; and verifying clean up of blood and other potentially infectious materials." More ways of prevention include wearing long sleeve shirts and sweatpants to limit the amount of skin to skin contact. A wrestler should also not share their equipment with other teammates and should regularly check their skin for any lesions or other signs of outbreaks. Body wipes are also common to see Coaches must also enforce the disinfecting and sanitary cleansing of the wrestling mats and other practice areas. This can greatly limit the spread of skin infections that can infect an individual indirectly.

One high school wrestling coach from Southern California described his methods of prevention using three simple procedures. "Keep the mats [clean]...you've got to bleach and mop them every day before practice. Along the same lines, gear should also be washed regularly, especially headgear...Most importantly, the wrestlers need to shower immediately after practices. If one kid doesn't, and he gets [infected], it can spread to everyone else on the team within a week. I've had it happen before, to the point where some schools won't allow any of our guys to wrestle in a meet. When this happens, it's a huge blow to the school's record and reputation. In the future, we are less likely to be invited to exclusive tournaments in the coming year."

Treatment

For every form of contagious infection, there is a readily available form of medication that can be purchased at any pharmacy. It is a commonly held belief among wrestlers, however, that these ointments do not treat symptoms Sometimes wrestlers who don't want to report an infection to their coach will resort to unusual and unhealthy treatments. Included among these 'home remedies' are nail polish remover, bleach, salt, and vinegar solutions, which are used to either suffocate or burn the infection, often leaving extensive scars. The remedies, while sometimes successful, are not guaranteed to actually kill the infection, often only eliminating visible symptoms temporarily. Even though the infection may no longer be symptomatic, it can still be easily transmitted to other individuals. Because of this, it is recommended that wrestlers attempting to treat skin infections use conventional medicine, as prescribed by a physician.

Significant Outbreaks

HSV-1 (July 1989) – An outbreak of Herpes Simplex was reported at a four-week high school wrestling camp in Minneapolis, which was attended by wrestlers from 26 states and 1 Canadian province. According to a report on the outbreak: "Wrestlers wore jerseys during practice sessions, but the use of headgear was optional. Wrestling mats were mopped twice each day with disinfectant. Epidemiologic and clinical data were collected during the final two days of the camp after officials alerted the Minnesota Department of Health, which, in turn, alerted the Centers for Disease Control. Results from 171 wrestlers (of 175 attendees) showed that 35 percent (60 boys) met the case definition for HSV-1 infection."

Sports-Related Traumatic Brain Injury

A sports-related traumatic brain injury is relatively uncommon, yet it is a serious accident which may lead to significant morbidity or mortality. Traumatic brain injuries (TBIs) have reduced in frequency and severity from years past due to the development of standardized rules and organized athletics. TBI in sports are usually a result of physical contact with another person or stationary object, these sports may include boxing, football, field/ice hockey, lacrosse, martial arts, rugby, soccer, wrestling, auto racing, cycling, equestrian, roller blading, skateboarding, skiing, or snowboarding.

A study was completed identifying the severity and frequency traumatic brain injuries occurred in high school sports:

"Of 23,566 reported injuries in the 10 sports during the 3-year study period, 1219 (5.5%) were MTBIs. Of the MTBIs, football accounted for 773 (63.4%) of cases; wrestling, 128 (10.5%); girls' soccer, 76 (6.2%); boys' soccer, 69 (5.7%); girls' basketball, 63 (5.2%); boys' basketball, 51 (4.2%); softball, 25 (2.1%); baseball, 15 (1.2%); field hockey, 13 (1.1%); and volleyball, 6 (0.5%). The injury rates per 100 player-seasons were 3.66 for football, 1.58 for wrestling, 1.14 for girls' soccer, 1.04 for girls' basketball, 0.92 for boys' soccer, 0.75 for boys' basketball, 0.46 for softball, 0.46 for field hockey, 0.23 for baseball, and 0.14 for volleyball. The median time lost from participation for all MTBIs was 3 days. There were 6 cases of subdural hematoma and intracranial injury reported in football. Based on these data, an estimated 62,816 cases of MTBI occur annually among high school varsity athletes participating in these sports, with football accounting for about 63% of cases."

The most common TBIs in sports are cerebral contusions, second impact syndrome concussions, dementia pugilistica, and hematomas.

Concussions

Epidemiology

A concussion is defined as a stunning, damaging, or shattering effect from a hard blow; especially: a jarring injury of the brain resulting in disturbance of cerebral function. Concussions are also sometimes referred to as mTBI (Mild Traumatic Brain Injury). Concussions are injuries to the head which cause a temporary lapse in the normal operation of brain function. Concussions have many symptoms which could be displayed in a physical, psychological or emotional manner. Concussions symptoms can sometimes be hard to determine because they present in a subtle manner. A symposium was held in 2008 in Zurich, Switzerland where a definition for concussions was developed. A concussion is now defined as "a complex pathophysiological process affecting the brain, induced by traumatic biomechanical forces."

There are five major features in conjunction with the definition:

- Concussion may be caused either by a direct blow to the head, face, or neck or elsewhere on the body with an "implosive" force transmitted to the head.

- Concussion typically results in the rapid onset of short-lived impairment of neurologic function that resolves spontaneously.

- Concussion may result in neuro-pathological changes, but the acute clinical symptoms largely reflect a functional disturbance rather than a structural injury.

- Concussion results in a graded set of clinical symptoms that may or may not involve loss of consciousness. Resolution of the clinical and cognitive symptoms typically follows a sequential course; however, it is important to note that in a small percentage of cases, post concussive symptoms may be prolonged.

- No abnormality on standard structural neuroimaging studies is seen in concussion.

Signs and Symptoms in Sports

Signs and symptoms of concussions can be hard to determine because they may not present strongly and because they may not present for several hours after the incident has occurred. There are 4 categories that symptoms of a concussion can be classified within: physical, cognitive, emotional and sleep disturbance. The most common symptom is a headache as well as the feeling of being "fog like". Other, more subtle symptoms that can accompany headaches are emotional changes, irritability, slowed reaction times and drowsiness. Accompanying symptoms can include sensitivity to light, and noise, fatigue, dizziness, nausea and vomiting. The loss of consciousness is another identifiable characteristic of concussions but it is not a required symptom to diagnose it. The loss of consciousness occurs in only 10% of concussions, so it cannot be a reliable sign of a concussion. Other distinguishing characteristics of concussions are retrograde amnesia (loss of memory just prior to injury) and posttraumatic amnesia (impaired recall of time between the injury or resumption of consciousness and the point at which new memories are stored and retrieved).

Diagnosis in Sports

There are many diagnostic tools and tests within sports. While the tests and scales may vary greatly from sport to sport, in the end, they effectively gain the same information regardless. The first initial assessment that should take place with every athlete found to be unconscious after head or neck trauma is the "ABC's" (airway, breathing, and circulation). There is an array of initial sideline evaluations that can be conducted after a possible concussive incident such as Maddocks questions, Standardized Assessment of Concussion (SAC), Balance Error Scoring System (BESS), or Sport Concussion Assessment Tool 2 (SCAT2). "The Maddocks questions are a brief set of questions to evaluate orientation as well as short and long-term memory related to the sport and current game. The questions are for sideline use only and are included in the SCAT2." The BESS test is a test based on an athlete's posture. There are 3 positions that the athlete tests in and a composite score of their errors over the 6 rounds of testing determines their scores. The SCAT2 uses both the BESS and SAC test. Limited research of the test since its release from the Zurich Concussion statement has not allowed it to be verified as a successful testing method. Many major professional sports organizations like the NFL, NHL, MLB and NBA have taken stronger looks at in game concussions through extensive studies to develop safer equipment and playing conditions for the players. In doing this they have developed their own initial sideline testing and concussion protocols. The NFL has adopted a standardized testing evaluation form based on the SCAT2 that it has implemented into all head and neck trauma incidents. In 2011 the NFL changed their concussion protocol and built upon their previous SCAT2 standardized test. "The new implementations include a focused screening neurological examination to exclude cervical spine and intracranial bleeding, assessment of orientation, immediate and delayed recall, concentration, as well as a balance evaluation."

Similarly in 2011, the NHL adopted a new league wide concussion protocol which would remove players from the bench, who may have possibly sustained head or neck trauma, and bring them back to an undisclosed quiet room. Players would be held there for a minimum of 15 minutes while completing tests similar of those to the NFL's testing protocol. In 2007 Major League Baseball also adopted a concussion program for umpires and players. In 2011 the policy was revised and 4 new features were added to the program. The first of which is that all umpires and players are to conduct base line testing during spring training or after a player signing. Secondly, the SCAT2 has been adopted as the official sideline test for all MLB teams. Thirdly, a 7-day disabled list has been set up for players with concussions; players on the list for 14 days are moved to the 15-day disabled list. Lastly, the leagues medical director must clear all players who have suffered a concussion before they can return to play. Of the four major professional sports in the U.S., the NBA is the only league to have not adopted a sideline concussion policy. Each team and their medical staff proceed differently with their policies.

Prognosis (Short/Long-Term Effects)

Short-Term Effects

Short-term effects deal mostly with Post-concussion Syndrome, which has no clearly defined definition. A person suffering from a single concussive incident typically has a strong recovery rate. The most common Post-concussion symptom is a persistent headache which usually disappears within 1–2 weeks. Other common short-term effects include dizziness, vomiting, nausea, sensitivity to light and sound, irritability, cognitive lapses and memory impairment. 20-90% of the persons affected develop one symptom within a month of the incident, after 3 months 40% of the affected persons show at least 3 symptoms.

Long-Term Effects

Receiving multiple concussive incidents has long been known to cause a cumulative effect on the brain. It is also known that each successive concussion makes it easier to obtain another concussion in the future. Receiving multiple concussions can lead to long-term memory loss, psychiatric disorders, brain damage and other neurological disorders. There are no clearly defined guidelines for the retirement of an athlete, but it has been proposed that an athlete who sustains 3 concussive incidents in a single season or has Post-concussion symptoms for more than 3 months should consider a lengthy period away from the sport. Especially with sports, when multiple concussions are received it is likely that a doctor will advise the player in question to avoid returning to sports where contact is possible.

Second-Impact Syndrome

Second-impact syndrome (SIS) occurs when an athlete sustains a second concussive incident before the symptoms of a prior concussive incident have fully healed. It does not take a severe concussion to cause SIS, even a mild grade concussion can lead to it. The condition is often fatal, and if death does not occur severe disability is probable. SIS is most often developed in young athletes, who are thought to be particularly vulnerable.

Prevention In Sports

Helmets

Throughout the progression of contact sports there have been continual innovations in protective gear, especially in terms of limiting head and neck traumas. The earliest known use of football helmets is documented in an 1893 Army-Navy game. Early helmets were typically only constructed of leather padding. Throughout the early 1900s helmets developed to include metal and plastics to better protect the player. In 1939 helmets became mandatory for college players, and a year later the NFL adopted the same policy. The increasing development and standardization of helmets along with rule changes that would protect players, would eventually cut down on head and neck traumas. In 2012 testing is being conducted on a new type of helmet which battles rotational acceleration which is linked closer to concussions than typical impacts. This helmet is called the Multidirectional Impact Protection System (MIPS). This new generation of helmet is shown to decrease rotational acceleration by 55% compared to the traditional football helmet. Like the NFL the NHL took steps to protecting players by mandating helmets in 1979. As of 2009 about 60% of NHL players currently wear a half visor for upper face protection.

Mouth Guards

Many sports including football, ice hockey, lacrosse, field hockey, and boxing implemented mandatory mouth guard policies during the 1960s and 70's. These policies were introduced to cut down on a player's chance of orofacial injury and concussions. Several studies conducted in many various professional and collegiate sports have yet to validate the claim that mouth guards cut down on concussions; although a study conducted by the NHL showed that symptom severity had significantly decreased with the use of mouth guards.

Cerebral Contusions

Epidemiology

Cerebral contusions are bruises to the brain caused by a direct blow to the head causing the brain to bounce against the inside of the skull and bruise brain tissue. The force of the blow causes either a tearing or twisting of the structure and blood vessels which hinders the ability of the receptors to send feedback to the brain. With the tearing or twisting of structure, the brain begins to swell and bleed. Since the brain cavity has no room to expand due to the swelling, bruises begin to form. Due to the nature of the injury, most of the contusive damage is found deeper in the brain.

In sports, most cerebral contusions are caused when the brain is either suddenly accelerated, decelerated, or strikes an immovable object. When the blow happens, brain tissue can be damaged, sometimes resulting in the need for hospitalization and surgery. A resection of the contused tissue is needed within surgery pending the severity of the incident. The highest rates of contusions occur in men between the ages of 15 to 24, somewhat due to their aggressive nature. If a person sustains a contusion one time, they are more likely to sustain a repeated one.

Signs And Symptoms In Sports

In the heat of a game, it may be hard to see or feel symptoms relating to cerebral contusions. If any of these signs are visible or as an athlete, you feel them, remove yourself from competition immediately. Cerebral contusions and other injuries can occur in any sport, not just in the traditional "collision" sports. According to the USCPSC, four of the top five sports that cause brain injuries are considered to have limited brain contact: basketball, bicycling, baseball, and playground activities. The most popular sport to cause cerebral contusions is American football due to the drastic acceleration/deceleration of the brain.

Immediate Signs of a Cerebral Contusion

- Headache
- Nausea
- Slurred speech
- Restlessness
- Pupil dilation
- Memory loss
- Personality shift
- Seizures

Post-Game Symptoms

- Loss of consciousness
- Severe headaches
- Coma (due to loss of consciousness)

If any of these symptoms are felt or noticed, a hospital visit is needed where further machine testing is done. In boxing, the rapid deceleration of the brain after an impact causes the symptoms to progress much faster or at a more traumatic rate. Doctors ringside monitor a boxer's attitude and brain function throughout the fight and are able to stop the match following startling news.

Diagnosis In Sports

Contusions are identified with two forms of diagnosis: acceleration of the brain and direct trauma. A direct trauma injury is much more severe than an acceleration injury (in most cases) and requires much more intensive diagnosis and testing. The full extent of the injury may not be known until testing done in a hospital is complete.

In football, medical trainers are well versed to diagnose symptoms pertaining to a traumatic brain injury. They are not, however, able to determine what type of injury it is or the extent the injury stems. Football trainers can medically clear or not clear players based on brain injury symptoms. If a trainer feels that certain symptoms exist that are similar to that of cerebral contusions, they will take the player out of the game and rush them to the hospital. Upon admission into the hospital, a CT scan will be ordered. A CT scan is the quickest method to diagnose cerebral contusions because it can be performed immediately and have fairly exact findings. The best method, as suggested by medical doctors, is an MRI because they present more sensitive and accurate findings. MRI's, however, must be scheduled and cannot be completed immediately following the injury. MRI's also take a long time to perform where the injury a player sustained may get worse within that time frame.

Case Study Example

History: The individual is possibly unconscious when examined by medical personnel on the field. A common symptom is prolonged unconsciousness (coma), however this player reports headache, dizziness, nausea, vomiting, and weakness of the extremities (paresis) and makes inappropriate responses to questions.

Physical exam: The individual's level of consciousness is disturbed. A neurological examination may not reveal any localizing signs. The individual with no other serious injuries than cerebral contusion will not have a fractured skull or any signs of opening or penetration of the skull.

Tests: Skull x-rays check for a fracture. CT or MRI detect any bleeding in the skull. The Glasgow Coma Scale classifies the severity of brain injury, with a score of 15 as normal and progressively lower scores indicating greater neurologic injury to the brain.

After testing is completed, doctors will make an estimate on the extent of the injury and possible recovery time. If cranial bleeding and swelling is minor, a short hospital stay (up to a week) is needed with close observation. If bleeding is severe, the player may be treated as a patient with a severe head injury (with surgery as the main option).

This process requires the patient to be admitted into an intinsive care unity with close monitoring of blood levels and brain activity.

Prognosis (Short/Long-Term Effects)

The effects of a cerebral contusion depend on the cause of the injury and what part of the brain was most affected. Outcomes vary from minor injuries that require short recovery times to severe injuries that can lead to death. Short-term effects of cerebral contusions can range from a mild headache to feeling lightheaded for a few days. Most short-term effects match that of a mild head injury while long-term effects can be much more serious. Most long-term injuries require surgery, rehabilitation, and close monitoring. In small cases, cerebral contusions can lead to death (about 15 per 100,000 people). If a cerebral contusion leads to a coma, recovery can be very long and rehabilitation extensive. If the coma is long, the probability of dying or permanent neurological damage is very possible.

Prevention in Sports

Rules exist within each sport to help prevent cerebral contusions and traumatic brain injuries. However, individual athletes are the best prevention against their own injuries. In a game, athletes notice when they have the symptoms of a cerebral contusion and should take themselves out of the game. It may be hard for medical personnel or coaches to notice when a player has a traumatic brain injury, so it is in the player's best interest to be removed from play. In hockey, traumatic brain injuries constitute 10%-15% of all head injuries. With the high percent of injuries being traumatic, extensive design improvements have been made to helmets. These improvements reduce the risk of cerebral contusions by providing more padding around the skull and a chin strap that keeps the helmet snug. In baseball, major improvements to helmets have been made to protect batters from the impact a baseball can have when hitting their head. Helmets, before this major improvement, were designed to withstand a velocity of 70 mph from a pitch or foul ball. Since the company Rawlings' new design, helmets can withstand a velocity of 100 mph and have further padding around the softer parts on the side of the skull.

Dementia Pugilistica (Punch-Drunk Syndrome)

Epidemiology

A syndrome affecting boxers that is caused by cumulative cerebral injuries and is characterized by impaired cognitive processes (as thinking and remembering), Parkinsonism, impaired and often slurred speech, and slow poorly coordinated movements especially of the legs. Dementia Pugilistica, more commonly known as "Punch Drunk Syndrome", is a degenerative brain disorder resulting from head trauma. Dementia Pugilistica (DP) is typically associated with the sport of boxing; although symptoms of DP may appear immediately after a single traumatic brain injury, they are typically described following the cessation of exposure to chronic brain injury.

Signs and Symptoms in Sports

Some of the subjective symptoms experienced after a Knockout are headaches, tinnitus, forgetfulness, impaired hearing, dizziness, nausea and impaired gait. Approximately ten percent of these active boxers reported constantly suffering from forgetfulness, headaches and other symptoms. Symptoms can be progressive and can develop late into a boxer's career or possibly years into retirement. Some of the earlier symptoms of "punch drunk syndrome" are noticeable in extremities; such as trembling hands or feet, or an instability in equilibrium. Signs of chronic brain damage can also affect irritability, paranoia and cause violent outbursts.

Diagnosis in Sports

Dementia pugilistica is difficult to diagnose until the later stages of a boxer's life. Symptoms are not apparent until boxer's are years into retirement. The damage is done in four primary sites of the brain: the septal regions, the cerebellum, the substantia nigra and the neurons. The septa end up separated and torn apart while the ventricles become enlarged. "The main motor pathways in the cerebellum and substantia nigra are affected, as well as the foramen magnum." Lastly, the neurons in the brains of boxer's have a "bizarre tendency for many neurons, mainly in the deep temporal grey matter, to develop abnormal neurofibrils called Alzheimer tangle. The most successful way to diagnose DP is through magnetic resonance imaging techniques, more commonly known as an MRI. Segmented inversion recovery ratio imaging technique is based on the ratio of a white matter suppressed image and gray matter suppressed image. "The (SIRRIM) technique improves the differentiation of gray matter from white matter and is sensitive to detect abnormalities of intracellular space, including changes during cellular death."

Prognosis (Short/Long-Term Effects)

Multiple studies have concluded that there is neurological evidence of damage to pyramidal, extrapyramidal and cerebellar systems with associated psychosis, memory loss or dementia, personality change and social instability. After fighting, boxers show raised levels of brain chemicals neurofilament light protein and total tau then they did after three months with no boxing.

Prevention in Sports

Protective measures have been taken especially in amateur boxing, such as the wearing of a head guard, more heavily cushioned gloves (weighing 10 ounces in amateur boxing and 8 ounces in professional boxing), shorter and fewer rounds, the addition of the 'outclassed rule' (where the point difference becomes greater than 20), and the option for the boxer to interrupt the fight itself.

Hematoma

Epidemiology

A hematoma is a localized collection of blood that gathers outside the blood vessels in an area it does not belong. Specifically a hematoma is tissue damage due to acceleration or deceleration from unrestricted movement, in which the result is shearing of the brain tissue. Two types of hematomas occurring within the brain are: subdural and extradural hematomas, which are classified as a traumatic brain injury (TBI). When a direct blow to the head occurs, there is bruising to the brain and damage to the internal tissue and blood vessels. Additionally, the jarring of the brain against the skull causes hematomas. Injuries commonly occur during contact sport such as boxing, football, basketball, motor cycling, scuba diving, mountaineering, hang gliding, skydiving, and horseback riding. Council on scientific affairs. Following a serve brain injury or a skull fracture one of the two hematomas may occur. An extradural hematoma is a TBI where blood collects between the inside of the skull and the dura, the thick outer covering of the brain. A subdural hematoma is when a localized collection of blood occurs under the surface of the dura matter. Blood collects on the outermost layer of the brain and creates an intracranial pressure.

Signs and Symptoms in Sports

Generally, symptoms for hematomas are confused speech, difficulty with balance or walking, headaches, lethargy or confusion, nausea or vomiting, numbness, seizures, slurred speech, visual disturbances, and weakness. For example, an athlete who experiences a subdural hematoma will experience loss of consciousness with little or no lucidity. Pupils are often dilated or unequal. Additionally, hemiparesis, seizure activity, and vomiting, may be apparent. An epidural hematoma typically results in serve a headache which is followed by a brief loss of consciousness and variable levels of lucidness. This may last for several hours while the brain function deteriorates. If untreated epidural hematoma causes increased blood pressure, shortness of breath, damage to brain function and may result in death.

Diagnosis in Sports

Subdural and epidural hematomas are serious conditions and should be immediately diagnosed and treated by a physician. Hematomas may not show the full extent of the problem initially after the head injury, but it may be revealed after comprehensive medical evaluation and diagnostic test. Diagnostic test may include: blood test, x-ray, computed tomography scan (CT/CAT scan), electroencephalogram (EEG), and magnetic resonance imaging (MRI). The two most important diagnostic tests are the CT scan and the MRI. The CT scan reveals evidence of blood within the skull, fractures, and signs of compression on the brain from the hematoma. The MRI is a more thorough evaluation of injuries to the brain tissue. Yet, a MRI cannot take place if the injured victim is in a confused state. Small hematomas may not require surgery if there is no pressure on the brain and minimal symptoms. Small hematomas may be monitored closely to ensure the hematoma is not enlarging and re- solved properly. A large hematoma larger than 1 cm at its thickest point produces severe headaches and brain function deterioration requires immediate surgery by a neurosur- geon. Surgery reduces the pressure within the brain and stops the bleeding.

Prognosis (Short/Long-Term Effects)

The most crutial aspect for recovery in patients with severe hematomas is rapid diag- nosis and appropriate treatment. Once the clot has been removed the intracranial pres- sure is monitored for several days. Conditions which are also monitored after surgery are seizures, clot accumulation, and infection. If complications do occur, sometime the hematoma needs to be re-drained. Additional complications following a surgical or nonsurgical treatment may include temporary or permanent weakness, numbness, difficulty speaking, memory loss, dizziness, headache, anxiety, difficulty concentrating, seizures, and/or brain herniation. The most helpful predictors of the treatment out- come is the glasgow coma scale (GCS). This is a standardized pupil response assess- ment of the neurologic status of the patient. GCS helps assess many different types of head injuries and predicts how a patient will recover following a hematoma. Factors such as elevated intracranial pressure, increased patients age, and abnormal GCS re- sults lead to a poor prognosis. The mortality rate following a hematoma could be as high as 80% and survivors many not regain the same pre-injury function. Subdural and epidural hematomas are serious injuries and recovery varies widely depending on the severity of the hematoma. Severity depends on type and location of the injury, the size of the blood collection, and how quickly treatment is obtained. Hence, it is difficult to determine when an athlete can return to sports after his/her injury. A variety of mul- tidisciplinary people such as sports medicine physicians, neurologist/neurosurgeons, athletic trainers, coaches, and family require input. If an athlete is approved to return, he or she is required to complete asymptomatic at rest and with exertion. The athlete also has to clear a CT scan indicating the hematoma has entirely resolved. Lastly, the athlete needs to be slowly brought back into the sport with close monitoring to be sure the symptoms do not recur.

Prevention in Sports

Preemptive measures include using safety equipment to reduce your risk of a head in- jury. Equipment examples are hard hats, bicycle or motorcycle helmets, and seat belts. To reduce the risk of hematomas, factors to avoid are taking anticoagulant medication (blood thinners, such as aspirin), long-term abuse of alcohol, repeated falls, and reoc- curring head injury

Sports Injury

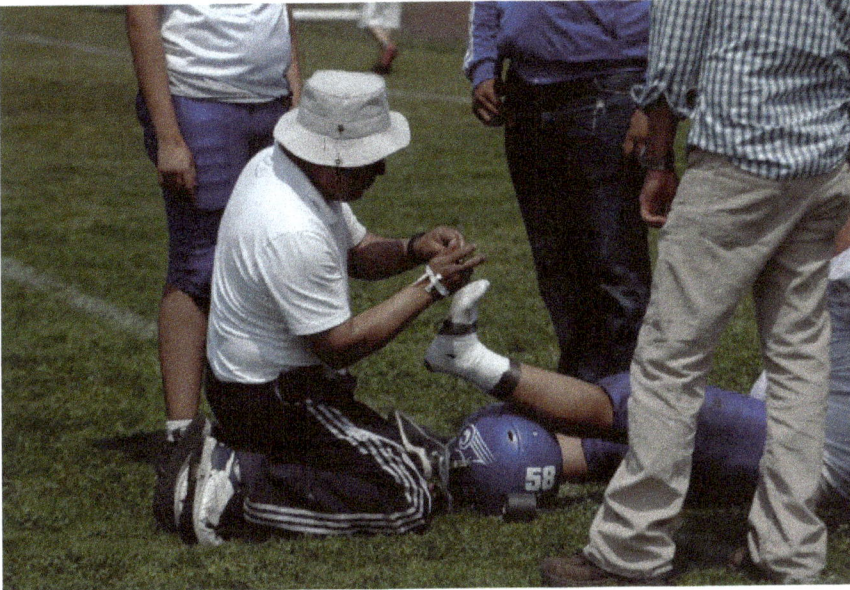

Player getting ankle taped at an American football game in Mexico

Sports injuries are injuries that occur in athletic activities or exercising. They can result from accidents, poor training technique in practice, inadequate equipment, and overuse of a particular body part. In the United States there are about 30 million teenagers and children alone that participate in some form of organized sport.

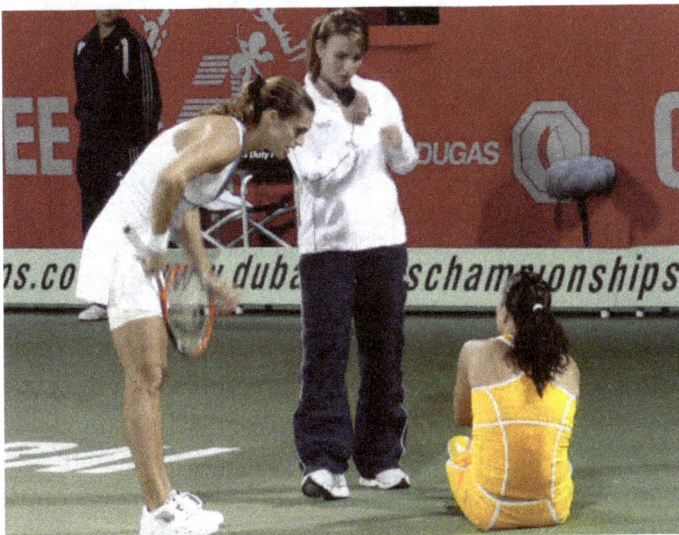

A tennis injury

About 3 million avid sports competitors 14 years of age and under experience sports injuries annually, which causes some loss of time of participation in the sport.

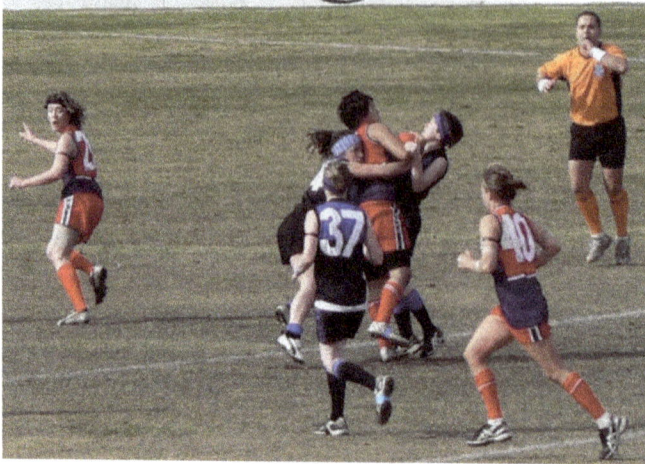

Tackles like this one in women's Australian rules football can cause injuries.

The leading cause of death involving sports-related injuries, although rare, is brain injuries. When injured the two main systems affected are the nervous and vascular systems. The origins in the body where numbness and tingling occurs upon sports injuries are usually the first signs of the body telling you that the body was impacted.

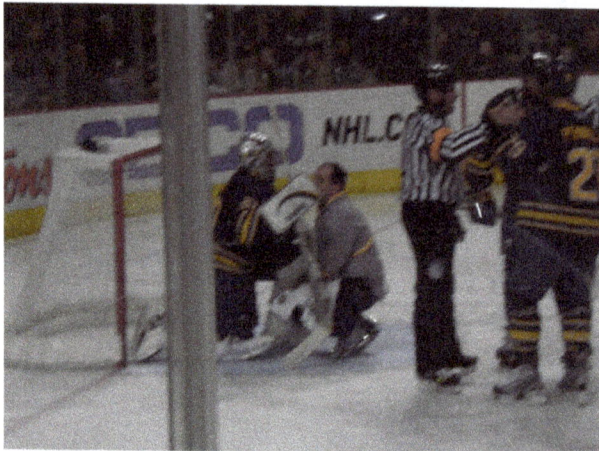

Ryan Miller of the Buffalo Sabres suffers an ankle sprain.

Thus, when an athlete complains of numbness and especially tingling, the key to a diagnosis is to obtain a detailed history of the athlete's acquired symptom perception, determine the effect the injury had on the body and its processes, and then establish the prime treatment method. In the process to determine what exactly happened in the body and the standing effects most medical professionals choose a method of technological medical devices to acquire a credible solution to the site of injury. Prevention helps reduce potential sport injuries. It is important to establish participation in warm-ups, stretching, and exercises that focus on main muscle groups commonly used in the sport of interest. Also, creating an injury prevention program as a team, which includes education on re-hydration, nutrition, monitoring team members "at risk", monitoring behavior, skills, and techniques. Season analysis reviews and preseason screenings are also beneficial reviews for preventing player sport injuries. One technique used in the process of preseason screening is the functional movement screen. The functional movement screen can assess movement patterns in athletes in order to find the at risk players. Following various researches about sport injuries shows that levels of anxiety, stress, and depression are elevated. A study in 2010 found that athletes with severe sports injuries would display higher levels of post-traumatic distress and the higher the levels of post-traumatic distress are linked with avoidant coping skills.

Classification

Traumatic injuries account for most injuries in contact sports such as ice hockey, association football, rugby league, rugby union, Australian rules football, Gaelic football and American football because of the dynamic and high collision nature of these sports. Collisions with the ground, objects, and other players are common, and unexpected dynamic forces on limbs and joints can cause injury.

Traumatic injuries can include:

- Contusion or bruise - damage to small blood vessels which causes bleeding within the tissues.

- Strain - trauma to a muscle due to overstretching and tearing of muscle fibers

- Sprain - an injury in a joint, caused by the ligament being stretched beyond its own capacity

- Wound - abrasion or puncture of the skin

- Bone fracture - break(s) in the bone

- Head injury - concussions or serious brain damage

- Spinal cord injury - damage to the central nervous system or spine

- Cramp-a strong muscle contraction that can be very painful lasting in few minutes but massaging the muscles can relieve the pain

In sports medicine, a catastrophic injury is defined as severe trauma to the human head, spine, or brain.

Concussions in sports became a major issue in the United States in the 2000s, as evidence connected repeated concussions and subconcussive hits with chronic traumatic encephalopathy (CTE) and increased suicide risk. CTE is a progressive degenerative disease of the brain found in people with a history of repetitive brain trauma, including symptomatic concussions as well as subconcussive hits to the head that do not cause symptoms. It is most pronounced in football, and a related ailment (dementia pugilistica) afflicts boxers, but is also seen in other sports, and in females and adolescents.

Overuse and repetitive stress injury problems associated with sports include:

- Runner's knee

- Tennis elbow

- Tendinosis

Some activities have particular risks:

- Bicycle safety

- Gun safety

- Sailing ship accidents

- Skateboarding#Safety

Sports Medicine

Injuries are a common occurrence in professional sports and most teams have a staff of athletic trainers and close connections to the medical community. Many retain team physicians.

Controversy has arisen at times when teams have made decisions that could threaten a players long-term health for short term gain. Sports medicine is the study and research of injuries in sport in order to prevent or reduce the severity of the injury.

Soft Tissue Injuries

When soft tissue experiences trauma, the dead and damaged cells release chemicals, which initiate an inflammatory response. Inflammation is characterized by pain, localized swelling, heat, redness and a loss of function. Small blood vessels are damaged and opened up, producing bleeding within the tissue. In the body's normal reaction, a small blood clot is formed in order to stop this bleeding and from this clot special cells (called fibroblasts) begin the healing process by laying down scar tissue.

The inflammatory stage is therefore the first phase of healing. However, too much of an inflammatory response in the early stage can mean that the healing process takes longer and a return to activity is delayed. Sports injury treatments are intended to minimize the inflammatory phase of an injury, so that the overall healing process is accelerated. Intrinsic and extrinsic factors are determinant for the healing process.

Prevention

Prevention helps reduce potential sport injuries and provides several benefits. Some benefits include a healthier athlete, longer duration of participation in the sport, potential for better performance, and reduced medical costs. Explaining the benefits to participate in sports injury prevention programs to coaches, team trainers, sports teams, and individual athletes will give them a glimpse at the likelihood for success by having the athletes feeling they are healthy, strong, comfortable, and capable to compete.

Primary, Secondary, and Tertiary Prevention

Prevention can be broken up into three broad categories of primary, secondary, and tertiary prevention. Primary prevention involves the avoidance of injury. An example is ankle braces being worn as a team, even those with no history of previous ankle injuries. If primary prevention activities were effective, there would be a lesser chance of injuries occurring in the first place. Secondary prevention involves an early diagnosis and treatment should be acquired once an injury has occurred. The goal of obtaining early diagnosis is to ensure that the injury is receiving proper care and recovering correctly, therefore limiting the concern for other medical problems to stem from the initial traumatic event. Lastly, tertiary prevention is solely focused on the rehabilitation to reduce and correct an existing disability resulting from the traumatic event. An example in the case of an athlete who has obtained an ankle injury the rehabilitation would consist of balance exercises to acquire the strength and mobility back as well as wearing an ankle brace, while gradually returning to the sport.

Season Analysis

It is most essential to establish participation in warm-ups, stretching, and exercises that focus on main muscle groups commonly used in the sport of interest. Participation in these events decreases the chances for getting muscle cramps, torn muscles, and stress fractures. A season analysis is one of the beneficial reviews for preventing player sport injuries. A season analysis is an attempt to identify risks before they occur by reviewing training methods, the competition schedule, traveling, and past injuries. If injuries have occurred in the past, the season analysis reviews the injury and looks for patterns to see if it may be related to a specific training event or competition program. For example, a stress fracture injury on a soccer team or cross country team may be correlated to a simultaneous increase in running and a change in running environment, like a transition from a soft to hard running surface. A season analysis can be documented as team-based results or individual athlete results. Other key program events that have been correlated to injury incidences are changes in training volume, changes in climate locations, selection for playing time in important matches, and poor sleep due to tight chaotic scheduling. It is important for team program directors and staff to implicate testing in order to ensure healthy, competitive, and confident athletes for their upcoming season.

Preseason Screening

Another beneficial review for preventing player sport injuries is preseason screenings. To prepare an athlete for the wide range of activities needed to partake in their sport pre-participation examinations are regularly completed on hundreds of thousands of athletes each year. It is extremely important that the physical exam is done properly in order to limit the risks of injury and also to diagnose early onsets of a possible injury. Preseason screenings consist of testing the mobility of joints (Ankles, wrists, hips, etc.), testing the stability of joints (knees, neck, etc.), testing the strength and power of muscles, and also testing breathing patterns. The objective of a preseason screening is to clear the athlete for participation and verify that there is no sign of injury or illness, which would represent a potential medical risk to the athlete (and risk of liability to the sports organization). Besides the physical examination and the fluidity of the movements of joints the preseason screenings often takes into account a nutrition aspect as well. It is important to maintain normal iron levels, blood pressure levels, fluid balance, adequate total energy intake, and normal glycogen levels. Nutrition can aid in injury prevention and rehabilitation, if one obtains the body's daily intake needs. Obtaining sufficient amount of calories, carbohydrates, fluids, protein, and vitamins and minerals is important for the overall health of the athlete and limits the risk of possible injuries. Iron deficiency, for example, is found in both male and female athletes; however 60 percent of female college athletes are affected by iron deficiency. There are many factors that can contribute to the loss in iron, like menstruation, gastrointestinal bleeding, inadequate iron intake from the diet, general fatigue, weakness, among others. The consequences of iron deficiency, if not solved, can be an impaired athletic performance and a decline in immune and cognitive function.

Functional Movement Screen

One technique used in the process of preseason screening is the Functional Movement Screen (FMS). Functional movement screening is an assessment used to evaluate movement patterns and asymmetries, which can provide insight into mechanical restrictions and potential risk for injury. Functional movement screening contains seven fundamental movement patterns that require a balance of both mobility and stability. These fundamental movement patterns provide an observable performance of basic locomotor, manipulative, and stabilizing movements. The tests place the individual athlete in extreme positions where weaknesses and imbalances become clear if proper stability and mobility is not functioning correctly. The seven fundamental movement patterns are a deep squat, hurdle step, in-line lunge, shoulder mobility, active straight-leg raise, trunk stability push-up, and rotary stability. For example, the deep squat is a test that challenges total body mechanics. It is used to gauge bilateral, symmetrical, and functional mobility of the hips, knees, and ankles. The dowel held overhead gauges bilateral and symmetrical mobility of the shoulders and the thoracic spine. The ability to perform the deep squat technique requires appropriate pelvic rhythm, closed-kinetic chain dorsiflexion of the ankles, flexion of the knees and hips, extension of the thoracic spine, as well as flexion and abduction of the shoulders. There is a scoring system applied to each movement as follows a score of 3 is given to the athlete if they can perform the movement without any compensations, a score of 2 is given to the athlete if they can perform the movement, but operate on poor mechanics and compensatory patterns to achieve the movement, a score of 1 is given to the athlete if they cannot perform the movement pattern even with compensations, and finally, a 0 is given to the athlete if one has pain during any part of the movement or test. Three of the seven fundamental tests including shoulder mobility, trunk stability push-up, and rotary stability have a clearance scoring associated with them meaning a pass or fail score. If the athlete fails this part of the test a score of 0 is given as the overall score. Once the scoring is complete the athlete and medical professional can review the documentation together and organize a set prevention program to help target and strengthen the areas of weakness in order to limit the risks of possible injuries.

Costs

Interventions targeted at decreasing the incidence of sports injuries can impact healthcare costs,as well as family and societal resources.

Sport Injury Prevention for Kids

There are approximately 8,000 children treated in emergency rooms each day for sports-related injures. Also, it is estimated that there are around 1.35 million kids suffering from sports-related injuries per year worldwide. This is why children need special attention and care when participating in sports.

Here's a list sports injury prevention tips for kids:

- Kids attending sports clinics tend to know the basic fundamentals of a particular sport. Injury awareness and prevention can also be learned in sports clinics.

- Warming up improves the blood flow in muscles. This brings more nutrients in different parts of the body, therefore bringing more energy throughout.

- Provide children the right equipment on a particular sport like helmets, shin guards, ankle braces, gloves and others to prevent injuries.

- Kids need to have breaks and drink water as well to keep them hydrated.

- Know certain first aid treatment on injuries to apply when there's an unforeseen accident.

Sports-Related Emotional Stress

Sport involvement can initiate both physical and mental demands on athletes. From youth little leagues to competing at a professional level, athletes are forced to learn ways to cope with stressors and frustrations that can arise from competition against others. Conducted research shows that levels of anxiety, stress, and depression are elevated following sports injuries. The pressure athletes experience is extensive; branching from coaches, parents, peers, and audiences. It is astonishing how one individual can endure so much pressure and remain so calm and collected. Positive mental motivation however is not experienced all the time. The pressure to win can cause significant emotional stress for an athlete. Many athletes experience the stressor involving winning as being the most important aspect of the match. If the match is not won, many athletes are punished and criticized for the loss, instead of being commended on their effort, sportsmanship, and hard work. Nearly two million people every year suffer sports-related injuries and receive treatment in emergency departments. Fatigue is a contributing factor that results in many sport injuries. As an athlete there are times where you may run on low energy leading to the deterioration in technique or form, which results in a slower reaction time, and finally a loss in stability of muscle joints and an injury. After an occurrence of an injury many athletes display self-esteem issues, athletic identity crises, and high levels of post-traumatic distress, which are linked to avoidant coping skills.

Psychological Stressors

- Self-esteem

- Athlete Identity Crisis

- Post-traumatic Distress

Treatment

Sports injuries can be treated and managed by using the P.R.I.C.E.S., D.R. A.B.C., T.O.T.A.P.S and R.I.C.E.R regimes:

P – Protect

R – Rest

I – Ice

C – Compression

E – Elevation

S - Stabilize

D – Danger

R – Response

A – Airway

B – Breathing

C – Circulation

T – Talk

O – Observe

T – Touch

A – Active movement

P – Passive movement

S – Skills test

R - Rest

I - Ice

C - Compression

E - Elevation

R - Referral

S - Stop

A - Ask

L - Look

T - Touch

A - Active movement

P - Passive movement

S - Stand up

The primary inflammatory stage typically lasts around 5 days and all treatment during this time is designed to address the cardinal signs of inflammation – pain, swelling, redness, heat and a loss of function.

Compression sportswear is becoming very popular with both professional and amateur athletes. These garments are thought to both reduce the risk of muscle injury and speed up muscle recovery.

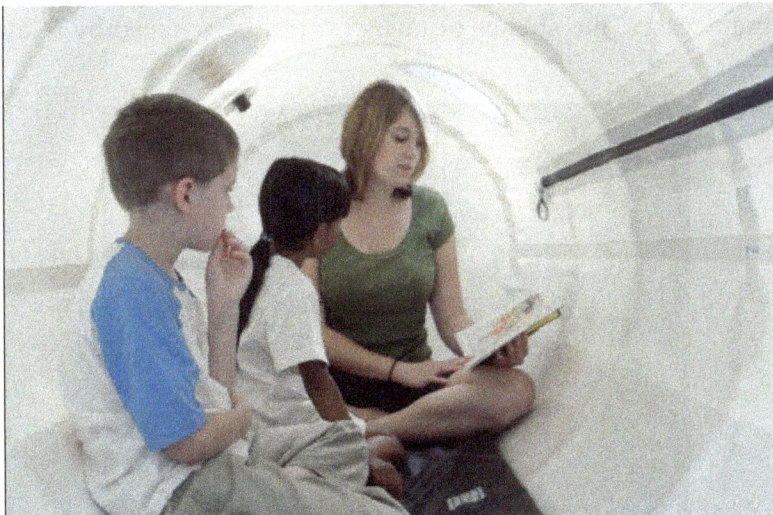

Portable Mild Hyperbaric Chamber 40" diameter

Although not proven some professional athletes use hyperbaric chambers to speed healing. Hines Ward of the Steelers sent his personal hyperbaric chamber (similar to the one pictured) to his hotel to sleep in believing it would help heal his sprained medial collateral ligament he suffered in their playoff win against the Ravens. Hines went on to play in Super Bowl XLIII.

Famous People Who had Sports Injuries

- Natasha Richardson (skiing accident),

- Christopher Reeve (horse-back riding)

Infectious Disease (Athletes)

Those involved in the care of athletes should be alert to the possibility of infectious disease for the following reasons:

- There is the chance, or even the expectation, of contact or collision with another player, or the playing surface, which may be a mat or artificial turf.

- The opportunities for skin breaks, obvious or subtle, are present and compromise skin defenses.

- Young people congregate in dormitories, locker rooms, showers, etc.

- There is the possibility of sharing personal toilet articles.

- Equipment, gloves and pads and protective gear, is difficult to sanitize and can become contaminated.

However, in many cases, the chance of infection can be reduced by relatively simple measures.

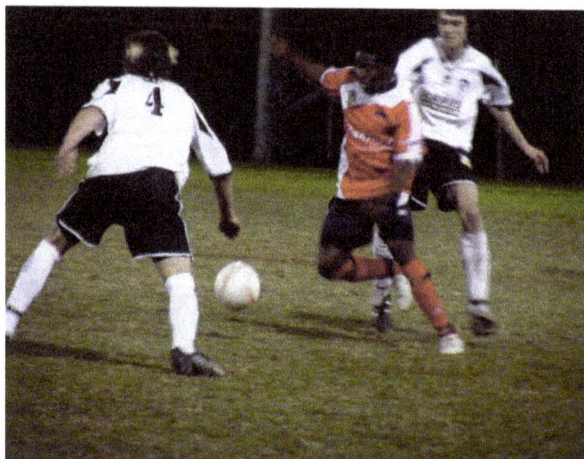

Herpes Gladiatorum

Wrestlers use mats which are abrasive and the potential for a true contagion is very real. The herpes simplex virus, type I, is very infectious and large outbreaks have been documented. A major epidemic threatened the 2007 Minnesota high school wrestling season, but was largely contained by instituting an eight-day isolation period during which time competition was suspended. Practices, such as 'weight cutting', which can at least theoretically reduce immunity, might potentiate the risk. In non-epidemic circumstances, herpes gladiatorum affects about 3% of high school wrestlers and 8% of collegiate wrestlers. There is the potential for prevention of infection, or at least containment, with antiviral agents which are effective in reducing the spread to other athletes when given to those who are herpes positive, or who have recurrent herpes gladiatorum.

The NCAA specifies that a wrestler must:
- be free of systemic symptoms (fever, malaise, etc.).
- have developed no new blisters for 72 hours before the examination.
- have no moist lesions; all lesions must be dried and have progressed to a FIRM ADHERENT CRUST.
- have been on appropriate systemic antiviral therapy for at least 120 hours before and at the time of the meet or tournament.

Active herpetic infections shall not be covered to allow participation.

Impetigo

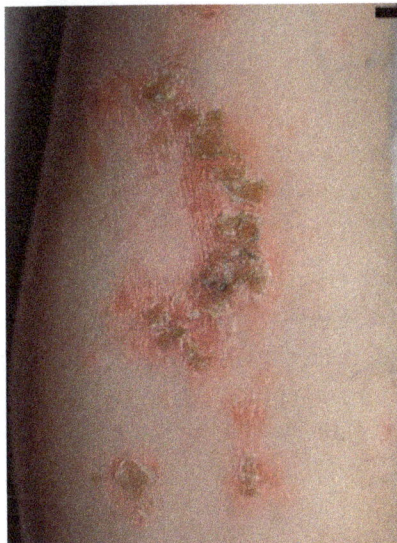

This superficial intra-dermal infection spreads by contact. A red, tender 'spot' quickly develops blisters or vesicles which rupture to develop a golden crust. Over the past 20

years, the pathogen has changed from being overwhelmingly hemolytic streptococcal to staphyloccocus aureus (80%), streptococcal (10%), and the remainder due to a combination of the two. The lesions appear most frequently on the face, around the mouth or nose, but there are often multiple sites that may include the buttocks and trunk. There is a seasonal predilection for summer and fall and contact sport is a definite risk factor. Amongst other regulations, the NCAA require an absence of new lesions for 48 hours before a meet or tournament, and at least 72 hours of completed antibiotic therapy.

The NCAA specifies that a wrestler must:
- not have developed any new skin lesion for 48 hours before a meet or tournament
- have no moist or exudative lesions at meet or tournament time
Gram stain of exudate from questionable lesions (if available) should be performed.
Active purulent lesions shall not be covered to allow participation.

Ringworm

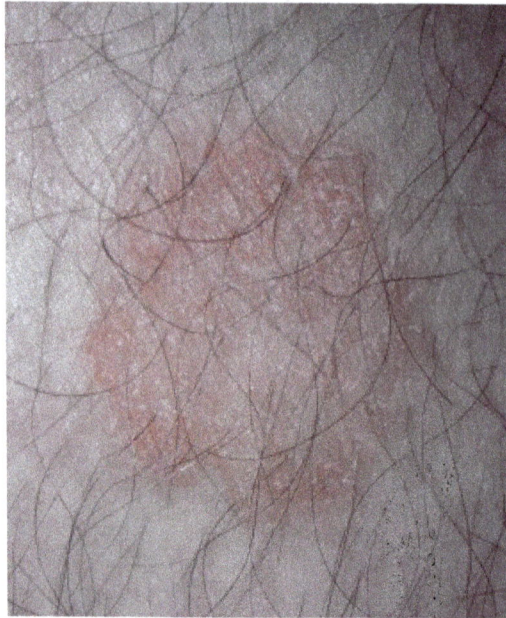

Ringworm, more properly called Tinea, presents as a reddish/brown raised or bumpy patch which may be lighter in the center, giving the appearance of a ring. It is caused by one of three parasitic fungi and is named after the body site involved. Consequently, the name does not indicate the fungal type, for example, Tinea corporis (body) and Tinea manum (hand). Ringworm spreads readily by direct skin-to-skin contact, and by using a contaminated hairbrush or other source. Some studies have indicated that spread may be reduced by prophylaxis with anti-fungal agents applied to the skin. Again, there are NCAA prohibitions on participation unless lesions are completely and securely covered in wrestling, or that one week of treatment has been completed in case of extensive involvement.

The NCAA specifies that to participate:
- at least 72 hours of topical therapy is required for skin lesions.
- at least two weeks of systemic antifungal therapy is required for scalp lesions.
- wrestlers with extensive and active lesions will be disqualified and those with local-
ized lesions will be disqualified if such lesions cannot be "properly covered".
- the disposition of tinea cases will be decided on an individual basis as determined
by the examining physician and/or certified athletic trainer.

Infectious Mononucleosis

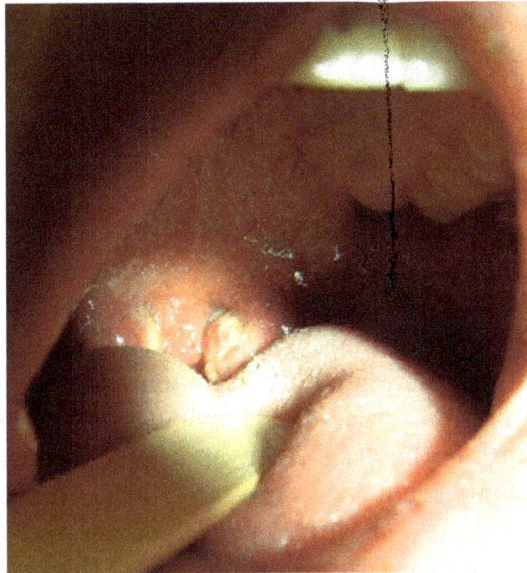

This was recognized as a clinical syndrome in the 1800s consisting of fever, pharyngitis and adenopathy. The term glandular fever was first used in 1889 and the association with Epstein-Barr virus infection in the late 1960s. Sprunt and Evans described the cynical characteristics of Epstein-Barr virus (EBV) infectious mononucleosis in 1920. It is primarily transmitted by oropharyngeal secretions. A study demonstrated that 13% of susceptible University freshmen developed EBV antibodies within nine months of enrollment. Seventy-four percent of those developed the clinical syndrome recognized as infectious mononucleosis.Of most interest in the care of the athlete is the enlargement of the spleen, which may extend beyond the protection normally offered by the lower ribs, and also be softer and consequently more vulnerable to rupture. Most patients do not have a palpable spleen on examination and the sensitivity of physical examination for splenic enlargement has been estimated at about 6%, (94% undetected). The risk of rupture during infectious mononucleosis has been estimated at one per thousand and one review indicated that almost all ruptures occurred in the first three weeks. This has led to the suggestion that athletes be withheld from exertion for a minimum of four weeks from the onset of IM. Others have suggested ultrasound examination at three weeks to assist with decision making concerning return to activity.

MRSA

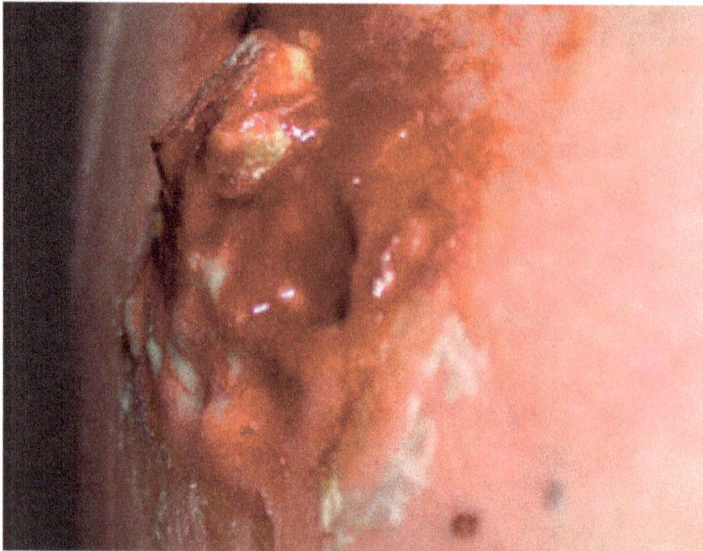

MRSA refers to a resistant variation of a common bacterium which has evolved to survive beta-lactam antibiotics, including Penicillin and Methicillin. First discovered in the UK in 1961, it is now worldwide. It is popularly referred to as a "superbug", more appropriately as multiple resistant Staphylococcus aureus. It most commonly colonizes the anterior third of the nasal cavity and otherwise healthy people may carry MRSA without symptoms, from weeks to years.There are three postulates relating to the development of multiple resistant 'staph'. One is the widespread, inappropriate use of antibiotics particularly for virus infections where they can do no good. Another is the inclusion of antibiotics in animal feed. A third is simply genetic selection of the "fittest bacteria". The commonest presentations include pustules, furuncles, carbuncles and abscesses, although misdiagnosis as a "spider bite" is not uncommon. The Centers for Disease Control have defined the five "C's" that make up the major risk factors as *Crowding*, frequent skin *Contact, Compromised* skin, sharing *Contaminated* personal care items, and lack of *Cleanliness*. Consequently, it is incumbent on those who look after athletes to stress adequate hygiene, cover open lesions completely with clean, dry dressings, advise against sharing of towels, bar soap, and personal care items, disinfect surfaces that contact bare skin and maintain equipment hygienically.

Hepatitides and HIV

Hepatitis B, Hepatitis C and HIV are classical examples of blood-borne disease. Unlike Hepatitis A, which is spread by the fecal-oral route and is indicative of a breakdown in food safety or potable water protection, Hepatitis B, C and HIV are spread by contact with bodily fluids, most frequently blood, although in the case of HIV, not exclusively so. Also, unlike Hepatitis A in which the sufferer almost always recovers completely, or rarely dies, both Hepatitis B and C give rise to chronic carrier state and indolent disease in many. At present, Hepatitis C is the commonest reason for liver transplantation in the US while HIV is currently incurable although its clinical course can be modified. In any case, between them, they have changed awareness of infectious disease in sports, and certainly changed management on the playing surface. Ironically, evidence for transmission of any of the three as a result of injury and/or contact on the playing surface is exceedingly limited and the greatest risk to the athlete surrounds behavior that may take place off court. A case report in 1982 described 5 of 10 members of a Japanese high school sumo wrestling club who contracted hepatitis. It was hypothesized that spread had occurred through skin cuts and abrasions. An outbreak of HBV in an American football team was reported in 2000. Eleven of 65 athletes were found to be HBV positive in a 19-month surveillance period. Contact with open wounds of an HBV carrier was again hypothesized. Interestingly, both of those case reports originated in Japan. HBV transmission has been estimated to be 50 to 100 times more likely than the risk of transmission of HIV. HBV is also more environmentally stable, is resistant to alcohol and some detergents, and to be capable of surviving on environmental surfaces for more than seven days. The risk of transmission in sport has been estimated at between one transmission in every 10,000 to 50,000 games to one transmission in every 850,000 to 4.25 million games. These calculations are based on the estimated prevalence of HBV among athletes and it should be appreciated that aggressive and successful HBV immunization programs have been promoted since. Another study has described the prevalence of HBV infection in athletes as being no different from blood donors of the same age. Regardless, prudent preventive measures as advocated by the Pediatrics Committee on Sports Medicine and Fitness and paraphrased as follows are in wide use:

- Athletes should not share personal items, such as razors, toothbrushes, and nail clippers.

- Athletes must cover areas of broken skin with an occlusive dressing before and during participation.

- Disposable vinyl or latex gloves should be worn to avoid contact with blood or other bodily fluids visibly tinged with blood and any object such as equipment, bandages or uniforms contaminated with these fluids.

- Athletes with active bleeding should be removed from competition as soon as possible and the bleeding stopped. Wounds should be cleaned with soap and water. Skin antiseptics may be used if soap and water are not available. Wounds must be covered with an occlusive dressing that remains intact during play before athletes return to competition.

- Minor cuts or abrasions that are not bleeding do not require interruption of play but can be cleaned and covered during scheduled breaks. During these breaks, if an athlete's equipment or uniform fabric is wet with blood, the equipment should be cleaned and disinfected, or the uniform should be replaced.

- Equipment and playing areas contaminated with blood must be cleaned until all visible blood is gone and then disinfected with an appropriate germicide such as a freshly-made bleach solution containing one part bleach in 10 parts of water. The decontaminated equipment or area should be in contact with the bleach solution for at least 30 seconds. The area may be wiped with a disposable cloth after the minimum contact time or be allowed to air dry.

These recommendations are basically echoed and expanded in the Sports Medicine Handbook of the National Collegiate Athletic Association.

References

- Page 42 in: *Weinzweig, Jeffrey (1999). Hand & Wrist Surgery Secrets (The Secrets Series). Philadelphia: Hanley & Belfus. ISBN 1-56053-364-1.*

- *Levangie, P. K., & Norkin, C. C. (2011). Joint structure and function: A comprehensive analysis (5th ed.). Philadelphia: F.A. Davis Co. ISBN 9780803623620.*

- *Bailes, Julian (2001). Neurological Sports Medicine: A Guide for Physicians and Athletic Trainers. Rolling Meadows, Illinois: Thieme. ISBN 1879284758.*

- *Unterharnscheidt, Friedrich (2003). Boxing: Medical Aspects. Academic Press. p. 294. ISBN 9780127091303.*

- *Terry R. Yochum; Lindsay J. Rowe (2004). Essentials of Skeletal Radiology (3rd ed.). Baltimore, MD: Lippincott Williams & Wilkins. ISBN 0781739462.*

- Page 42 in: *Weinzweig, Jeffrey (1999). Hand & Wrist Surgery Secrets (The Secrets Series). Philadelphia: Hanley & Belfus. ISBN 1-56053-364-1.*

- *Herring, Stanley A.; Akuthota, Venu (2009). Nerve and Vascular Injuries in Sports Medicine. London; New York: Springer. ISBN 9780387765990. Retrieved 28 March 2016.*

- *Bager, Roald; Engebretsen, Lars (2009). Sports Injury Prevention. Chichester, UK; Hoboken, NJ: Wiley-Blackwell. ISBN 9781405162449. Retrieved 28 March 2016.*

- *"Little League Implements New Rule to Protect Pitchers' Arms". Little League. Retrieved 21 April2015."Sports Injury Statistics". Children's Hospital of Wisconsin. Retrieved 28 March 2016.*

- *O'Connor, John William (2010). "Emotional Trauma in Athletic Injury and the Relationship Among Coping Skills, Injury Severity, and Post Traumatic Stress". ProQuest Dissertations Publishing. Retrieved 28 March 2016.*

- *Rowland, Thomas (2012). "Iron Deficiency in Athletes". American Journal of Lifestyle Medicine. SAGE Publications. Retrieved 24 April 2016.*

- *Beardsley, Chris; Contreras, Bret (2014). "The Functional Movement Screen". Strength and Conditioning Journal. ISSN 1524-1602. Retrieved 25 April 2016.*

- *Misra, Arpit (March 17, 2014). "Common Sports Injuries: Incidence and Average Charges" (PDF). U.S. Department of Health and Human Services. ASPE Office of Health Policy. Retrieved 28 March 2016.*

- *Smith, A.M.; Nippert, A.H. (2008). "Psychologic Stress Related to Injury and Impact on Sport Performance". Department of Kinesiology and Health Sciences. Concordia University- St. Paul, MN. : 399–418, x. doi:10.1016/j.pmr.2007.12.003. PMID 18395654. Retrieved 28 March 2016.*

Various Sports Injuries

This chapter is the further classification of injuries that are listed in chapter two. The following topics will provide the reader an elaborate understanding of the other major types of injuries that are prevalent in sports like tennis elbow, shin splints and saddle sore to name a few. The chapter will offer new perspectives and insights into the field.

Tennis Elbow

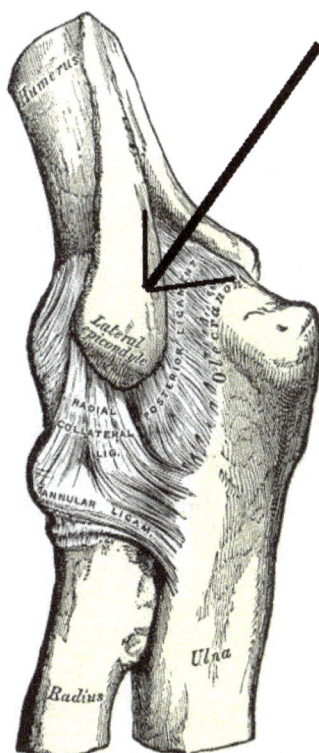

Left elbow-joint, showing posterior and radial collateral ligaments.
(Lateral epicondyle visible at center.)

Tennis elbow or lateral epicondylitis is a condition in which the outer part of the elbow becomes sore and tender. The forearm muscles and tendons become damaged from overuse — repeating the same strenuous motions again and again. This leads to pain and tenderness on the outside of the elbow.

Any activity, including playing tennis, which involves the repetitive use of the extensor muscles of the forearm can cause acute or chronic tendonitis of the tendinous insertion of these muscles at the lateral epicondyle of the elbow. The condition is common in carpenters and other laborers who swing a hammer or other tool with the forearm, continuing activity after onset of the condition and avoiding mandatory rest may lead to permanent onset of pain and only treatable via surgery. Dr. F. Runge (a German physician) is usually credited for the first description of the condition in 1873; he called it "writer's cramp" (*Schreibekrampfes*). Later, it was called "washer women's elbow". As it also occurred in tennis, it soon was called "tennis elbow" after British surgeon Henry Morris published an article in *The Lancet* describing "the lawn tennis arm," 1883. The term "tennis elbow" first appeared in an 1883 paper by H.P. Major as "lawn-tennis elbow".

Signs and Symptoms

- Pain on the outer part of the elbow (lateral epicondyle)

- Point tenderness over the lateral epicondyle—a prominent part of the bone on the outside of the elbow

- Pain from gripping and movements of the wrist, especially wrist extension and lifting movements

- Pain from activities that use the muscles that extend the wrist (e.g. pouring a container of liquid, lifting with the palm down, sweeping, especially where wrist movement is required)

Symptoms associated with tennis elbow include, but are not limited to: radiating pain from the outside of the elbow to the forearm and wrist, pain during extension of wrist, weakness of the forearm, a painful grip while shaking hands or torquing a doorknob, and not being able to hold relatively heavy items in the hand. The pain is similar to the condition known as *golfer's elbow*, but the latter occurs at the medial side of the elbow.

Causes

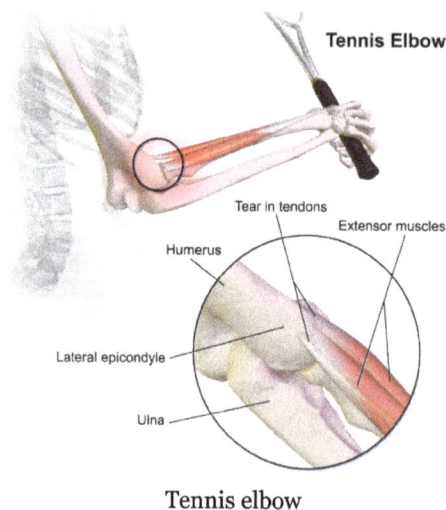

Tennis elbow

Tennis elbow is a type of repetitive strain injury, resulting from tendon overuse and failed healing of the tendon. In addition, the extensor carpi radialis brevis muscle plays a key role.

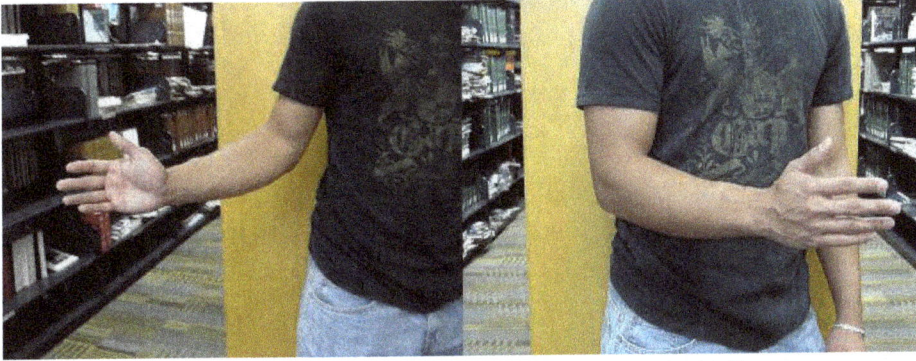

Example of repetitive movement that may cause tennis elbow

Early experiments suggested that tennis elbow was primarily caused by overexertion. However, studies show that trauma such as direct blows to the epicondyle, a sudden forceful pull, or forceful extension cause more than half of these injuries. It has also been known that incorrectly playing tennis may cause early stages of tennis elbow as shock is received when mishitting the ball.

Cyriax proposes one explanation of how tennis elbow may come about. The hypothesis states that there are microscopic and macroscopic tears between the common extensor tendon and the periosteum of the lateral humeral epicondyle. An operation conducted in this study showed that 28 out of 39 patients showed tearing at the tendon cuff. Kaplan stated that the radial nerve was significantly involved in tennis elbow. He noted the constriction of the radial nerve by adhesions to the capsule of the radiohumeral joint and the short extensor muscle of the wrist. He found evidence that many differed in how they contracted tennis elbow. Disorders such as calcification of the rotator cuff, bicipital tendinitis, or carpal tunnel syndrome may increase chances of tennis elbow.

Pathophysiology

Histological findings include granulation tissue, microrupture, degenerative changes, and there is no traditional inflammation. As a consequence, "lateral elbow tendinopathy or tendinosis" is used instead of "lateral epicondylitis".

Examination of tennis elbow tissue reveals noninflammatory tissue, and therefore, the term "angio-fibroblastic tendinosis" is used.

Longitudinal sonogram of the lateral elbow displays thickening and heterogeneity of the common extensor tendon that is consistent with tendinosis, as the ultrasound reveals calcifications, intrasubstance tears, and marked irregularity of the lateral epicondyle. Although the term "epicondylitis" is frequently used to describe this disorder, most histopathologic findings of studies have displayed no evidence of an acute, or a chronic inflammatory process. Histologic studies have demonstrated that this condition is the result of tendon degeneration, which causes normal tissue to be replaced by a disorganized arrangement of collagen. Therefore, the disorder is more appropriately referred to as "tendinosis" or "tendinopathy" rather than "tendinitis."

Colour Doppler ultrasound reveals structural tendon changes, with vascularity and hypo-echoic areas that correspond to the areas of pain in the extensor origin.

The pathophysiology of lateral epicondylitis is degenerative. Non-inflammatory, chronic degenerative changes of the origin of the extensor carpi radialis brevis (ECRB) muscle are identified in surgical pathology specimens. It is unclear if the pathology is affected by prior injection of corticosteroid.

Tennis players generally believe tennis elbow is caused by the repetitive nature of hitting thousands of tennis balls, which leads to tiny tears in the forearm tendon attachment at the elbow.

The extensor digiti minimi also has a small origin site medial to the elbow that this condition can affect. The muscle involves the extension of the little finger and some extension of the wrist allowing for adaption to "snap" or flick the wrist—usually associated with a racquet swing. Most often, the extensor muscles become painful due to tendon breakdown from over-extension. Improper form or movement allows for power in a swing to rotate through and around the wrist—creating a moment on that joint instead of the elbow joint or rotator cuff. This moment causes pressure to build impact forces to act on the tendon causing irritation and inflammation.

The following speculative rationale is offered by proponents of an overuse theory of etiology: The extensor carpi radialis brevis has a small origin and does transmit large forces through its tendon during repetitive grasping. It has also been implicated as being vulnerable during shear stress during all movements of the forearm.

While it is commonly stated that lateral epicondylitis is caused by repetitive micro-trauma/overuse, this is a speculative etiological theory with limited scientific support that is likely overstated. Other speculative risk factors for lateral epicondylitis include taking up tennis later in life, unaccustomed strenuous activity, decreased mental chronometry and speed and repetitive eccentric contraction of muscle (controlled lengthening of a muscle group).

Prevention

Another factor of tennis elbow injury is experience and ability. The proportion of players who reported a history of tennis elbow had an increased number of playing years. As for ability, poor technique increases the chance for injury much like any sport. Therefore, an individual must learn proper technique for all aspects of their sport. The competitive level of the athlete also affects the incidence of tennis elbow. Class A and B players had a significantly higher rate of tennis elbow occurrence compared to class C and novice players. However, an opposite, but not statistically significant, trend is observed for the recurrence of previous cases, with an increasingly higher rate as ability level decreases.

Other ways to prevent tennis elbow:

- Decrease the amount of playing time if already injured or feeling pain in outside part of the elbow.

- Stay in overall good physical shape.

- Strengthen the muscles of the forearm: (pronator quadratus, pronator teres, and supinator muscle)—the upper arm: (biceps, triceps)—and the shoulder (deltoid muscle) and upper back (trapezius). Increased muscular strength increases stability of joints such as the elbow.

- Like other sports, use equipment appropriate to your ability, body size, and muscular strength.

- Avoid any repetitive lifting or pulling of heavy objects (especially over your head)

Vibration dampeners (otherwise known as "gummies") are not believed to be a reliable preventative measure. Rather, proper weight distribution in the racket is thought to be a more viable option in negating shock.

Diagnosis

To diagnose tennis elbow, the physician performs a battery of tests in which he places pressure on the affected area while asking the patient to move the elbow, wrist, and fingers. X-rays can confirm and distinguish possibilities of existing causes of pain that are unrelated to tennis elbow, such as fracture or arthritis. Medical ultrasonography and magnetic resonance imaging (MRI) are other valuable tools for diagnosis but are frequently avoided due to the high cost. MRI screening can confirm excess fluid and swelling in the affected region in the elbow, such as the connecting point between the forearm bone and the extensor carpi radialis brevis.

Diagnosis is made by clinical signs and symptoms that are discrete and characteristic. With the elbow fully extended, the patient feels points of tenderness over the affected point on the elbow—which is the origin of the extensor carpi radialis brevis muscle from the lateral epicondyle (extensor carpi radialis brevis origin). There is also pain with passive wrist flexion and resistive wrist extension (Cozen's test). Resisted middle finger extension might indicate the involvement of Extensor Digitorum also. These tests shall be used to measure the prognosis of the condition.

Depending upon severity and quantity of multiple tendon injuries that have built up, the extensor carpi radialis brevis may not be fully healed by conservative treatment.

Nirschl defines four stages of lateral epicondylitis, showing the introduction of permanent damage beginning at Stage 2.

1. Inflammatory changes that are reversible

2. Nonreversible pathologic changes to origin of the extensor carpi radialis brevis muscle

3. Rupture of ECRB muscle origin

4. Secondary changes such as fibrosis or calcification.

Treatment

Evidence for the treatment of lateral epicondylitis before 2010 was poor. There were clinical trials addressing many proposed treatments, but the trials were of poor quality.

A 2009 study looked at using eccentric exercise with a rubber bar in addition to standard treatment: the trial was stopped after 8 weeks because the improvement using the bar for therapy was so significant. Based on small sample size and a follow-up only 7 weeks from commencement of treatment, the study shows short-term improvements. This along with other studies allowed doctors to conclude that approximately 80-95% of all tennis elbow cases can be treated without surgery. However, long-term results have not yet been determined.

In some cases, severity of tennis elbow symptoms mend without any treatment, within six to 24 months. Tennis elbow left untreated can lead to chronic pain that degrades quality of daily living.

Physical

There are several recommendations regarding prevention, treatment, and avoidance of recurrence that are largely speculative including stretches and progressive strengthening exercises to prevent re-irritation of the tendon and other exercise measures.

One way to help treat minor cases of tennis elbow is to simply relax the affected arm. The rest will allow the stress and tightness within the forearm to slowly relax and eventually have the arm in working condition once again in a day or two, depending on the case.

Evidence from the Tyler study suggests that eccentric exercise using a rubber bar is highly effective at eliminating pain and increasing strength. Highlights of the study were described in The New York Times. The exercise involves grasping a rubber bar, twisting it, then slowly untwisting it.

Moderate evidence exists demonstrating that joint manipulation directed at the elbow and wrist and spinal manipulation directed at the cervical and thoracic spinal regions results in clinical changes to pain and function. There is also moderate evidence for short-term and mid-term effectiveness of cervical and thoracic spine manipulation as an add-on therapy to concentric and eccentric stretching plus mobilisation of wrist and forearm. Although not yet conclusive, the short-term analgesic effect of manipulation techniques may allow more vigorous stretching and strengthening exercises, resulting in a better and faster recovery process of the affected tendon in lateral epicondylitis.

Low level laser therapy, administered at specific doses and wavelengths directly to the lateral elbow tendon insertions, offers short-term pain relief and less disability in tennis elbow, both alone and in conjunction with an exercise regimen. Of late, dry needling has been gaining popularity in various types of tendinopathies and pain of muscular origin. Even in lateral epicondylitis, dry needling is widely employed by many physical therapists across the world. It is believed that dry needling would cause a tiny local injury in order to bring about various desirable growth factors in the vicinity. Dry needling is also aimed at eliciting local twitch response (LTR) in the extensor muscles, as in some cases of tennis elbow the extensor muscles of the forearm would harbor trigger points, which itself could be a major source of pain.

Orthotic Devices

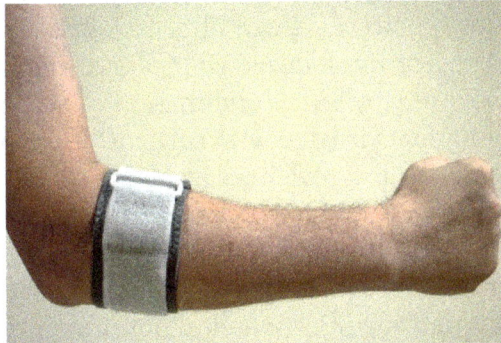

Counterforce orthosis reduces the elongation within the musculotendinious fibers

Orthosis is a device externally used on the limb to improve the function or reduce the pain. Orthotics are useful therapeutic interventions for initial therapy of tennis elbow. There are two main types of orthoses prescribed for this problem: counterforce elbow orthoses and wrist extension orthoses.

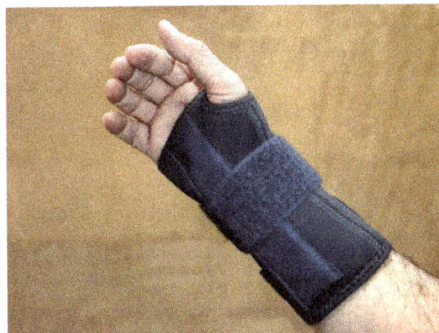

Wrist extensor orthosis reduces the overloading strain at the lesion area

Counterforce orthosis has a circumferential structure surrounding the arm. This orthosis usually has a strap which applies a binding force over the origin of the wrist extensors. The applied force by orthosis reduces the elongation within the musculotendinious fibers. Wrist extensor orthosis maintains the wrist in the slight extension. This position reduces the overloading strain at the lesion area.

Studies indicated both type of orthoses improve the hand function and reduce the pain in people with tennis elbow.

Medication

Although anti-inflammatories are a commonly prescribed treatment for tennis elbow, the evidence for their effect is usually anecdotal with only limited studies showing a benefit. A systematic review found that topical non-steroidal anti-inflammatory drugs (NSAIDs) may improve pain in the short term (up to 4 weeks) but was unable to draw firm conclusions due to methodological issues. Evidence for oral NSAIDs is mixed.

Evidence is poor for an improvement from injections of any type, be it corticosteroids, botulinum toxin, prolotherapy or other substances. Corticosteroid injection may be effective in the short term however are of little benefit after a year, compared to a wait-and-see approach. A recent randomized control trial comparing the effect of corticosteroid injection, physiotherapy, or a combination of corticosteroid injection and physiotherapy found that patients treated with corticosteroid injection versus placebo had lower complete recovery or improvement at 1 year (Relative risk 0.86). Patients that received corticosteroid injection also had a higher recurrence rate at 1 year versus placebo (54% versus 12%, relative risk 0.23). Complications from repeated steroid injections include skin problems such as hypopigmentation and fat atrophy leading to indentation of the skin around the injection site. Botulinum toxin type A to paralyze the forearm extensor muscles in those with chronic tennis elbow that has not improved with conservative measures may be reasonable.

Surgery

In recalcitrant cases, surgery may be an option. Surgical methods include:

- Lengthening, release, debridement, or repair of the origin of the extrinsic extensor muscles of the hand at the lateral epicondyle
- Rotation of the anconeus muscle
- Denervation of the lateral epicondyle
- Decompression of the posterior interosseous nerve

Surgical techniques for lateral epicondylitis can be done by open surgery, percutaneous surgery or arthroscopic surgery, with no evidence that any particular type is better or worse than another.

Prognosis

Response to initial therapy is common, but so is relapse (25% to 50%) and/or prolonged, moderate discomfort (40%).

Epidemiology

In tennis players, about 39.7% have reported current or previous problems with their elbow. Less than one quarter (24%) of these athletes under the age of 50 reported that the tennis elbow symptoms were "severe" and "disabling," while 42% were over the age of 50. More women (36%) than men (24%) considered their symptoms severe and disabling. Tennis elbow is more prevalent in individuals over 40, where there is about a four-fold increase among men and two-fold increase among women. Tennis elbow equally affects both sexes and, although men have a marginally higher overall prevalence rate as compared to women, this is not consistent within each age group, nor is it a statistically significant difference.

Playing time is a factor in tennis elbow occurrences. However, increased incidence with increased playing time is statistically significant only for respondents under 40. Individuals over 40 who played over two hours had a two-fold increase in chance of injury. Those under 40 had a 3.5 times increase compared to those who played less than two hours per day.

Shin Splints

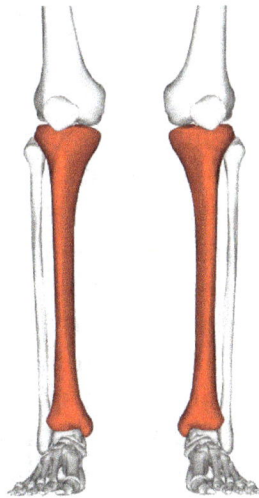

Red area represents tibia. MTSS pain found on inner and lower 2/3rds of tibia.

Shin splints, also known as medial tibial stress syndrome (MTSS), is defined by the American Academy of Orthopaedic Surgeons as "pain along the inner edge of the shinbone (tibia)." Shin splints are usually caused by repeated trauma to the connective muscle tissue surrounding the tibia. They are a common injury affecting athletes who engage in running sports or other forms of physical activity, including running and jumping. They are characterized by general pain in the lower region of the leg between the knee and the ankle. Shin splints injuries are specifically located in the middle to lower thirds of the outside or lateral part of the tibia, which is the larger of two bones comprising the lower leg.

Shin splints are the most prevalent lower leg injury and affect a broad range of individuals. It affects mostly runners and accounts for approximately 13% to 17% of all running-related injuries. High school age runners see shin splints injury rates of approximately 13%. Aerobic dancers have also been known to suffer from shin splints, with injury rates as high as 22%. Military personnel undergoing basic training experience shin splints injury rates between 4%-6.4% and 7.9%.

Signs and Symptoms

Shin splint pain is described as a recurring dull ache along the inner part of the lower two-thirds of the tibia. In contrast, stress fracture pain is localized to the fracture site.

Biomechanically, over-pronation is the common cause for shin splints and action should be taken to offset the biomechanical irregularity. Pronation occurs when the ankle bone moves downward and towards the middle to create a more stable point of contact with the ground. In other words, the ankle rolls inwards so that more of the arch has contact with the ground. This abnormal movement causes muscles to fatigue more quickly and to be unable to absorb any shock from the foot hitting the ground.

Causes

While the exact cause is unknown, shin splints can be attributed to the overloading of the lower leg due to biomechanical irregularities resulting in an increase in stress exerted on the tibia. A sudden increase in intensity or frequency in activity level fatigues muscles too quickly to properly help absorb shock, forcing the tibia to absorb most of that shock. This stress is associated with the onset of shin splints. Muscle imbalance, including weak core muscles, inflexibility and tightness of lower leg muscles, including the gastrocnemius, soleus, and plantar muscles (commonly the flexor digitorum longus) can increase the possibility of shin splints. The pain associated with shin splints is caused from a disruption of Sharpey's fibres that connect the medial soleus fascia through the periosteum of the tibia where it inserts into the bone. With repetitive stress, the impact forces eccentrically fatigue the soleus and create repeated tibial bending or bowing, contributing to shin splints. The impact is made worse by running uphill, downhill, on uneven terrain, or on hard surfaces. Improper footwear, including worn-out shoes, can also contribute to shin splints.

Diagnosis

Shin splints can be diagnosed by a physician after taking a thorough history and performing a complete physical examination. The physical examination focuses on palpable, or gentle pressure, tenderness over a 4–6 inch section on the lower, inside shin area. The pain has been described as a dull ache to an intense pain that increases during exercise, and some individuals experience swelling in the pain area. Clinical history focuses on an individual's previous history with shin splints. People who have previously had shin splints are more likely to have it again.

Vascular and neurological examinations produce normal results in patients with shin splints. Radiographies and three-phase bone scans are recommended to differentiate between shin splints and other causes of chronic leg pain. Bone sctintigraphy and MRI scans can be used to differentiate between stress fractures and shin splints.

It is important to differentiate between different lower leg pain injuries, including shin splints, stress fractures, compartment syndrome, nerve entrapment, and popliteal artery entrapment syndrome. These conditions often have many overlapping symptoms which makes a final diagnosis difficult, and correct diagnosis is needed to determine the most appropriate treatment.

Treatment

Typical treatments include rest, ice, strengthening and gradually returning to activity. Rest and ice work to allow the tibia to recover from sudden, high levels of stress and reduce inflammation and pain levels. It is important to significantly reduce any pain or swelling before returning to activity. Strengthening exercises should be performed after pain has subsided, focusing on lower leg and hip muscles. Individuals should gradually return to activity, beginning with a short and low intensity level. Over multiple weeks, they can slowly work up to normal activity level. It is important to decrease activity level if any pain returns. Individuals should consider running on other surfaces besides asphalt, such as grass, to decrease the amount of force the lower leg must absorb. Orthoses and insoles help to offset biomechanical irregularities, like pronation, and help to support the arch of the foot.

Less common forms of treatment for more severe cases of shin splints include extracorporeal shockwave therapy (ESWT) and surgery. Surgery is only performed in extreme cases where more conservative options have been tried for at least a year. However, surgery does not guarantee 100% recovery.

Epidemiology

Risk factors for developing shin splints include:

- Excessive pronation at subtalar joint

- Excessively tight calf muscles (which can cause excessive pronation)

- Engaging the medial shin muscle in excessive amounts of eccentric muscle activity

- Undertaking high-impact exercises on hard, noncompliant surfaces (ex: running on asphalt or concrete)

- Smoking and low fitness level

While medial tibial stress syndrome is the most common form of shin splints, compartment syndrome and stress fractures are also common forms of shin splints. Females are 1.5 to 3.5 times more likely to progress to stress fractures from shin splints. This is due in part to females having a higher incidence of diminished bone density and osteoporosis.

Achilles Tendon Rupture

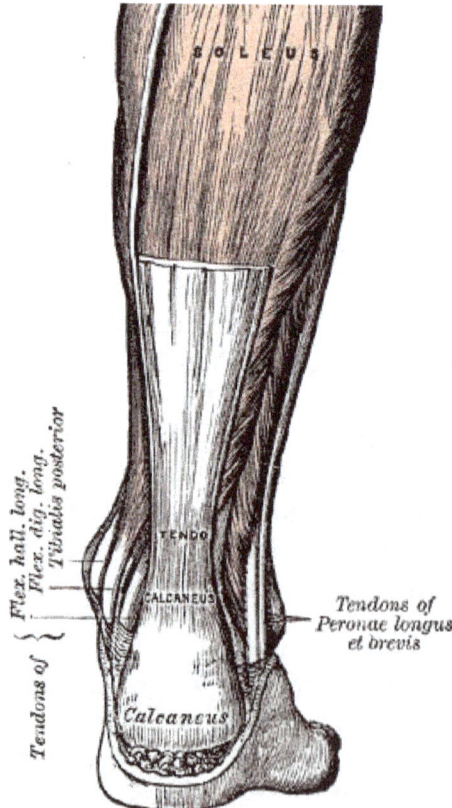

The achilles tendon

Achilles tendon rupture is when the achilles tendon breaks. The achilles is the most commonly injured tendon. Rupture can occur while performing actions requiring explosive acceleration, such as pushing off or jumping. The male to female ratio for Achilles tendon rupture varies between 7:1 and 4:1 across various studies.

Causes

The Achilles tendon is most commonly injured by sudden plantarflexion or dorsiflexion of the ankle, or by forced dorsiflexion of the ankle outside its normal range of motion.

Other mechanisms by which the Achilles can be torn involve sudden direct trauma to the tendon, or sudden activation of the Achilles after atrophy from prolonged periods of inactivity. Some other common tears can occur from overuse while participating in intense sports. Twisting or jerking motions can also contribute to injury.

Fluoroquinolone antibiotics, famously ciprofloxacin, are known to increase the risk of tendon rupture, particularly Achilles.

People who commonly fall victim to Achilles rupture or tear include recreational athletes, people of old age, individuals with previous Achilles tendon tears or ruptures, previous tendon injections or quinolone use, extreme changes in training intensity or activity level, and participation in a new activity.

Most cases of Achilles tendon rupture are traumatic sports injuries. The average age of patients is 29–40 years with a male-to-female ratio of nearly 20:1. Fluoroquinolone antibiotics, such as ciprofloxacin, and glucocorticoids have been linked with an increased risk of Achilles tendon rupture. Direct steroid injections into the tendon have also been linked to rupture.

Quinolone has been associated with Achilles tendinitis and Achilles tendon ruptures for some time. Quinolones are antibacterial agents that act at the level of DNA by inhibiting DNA Gyrase. DNA Gyrase is an enzyme used to unwind double stranded DNA which is essential to DNA Replication. Quinolone is specialized in the fact that it can attack bacterial DNA and prevent them from replicating by this process, and are frequently prescribed to the elderly. Approximately 2% to 6% of all elderly people over the age of 60 who have had Achilles ruptures can be attributed to the use of quinolones.

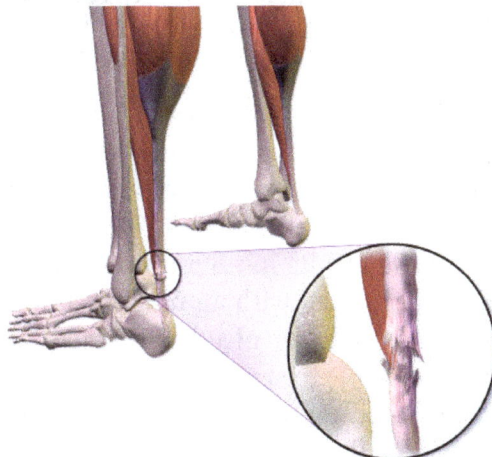

Achilles Tendon Tear

Anatomy

The Achilles tendon is the strongest and thickest tendon in the body, connecting the gastrocnemius, soleus and plantaris to the calcaneus. It is approximately 15 centimeters (5.9 inches) long and begins near the middle portion of the calf. Contraction of the gastrosoleus plantar flexes the foot, enabling such activities as walking, jumping, and running. The Achilles tendon receives its blood supply from its musculotendinous junction with the triceps surae and its innervation from the sural nerve and to a lesser degree from the tibial nerve.

Diagnosis

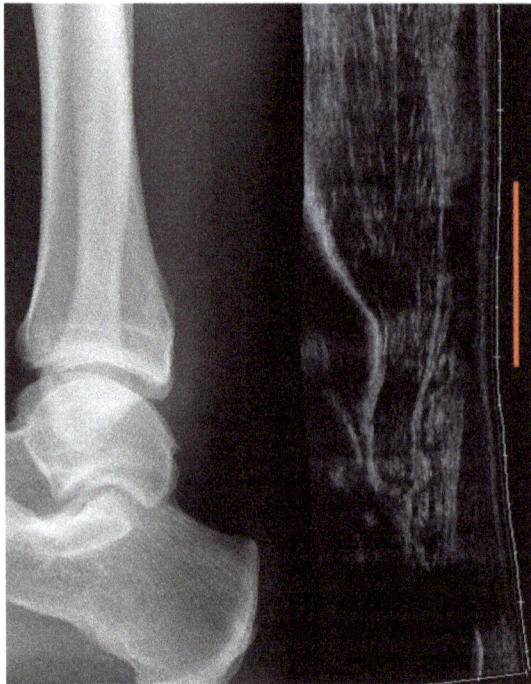

Achilles tendon rupture seen at sonography: discontinuity over several centimeters (red line).
No fracture or avulsion (radiograph).

Diagnosis is made by clinical history; typically people say it feels like being kicked or shot behind the ankle. Upon examination a gap may be felt just above the heel unless swelling has filled the gap and the Simmonds' test (aka Thompson test) will be positive; squeezing the calf muscles of the affected side while the patient lies prone, face down, with his feet hanging loose results in no movement (no passive plantarflexion) of the foot, while movement is expected with an intact Achilles tendon and should be observable upon manipulation of the uninvolved calf. Walking will usually be severely impaired, as the patient will be unable to step off the ground using the injured leg. The patient will also be unable to stand up on the toes of that leg, and pointing the foot downward (plantarflexion) will be impaired. Pain may be severe, and swelling is common.

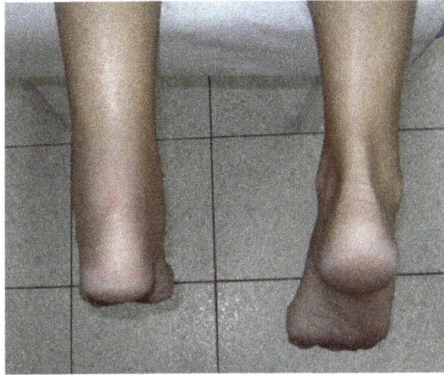

Left Achilles tendon rupture

Sometimes an ultrasound scan may be required to clarify or confirm the diagnosis. MRI can also be used to confirm the diagnosis.

Imaging

Musculoskeletal ultrasonography can be used to determine the tendon thickness, character, and presence of a tear. It works by sending extremely high frequencies of sound through the body. Some of these sounds are reflected back off the spaces between interstitial fluid and soft tissue or bone. These reflected images can be analyzed and computed into an image. These images are captured in real time and can be very helpful in detecting movement of the tendon and visualising possible injuries or tears. This device makes it very easy to spot structural damages to soft tissues, and consistent method of detecting this type of injury. This imaging modality is inexpensive, involves no ionizing radiation and, in the hands of skilled ultrasonographers, may be very reliable.

Magnetic resonance imaging (MRI) can be used to discern incomplete ruptures from degeneration of the Achilles tendon, and MRI can also distinguish between paratenonitis, tendinosis, and bursitis. This technique uses a strong uniform magnetic field to align millions of protons running through the body. these protons are then bombarded with radio waves that knock some of them out of alignment. When these protons return they emit their own unique radio waves that can be analysed by a computer in 3D to create sharp cross sectional image of the area of interest. MRI can provide unparalleled contrast in soft tissue for an extremely high quality photograph making it easy for technicians to spot tears and other injuries.

Radiography can also be used to indirectly identify Achilles tears. Radiography uses X-rays to analyse the point of injury. This is not very effective at identifying injuries to soft tissue. X-rays are created when high energy electrons hit a metal source. X-ray images are acquired by utilising the different attenuation characteristics of dense (e.g. calcium in bone) and less dense (e.g. muscle) tissues when these rays pass through tissue and are captured on film. X-rays are generally exposed to optimise visualisation of dense objects such as bone while soft tissue remains relatively undifferentiated in the background. Radiography has little role in assessment of Achilles' tendon injury and is more useful for ruling out other injuries such as calcaneal fractures.

Treatment

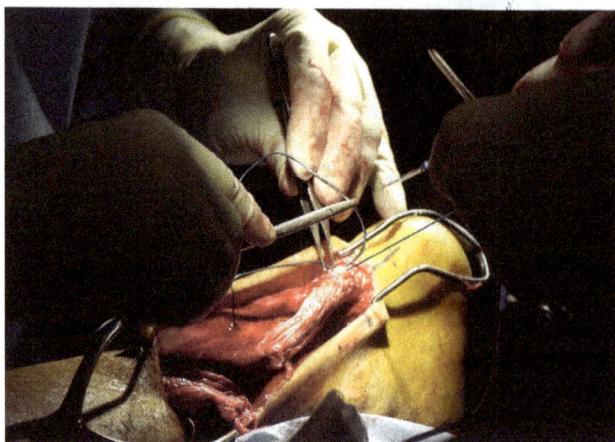

Surgical repair of a ruptured Achilles tendon.

Treatment options for an Achilles tendon rupture include surgical and non-surgical approaches. Among the medical profession opinions are divided what is to be preferred.

Non-surgical management traditionally was selected for minor ruptures, less active patients, and those with medical conditions that prevent them from undergoing surgery. It traditionally consisted of restriction in a plaster cast for six to eight weeks with the foot pointed downwards (to oppose the ends of the ruptured tendon). But recent studies have produced superior results with much more rapid rehabilitation in fixed or hinged boots.

Some surgeons feel an early surgical repair of the tendon is beneficial. The surgical option was long thought to offer a significantly smaller risk of *re-rupture* compared to traditional non-operative management (5% vs 15%). Of course, surgery imposes higher relative risks of perioperative mortality and morbidity e.g. infection including MRSA, bleeding, deep vein thrombosis, lingering anesthesia effects, etc.

However, four recent studies have scientifically tested the benefits of surgery, using randomized streaming of patients into surgical and non-surgical protocols, and applying virtually identical (and aggressive) rehabilitation protocols to both types of patients. All four such studies completed to date have found only small, but statistically significant benefits from the surgery, separated from the other confounding variables. They have all produced reasonably comparable results in re-rupture rates (with each study adding a cautious note about small sample size, one study showing 12% re-rupture in non-surgical treatment versus 4% re-rupture in surgical treatment, which is statistically insignificant), strength, and range of motion, while most have reaffirmed the greater complication rate from surgery. Two studies showed small, but statistically significant differences in plantarflexion strength. The surgical group had significantly better results in the heel-rise work, heel-rise height, concentric power, and hopping tests at the 6-month evaluation than did the nonsurgical group. However, at the 12-month evaluation, there was a significant between-groups difference only in the heel-rise work test.

The relative benefits of surgical and nonsurgical treatments remains a subject of debate; authors of studies are cautious about the preferred treatment. It should be noted that in centers that do not have early range of motion rehabilitation available, surgical repair is preferred to decrease re-rupture rates.

Surgery

There are two different types of surgeries; open surgery and percutaneous surgery.

During an open surgery an incision is made in the back of the leg and the Achilles tendon is stitched together. In a complete or serious rupture the tendon of plantaris or another vestigial muscle is harvested and wrapped around the Achilles tendon, increasing the strength of the repaired tendon. If the tissue quality is poor, e.g. the injury has been neglected, the surgeon might use a reinforcement mesh (collagen, Artelon or other degradable material).

In percutaneous surgery, the surgeon makes several small incisions, rather than one large incision, and sews the tendon back together through the incision(s). Surgery may be delayed for about a week after the rupture to let the swelling go down. For sedentary patients and those who have vasculopathy or risks for poor healing, percutaneous surgical repair may be a better treatment choice than open surgical repair.

Rehabilitation

Non-surgical treatment used to involve very long periods in a series of casts, and took longer to complete than surgical treatment. But both surgical and non-surgical rehabilitation protocols have recently become quicker, shorter, more aggressive, and more successful. It used to be that patients who underwent surgery would wear a cast for approximately 4 to 8 weeks after surgery and were only allowed to gently move the ankle once out of the cast. Recent studies have shown that patients have quicker and more successful recoveries when they are allowed to move and lightly stretch their ankle immediately after surgery. To keep their ankle safe these patients use a removable boot while walking and doing daily activities. Modern studies including non-surgical patients generally limit non-weight-bearing (NWB) to two weeks, and use modern removable boots, either fixed or hinged, rather than casts. Physiotherapy is often begun as early as two weeks following the start of either kind of treatment.

There are three things that need to be kept in mind while rehabilitating a ruptured Achilles: range of motion, functional strength, and sometimes orthotic support. Range of motion is important because it takes into mind the tightness of the repaired tendon. When beginning rehab a patient should perform stretches lightly and increase the intensity as time and pain permits. Putting linear stress on the tendon is important because it stimulates connective tissue repair, which can be achieved while performing the "runners stretch," (putting your toes a couple inches up the wall while your heel is on the ground). Doing stretches to gain functional strength are also important because it improves healing in the tendon, which will in turn lead to a quicker return to activities. These stretches should be more intense and should involve some sort of weight bearing, which helps reorient and strengthen the collagen fibers in the injured ankle. A popular stretch used for this phase of rehabilitation is the toe raise on an elevated surface. The patient is to push up onto the toes and lower his or her self as far down as possible and repeat several times. The other part of the rehab process is orthotic support. This doesn't have anything to do with stretching or strengthening the tendon, rather it is in place to keep the patient comfortable. These are custom made inserts that fit into the patients shoe and help with proper pronation of the foot, which is otherwise a problem that can lead to problems with the Achilles.

To briefly summarize the steps of rehabilitating a ruptured Achilles tendon, you should begin with range of motion type stretching. This will allow the ankle to get used to moving again and get ready for weight bearing activities. Then there is functional strength, this is where weight bearing should begin in order to start strengthening the tendon and getting it ready to perform daily activities and eventually in athletic situations.

Athletic Heart Syndrome

Athletic heart syndrome, (AHS) also known as athlete's heart, athletic bradycardia, or exercise-induced cardiomegaly is a nonpathological condition commonly seen in sports medicine, in which the human heart is enlarged, and the resting heart rate is lower than normal.

Athlete's heart is common in athletes who routinely exercise more than an hour a day, and occurs primarily in endurance athletes, though it can occasionally arise in heavy weight trainers. The condition is generally considered benign, but may occasionally hide a serious medical condition, or may even be mistaken for one.

Athlete's heart most often does not have any physical symptoms, although an indicator would be a consistently low resting heart rate. Athletes with AHS often do not realize they have the condition unless they undergo specific medical tests, because athlete's heart is a normal, physiological adaptation of the body to the stresses of physical conditioning and aerobic exercise. People diagnosed with athlete's heart commonly display three signs that would usually indicate a heart condition when seen in a regular person: bradycardia, cardiomegaly, and cardiac hypertrophy. Bradycardia is a slower than normal heartbeat, at around 40–60 beats per minute. Cardiomegaly is the state of an enlarged heart, and cardiac hypertrophy the thickening of the muscular wall of the heart, specifically the left ventricle, which pumps oxygenated blood to the aorta. Especially during an intensive workout, more blood and oxygen are required to the peripheral tissues of the arms and legs in highly trained athletes' bodies. A larger heart results in higher cardiac output, which also allows it to beat more slowly, as more blood is pumped out with each beat.

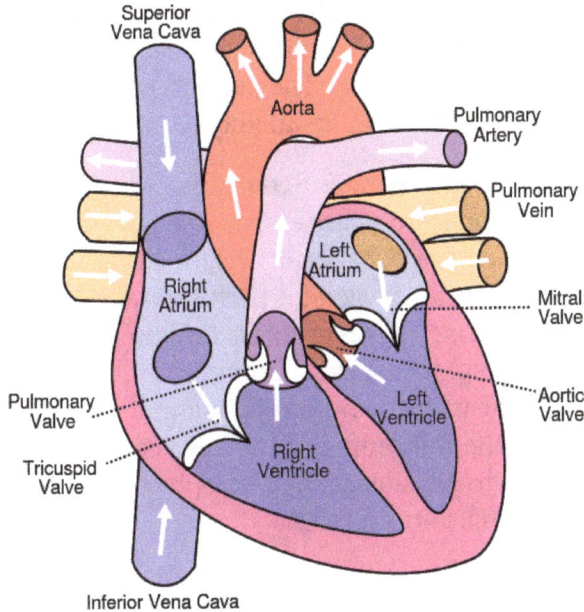

The human heart

Another sign of athlete's heart syndrome is an S3 gallop, which can be heard through a stethoscope. This sound can be heard as the diastolic pressure of the irregularly shaped heart creates a disordered blood flow. However, if an S4 gallop is heard, the patient should be given immediate attention. An S4 gallop is a stronger and louder sound created by the heart, if diseased in any way, and is typically a sign of a serious medical condition.

Cause

Athlete's heart is a result of dynamic physical activity such as (more than 5 hours a week) aerobic training, rather than static training such as weight lifting. During intensive prolonged endurance or strength training, the body signals the heart to pump more blood through the body to counteract the oxygen deficit building in the skeletal muscles. Enlargement of the heart is a natural physical adaptation of the body to deal with the high pressures and large amounts of blood that can affect the heart during these periods of time. Over time, the body will increase both the chamber size of the left ventricle, and the muscle mass and wall thickness of the heart.

Cardiac output, the amount of blood that leaves the heart in a given time period (i.e. liters per minute), is proportional to both the chamber sizes of the heart and the rate at which the heart beats. With a larger left ventricle, the heart rate can decrease and still maintain a level of cardiac output necessary for the body. Therefore, athletes with AHS commonly have lower resting heart rates than nonathletes.

The heart becomes enlarged, or hypertrophic, due to intense cardiovascular workouts, creating an increase in stroke volume, an enlarged left ventricle (and right ventricle), and a decrease in resting pulse along with irregular rhythms. The wall of the left ventricle increases in size by about 15–20% of its normal capacity. No decrease of the diastolic function of the left ventricle occurs. The patient may also experience an irregular heartbeat and a resting pulse rate between 40 and 60 beats per minute (bradycardia).

The level of physical activity in a person determines what physiological changes the heart makes. The two types of exercise are static (strength-training) and dynamic (endurance-training). Static exercise consists of weight lifting and is mostly anaerobic, meaning the body does not rely on oxygen for performance. It also moderately increases heart rate and stroke volume (oxygen debt). Dynamic exercises include running, swimming, skiing, and cycling, which rely on oxygen from the body. This type of exercise also increases both heart rate and stroke volume of the heart. Both static and dynamic exercises involve the thickening of the left ventricular wall due to increased cardiac output, which leads to physiologic hypertrophy of the heart. Once athletes stop training, the heart returns to its normal size.

Diagnosis

Athlete's heart is usually an incidental finding during a routine screening or during tests for other medical issues. An enlarged heart can be seen at echocardiography or sometimes on a chest X-ray. Similarities at presentation between athlete's heart and clinically relevant cardiac problems may prompt electrocardiography (ECG)and exercise cardiac stress tests. The ECG can detect sinus bradycardia, a resting heart rate of fewer than 60 beats per minute. This is often accompanied by sinus arrhythmia. The pulse of a person with athlete's heart can sometimes be irregular while at rest, but usually returns to normal after exercise begins.

Regarding differential diagnosis, left ventricular hypertrophy is usually indistinguishable from athlete's heart and at ECG, but can usually be discounted in the young and fit.

It is important to distinguish between athlete's heart and hypertrophic cardiomyopathy, a serious cardiovascular disease characterised by thickening of the heart's walls, which produces a similar ECG pattern at rest. This genetic disorder is found in one of 500 Americans and is a leading cause of sudden cardiac death in young athletes (although only about 8% of all cases of sudden death are actually exercise-related). The following table shows some key distinguishing characteristics of the two conditions.

Feature	Athletic heart syndrome	Cardiomyopathy
Left ventricular hypertrophy	< 13 mm	> 15 mm
Left ventricular end-diastolic diameter	< 60 mm	> 70 mm
Diastolic function	Normal (E:A ratio > 1)	Abnormal (E:A ratio < 1)
Septal hypertrophy	Symmetric	Asymmetric (in hypertrophic cardiomyopathy)
Family history	None	May be present
BP response to exercise	Normal	Normal or reduced systolic BP response
Deconditioning	Left ventricular hypertrophy regression	No left ventricular hypertrophy regression

The medical history of the patient (endurance sports) and physical examination (bradycardia, and maybe a third or fourth heart sound), can give important hints.

- ECG - typical findings in resting position are, for example, sinus bradycardia, atrioventricular block (primary and secondary) and right bundle branch block - all those findings normalize during exercise.

- Echocardiography - differentiation between physiological and pathological increases of the heart's size is possible, especially by estimating the mass of the wall (not over 130 g/m²) and its end diastolic diameter (not much less 60 mm) of the left ventricle.

- X-ray examination of the chest may show increased heart size (mimicking other possible causes of enlargement).

Clinical Relevance

Athlete's heart is not dangerous for athletes (though if a nonathlete has symptoms of bradycardia, cardiomegaly, and cardiac hypertrophy, another illness may be present). Athlete's heart is not the cause of sudden cardiac death during or shortly after a workout, which mainly occurs due to hypertrophic cardiomyopathy, a genetic disorder.

No treatment is required for people with athletic heart syndrome; it does not pose any physical threats to the athlete, and despite some theoretical concerns that the ventricular remodeling might conceivably predispose for serious arrhythmias, no evidence has been found of any increased risk of long-term events. Athletes should see a physician and receive a clearance to be sure their symptoms are due to athlete's heart and not another heart disease, such as cardiomyopathy. If the athlete is uncomfortable with having athlete's heart or if a differential diagnosis is difficult, deconditioning from exercise for a period of three months allows the heart to return to its regular size. However, one long-term study of elite-trained athletes found that dilation of the left ventricle was only partially reversible after a long period of deconditioning. This deconditioning is often met with resistance to the accompanying lifestyle changes. The real risk attached to athlete's heart is if athletes or nonathletes simply assume they have the condition, instead of making sure they do not have a life-threatening heart illness.

Screening for Related Conditions

Because several well-known and high-profile cases of athletes experiencing sudden unexpected death due to cardiac arrest, such as Reggie White and Marc-Vivien Foé, a growing movement is making an effort to have both professional and school-based athletes screened for cardiac and other related conditions, usually through a careful medical and health history, a good family history, a comprehensive physical examination including auscultation of heart and lung sounds and recording of vital signs such as heart rate and blood pressure, and increasingly, for better efforts at detection, such as an electrocardiogram.

An electrocardiogram (ECG) is a relatively straightforward procedure to administer and interpret, compared to more invasive or sophisticated tests; it can reveal or hint at many circulatory disorders and arrhythmias. Part of the cost of an ECG may be covered by some insurance companies, though routine use of ECGs or other similar procedures such as echocardiography (ECHO) are still not considered routine in these contexts. Widespread routine ECGs for all potential athletes during initial screening and then during the yearly physical assessment could well be too expensive to implement on a wide scale, especially in the face of the potentially very large demand. In some places, a shortage of funds, portable ECG machines, or qualified personnel to administer and interpret them (medical technicians, paramedics, nurses trained in cardiac monitoring, advanced practice nurses or nurse practitioners, physician assistants, and physicians in internal or family medicine or in some area of cardiopulmonary medicine) exist.

If sudden cardiac death occurs, it is usually because of pathological hypertrophic enlargement of the heart that went undetected or was incorrectly attributed to the benign "athletic" cases. Among the many alternative causes are episodes of isolated arrhythmias which degenerated into lethal VF and asystole, and various unnoticed, possibly asymptomatic cardiac congenital defects of the vessels, chambers, or valves of the heart. Other causes include carditis, endocarditis, myocarditis, and pericarditis whose symptoms were slight or ignored, or were asymptomatic.

The normal treatments for episodes due to the pathological look-alikes are the same mainstays for any other episode of cardiac arrest: Cardiopulmonary resuscitation, defibrillation to restore normal sinus rhythm, and if initial defibrillation fails, administration of intravenous epinephrine or amiodarone. The goal is avoidance of infarction, heart failure, and/or lethal arrhythmias (ventricular tachycardia, ventricular fibrillation, asystole, or pulseless electrical activity), so ultimately to restore normal sinus rhythm.

History

The athlete's heart syndrome was first described in 1899 by S. Henschen. He compared the heart size of cross-country skiers to those who lived sedentary lives. He noticed that those who participated in competitive sports displayed symptoms of athlete's heart syndrome. Henschen believed the symptoms were a normal adjustment to exercise, and felt concern was not needed. Henschen believed that the entire heart became enlarged, when in fact, only the left side becomes hypertrophic. He also believed athletes with AHS lived shorter lives than those who did not acquire the syndrome. Because his research occurred throughout the 19th century, technology was limited, and it became difficult to come up with appropriate ways to measure the hearts of athletes. Few believed in Henschen's theory about athletes having larger hearts than those who did not participate in sports. Today, Henschen's original theory has proved to be correct.

Patellar Tendinitis

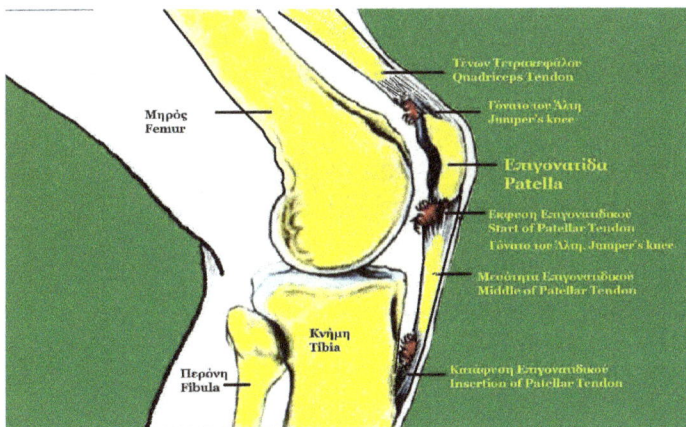

Τένων Τετρακεφάλου / Quadriceps Tendon

Γόνατο του Άλτη / Jumper's knee

Μηρός / Femur

Επιγονατίδα / Patella

Έκφυση Επιγονατιδικού / Start of Patellar Tendon / Γόνατο του Άλτη Jumper's knee

Μεσότητα Επιγονατιδικού / Middle of Patellar Tendon

Κνήμη / Tibia

Περόνη / Fibula

Κατάφυση Επιγονατιδικού / Insertion of Patellar Tendon

Patellar tendinitis (patellar tendinopathy, also known as jumper's knee), is a relatively common cause of pain in the inferior patellar region in athletes. It is common with frequent jumping and studies have shown it may be associated with stiff ankle movement and ankle sprains.

Presentation

Jumper's knee (patellar tendinopathy, patellar tendinosis, patellar tendinitis) commonly occurs in athletes who are involved in jumping sports such as basketball and volleyball. Patients report anterior knee pain, often with an aching quality. The symptom onset is insidious. Rarely is a discrete injury described. Usually, involvement is infrapatellar at or near the infrapatellar pole, but it may also be suprapatellar.

Depending on the duration of symptoms, jumper's knee can be classified into 1 of 4 stages, as follows:

Stage 1 – Pain only after activity, without functional impairment

Stage 2 – Pain during and after activity, although the patient is still able to perform satisfactorily in his or her sport

Stage 3 – Prolonged pain during and after activity, with increasing difficulty in performing at a satisfactory level

Stage 4 – Complete tendon tear requiring surgical repair

It begins as inflammation in the patellar tendon where it attaches to the patella and may progress by tearing or degenerating the tendon. Patients present with an ache over the patella tendon. Most patients are between 10 and 16 years old. Magnetic resonance imaging can reveal edema (increased T2 signal intensity) in the proximal aspect of the patellar tendon.

Causes

It is an overuse injury from repetitive overloading of the extensor mechanism of the knee. The microtears exceed the body's healing mechanism unless the activity is stopped.

Among the risk factors for patellar tendonitis are low ankle dorsiflexion, weak gluteal muscles, and muscle tightness, particularly in the calves, quadriceps muscle, and hamstrings.

The injury occurs to athletes in many sports.

Treatment

Early stages may be treated conservatively using the R.I.C.E methods.

1. Rest

2. Ice

3. Compression

4. Elevation

Exercises involving eccentric muscle contractions of the quadriceps on a decline board are strongly supported by extant literature. A physical therapist may also recommend specific exercises and stretches to strengthen the muscles and tendons.

Should this fail, autologous blood injection, or platelet-rich plasma injection may be performed and is typically successful though not as successful as high volume saline injection (Crisp *et al.*). Uncommonly it may require surgery to remove myxoid degeneration in the tendon. This is reserved for patients with debilitating pain for 6–12 months despite conservative measures. Novel treatment modalities targeting the abnormal blood vessel growth which occurs in the condition are currently being investigated.

Commotio Cordis

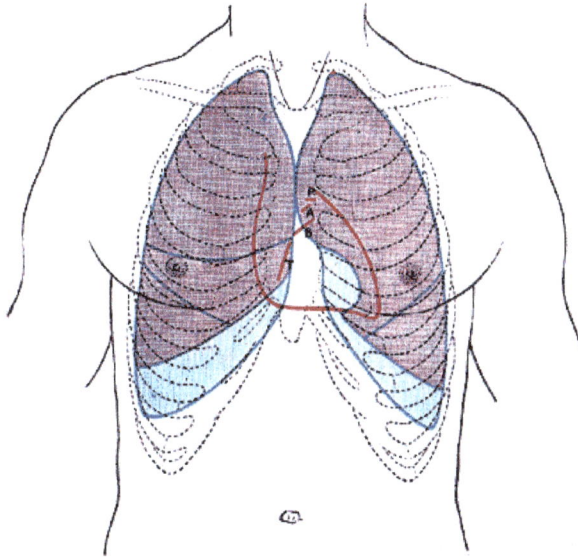

Human adult thorax, showing the outline of the heart (in red). The sensitive zone for mechanical induction of heart rhythm disturbances lies between the 2nd and the 4th ribs, to the left of the sternum

Commotio cordis (Latin, "agitation of the heart") is an often lethal disruption of heart rhythm that occurs as a result of a blow to the area directly over the heart (the precordial region), at a critical time during the cycle of a heart beat causing cardiac arrest. It is a form of ventricular fibrillation (V-Fib), not mechanical damage to the heart muscle or surrounding organs, and not the result of heart disease. The fatality rate is about 65%. It can sometimes, but not always, be reversed by defibrillation.

Commotio cordis occurs mostly in boys and young men (average age 15), usually during sports, most often baseball, often despite a chest protector. It is most often caused by a projectile, but can also be caused by the blow of an elbow or other body part. Being less developed, the thorax of an adolescent is likely more prone to this injury given the circumstances.

The phenomenon was confirmed experimentally in the 1930s, with research in anaesthetized rabbits, cats and dogs.

Incidence

Commotio cordis is a very rare event, but nonetheless is often considered when an athlete presents with sudden cardiac death. Some of the sports which have a risk for this cause of trauma are baseball, association football, ice hockey, polo, rugby football, cricket, softball, pelota, fencing, lacrosse, boxing, karate, kung fu, and other martial arts. Children are especially vulnerable, possibly due to the mechanical properties of their thoracic skeleton. From 1996 to spring 2007, the USA National Commotio Cordis Registry had 188 cases recorded, with about half occurring during organized sports Almost all (96%) of the victims were male, the mean age of the victims during that period was 14.7 years, and fewer than one in five survived the incident.

Other Situations

Commotio cordis may also occur in other situations, such as in children who are punished with blows over the precordium, cases of torture, and frontal collisions of motor vehicles (the impact of the steering wheel against the thorax, although this has decreased substantially with the use of safety belts and air bags).

In contrast, the precordial thump (hard blows given over the precordium with a closed fist to revert cardiac arrest) is a sanctioned procedure for emergency resuscitation by trained health professionals witnessing a monitored arrest when no equipment is at hand, endorsed by the latest guidelines of the International Liaison Committee on Resuscitation. It has been discussed controversially, as—in particular in severe hypoxia—it may cause the opposite effect (i.e., a worsening of rhythm—commotio cordis). In a normal adult, the energy range involved in the precordial thump is five to 10 times below that associated with commotio cordis.

Mechanism of Injury

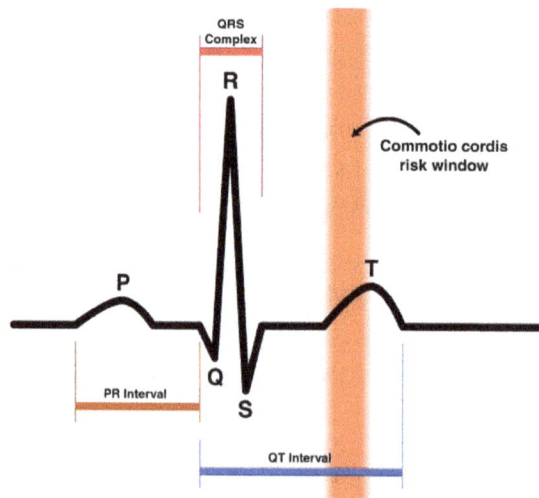

Diagram showing the portion of normal sinus rhythm during which commotio cordis is a risk

These factors influence the chance of commotio cordis:

- Direction of impact over the precordium (precise area, angle of impact)

- Total applied energy (area of impact versus energy, i.e., the kinetic energy of the projectile $E_k = \frac{1}{2}mv^2$)

- Impact occurring within a specific 10– to 30-millisecond portion of the cardiac cycle. This period occurs in the ascending phase of the T wave, when the ventricular myocardium is repolarizing, moving from systole to diastole (relaxation).

The small window of vulnerability explains why it is a rare event. Considering that the total cardiac cycle has a duration of 1 second (for a base cardiac frequency of 60 beats per minute), the probability of a mechanical trauma within the window of vulnerability is 1 to 3% only. That also explains why the heart becomes more vulnerable when it is physically strained by sports activities:

1. The increase in heart rate (exercise tachycardia) may double the probability above (e.g., with 120 beats per minute the cardiac cycle shortens to 500 milliseconds without fundamentally altering the window-of-vulnerability's size)

2. Relative exercise-induced hypoxia and acceleration of the excitoconductive system of the heart make it more susceptible to stretch-induced ventricular fibrillation.

The cellular mechanisms of commotio cordis are still poorly understood, but probably related to the activation of mechanosensitive proteins, ion channels.

Impact energies of at least 50 joules are estimated to be required to cause cardiac arrest, when applied in the right time and spot of the precordium of an adult. Impacts up to 130 joules have already been measured with hockey pucks and lacrosse balls, 450 joules in karate punches, and 1028 joules in boxer Rocky Marciano's punch. The 50-joule threshold, however, can be considerably lowered when the victim's heart is under ischemic conditions, such as in coronary artery insufficiency.

Also an upper limit of impact energy is applied to the heart; too much energy will create structural damage to the heart muscle, as well as causing electrical upset. This condition is referred to as contusio cordis (from Latin for bruising of the heart). On isolated guinea pig hearts, as little as 5 mJ were needed to induce release of creatine kinase, a marker for muscle cell damage. Obviously, this figure does not include the dissipation of energy through the chest wall, and is not scaled up for humans, but it is indicative that relatively small amounts of energy are required to reach the heart before physical damage is done.

Outcome and Treatment

Most cases are fatal. Automated external defibrillators have helped increase the survival rate to 35%. Defibrillation must be started as soon as possible (within 3 minutes) for maximal benefit. Commotio cordis is the leading cause of fatalities in youth baseball in the US, with two to three deaths per year. It has been recommended that "communities and school districts reexamine the need for accessible automatic defibrillators and cardiopulmonary resuscitation-trained coaches at organized sporting events for children."

Prevention

The risk would probably be reduced by improved coaching techniques, such as teaching young batters to turn away from the ball to avoid errant pitches, according to doctors. Defensive players in lacrosse and hockey are now taught to avoid using their chest to block the ball or puck. Chest protectors and vests are designed to reduce trauma from blunt bodily injury, but this does not offer protection from commotio cordis and may offer a false sense of security. Almost 20% of the victims in competitive football, baseball, lacrosse and hockey were wearing protectors. This ineffectiveness has been confirmed by animal studies. Development of adequate chest protectors may prove difficult.

Legal Issues

Several people have been convicted of involuntary manslaughter in cases involving insufficient and slow medical help to athletes who experienced commotio cordis during sports events, as well as in cases of intentional delivery of contusive blows. In 1992, Italian hockey player Miran Schrott died after a blow to his chest from the stick of Canadian-Italian player Jimmy Boni. Boni was charged with culpable homicide, and eventually pleaded guilty to manslaughter, paying a $1,300 fine and $175,000 restitution to Schrott's family.

Patellar Dislocation

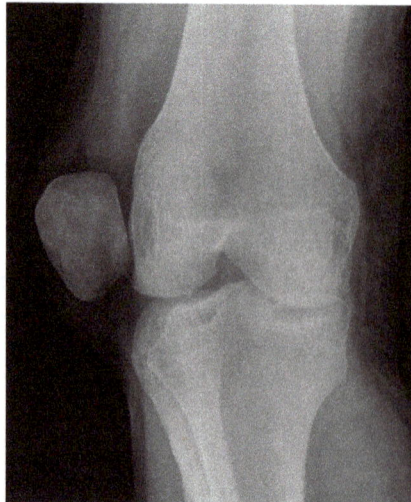

Radiograph of a patient with patellar dislocation. Normally the patella projects over the distal femur.

Patellar dislocation is an injury of the knee, typically caused by a direct blow or a sudden twist of the leg. It occurs when the patella (kneecap) slips out of its normal position in the patellofemoral groove, and generally causes intense pain with swelling of the knee. Open or arthroscopic surgery may be used to repair damage, but are typically avoided since rates of re-injury, knee function, and patients' opinions do not differ much from conservative treatment.

The patella generally dislocates laterally, and can be accompanied by acute pain and disability. Immediate reduction can be accomplished by hyperextension of the knee, and by providing a medialward pressure to move the patella back into the patellofemoral groove. Hyperextension of the knee on its own could possibly move the patella into place, because this motion locks the knee in place. When the knee is locked the ligaments are twisted and taut, allowing the muscles involved to relax and the patella to slide back into place. If that does not work, a medical professional must manually perform an orthopedic reduction. Swelling and impaired mobility follow patellar dislocation, and a rehabilitation program of six to sixteen weeks is recommended whether or not the patient undergoes surgery.

Young athletes suffer patellar dislocations more commonly than any other group, and the average age of occurrences is 16–20 years. Sports commonly associated with the injury involve sudden twisting motions of the knee and/or impact, such as soccer, gymnastics and ice hockey. It can also occur when a person trips over an object or slips on a slick surface, especially if that person has predisposing factors.

Signs and Symptoms

People often describe pain as being "inside the knee cap." The leg tends to flex even when relaxed. In some cases, the injured ligaments involved in patellar dislocation do not allow the leg to flex almost at all.

Risk Factors

A predisposing factor is tightness in the tensor fasciae latae muscle and iliotibial tract in combination with a quadriceps imbalance between the vastus lateralis and vastus medialis muscles can play a large role. However individuals with larger Q angles are genetically more predisposed to this type of injury due to the increased lateral angle at which the femur and tibia meet.

Another cause of patellar symptoms is *lateral patellar compression syndrome*, which can be caused from lack of balance or inflammation in the joints. The pathophysiology of the kneecap is complex, and deals with the osseous soft tissue or abnormalities within the patellofemoral groove. The patellar symptoms cause knee extensor dysplasia, and sensitive small variations affect the muscular mechanism that controls the joint movements.

24% of patients whose patellas have dislocated have relatives who have experienced patellar dislocations.

Athletic Population

Patellar dislocation occurs in sports that involve rotating the knee. Direct trauma to the knee can knock the patella out of joint.

Anatomical Factors

People who have larger Q angles tend to be more prone to having knee injuries such as dislocations, due to the central line of pull found in the quadriceps muscles that run from the anterior superior iliac spine to the center of the patella. The range of a normal Q angle for men ranges from <15 degrees and for females <20 degrees, putting females at a higher risk for this injury. An angle greater than 25 degrees between the patellar tendon and quadriceps muscle can predispose a person to patellar dislocation.

In patella alta, the patella sits higher on the knee than normal. Normal function of the VMO muscle stabilizes the patella. Decreased VMO function results in instability of the patella.

Forces

When there is too much tension on the patella, the ligaments will weaken and be susceptible to tearing ligaments or tendons due to shear force or torsion force, which then displaces the kneecap from its origination. Another cause that patellar dislocation can occur is when the trochlear groove that has been completely flattened is defined as trochlear dysplasia. Not having a groove because the trochlear bone has flattened out can cause the patella to slide because nothing is holding the patella in place.

Mechanism of Injury

Patellar dislocations occur by:

- A direct impact that knocks the patella out of joint
- A twisting motion of the knee, or ankle
- A sudden lateral cut

Anatomy of the Knee

The patella is a triangular sesamoid bone which is embedded in tendon. It rests in the patellofemoral groove, an articular cartilage-lined hollow at the end of the thigh bone (femur) where the thigh bone meets the shin bone (tibia). Several ligaments and tendons hold the patella in place and allow it to move up and down the patellofemoral groove when the leg bends. The top of the patella attaches to the quadriceps muscle via the quadriceps tendon, the middle to the vastus medialis obliquus and vastus lateralis

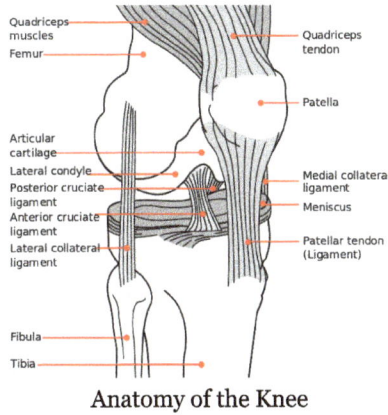

Anatomy of the Knee

muscles, and the bottom to the head of the tibia (tibial tuberosity) via the patellar tendon, which is a continuation of the quadriceps femoris tendon. The medial patellofemoral ligament attaches horizontally in the inner knee to the adductor magnus tendon and is the structure most often damaged during a patellar dislocation. Finally, the lateral collateral ligament and the medial collateral ligament stabilize the patella on either side. Any of these structures can sustain damage during a patellar dislocation.

Diagnosis

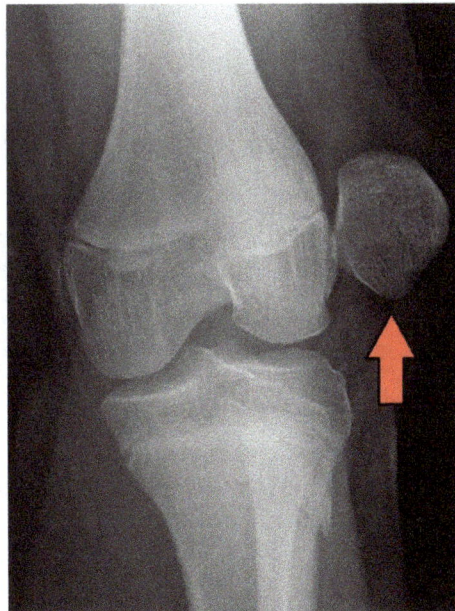

Petellar dislocation

To assess the knee, a clinician can perform the patellar apprehension test by moving the patella back and forth while the patient flexes the knee at approximately 30 degrees.

The patient can do the *patella tracking assessment* by making a single leg squat and standing, or by lying on his or her back with knee extended from flexed position. A patella that slips medially on early flexion is called the J sign, and indicates imbalance between the VMO and lateral structures.

Prevention

The patella is a floating sesamoid bone held in place by the quadriceps muscle tendon and patellar tendon ligament. Exercises should strengthen quadriceps muscles such as rectus femoris, vastus intermedius, and vastus lateralis. However, tight and strong lateral quadriceps can be an underlying cause of patellar dislocation. If this is the case, it is advisable to strengthen the medial quadriceps, vastus medialis (VMO), and stretch the lateral muscles. Exercises to strengthen quadriceps muscles include, but are not limited to, squats and lunges. Adding extra external support around the knee by using devices such as knee [orthotics] or athletic tape can help to prevent patellar dislocation and other knee-related injuries. External supports, such as knee braces and athletic tape, work by providing movement in only the desired planes and help hinder movements that can cause abnormal movement and injuries. Women who wear high heels tend to develop short calf muscles and tendons. Exercises to stretch and strengthen calf muscles are recommended on a daily basis.

Treatment

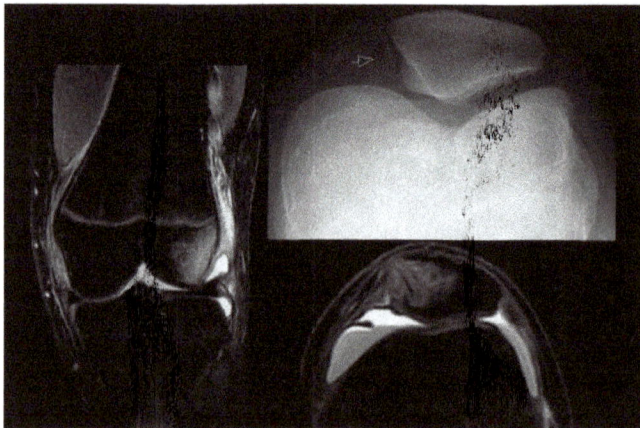

X-ray and MRI after luxation of the patella. There is a fragment and bone bruise at the medial surface of the patella and in the corresponding surface of the lateral condyle of the femur. The medial retinaculum of the patella is disrupted.

Two types of treatment options are typically available:

- Surgery

- Conservative treatment (rehabilitation and physical therapy)

Surgery may impede normal growth of structures in the knee, so doctors generally do not recommend knee operations for young people who are still growing. There are also risks of complications, such as an adverse reaction to anesthesia or an infection.

When designing a rehabilitation program, clinicians consider associated injuries such as chipped bones or soft tissue tears. Clinicians take into account the patient's age, activity level, and time needed to return to work and/or athletics. Doctors generally only recommend surgery when other structures in the knee have sustained severe damage, or specifically when there is:

- Concurrent osteochondral injury

- Continued gross instability

- Palpable disruption of the medial patellofemoral ligament and the vastus medialis obliquus

- High-level athletic demands coupled with mechanical risk factors and an initial injury mechanism not related to contact

Supplements like glucosamine and NSAIDs can be used to minimize bothersome symptoms.

Rehabilitation

An effective rehabilitation program reduces the chances of reinjury and of other knee-related problems such as patellofemoral pain syndrome and osteoarthritis. Rehabilitation focuses on maintaining strength and range of motion to reduce pain and maintain the health of the muscles and tissues around the knee joint.

Epidemiology

Rate in the United States have been estimated to occur among an at-risk population of 1,774,210,081 people each year. Incidence rates published in the American Journal of Sports Medicine for ages 10–17 were found to be about 29 per 100,000 persons per year, while the adult population average for this type of injury ranged between 5.8 and 7.0 per 100,000 persons per year. The highest rates of patellar dislocation were found in the youngest age groups, while the rates declined with increasing ages. Females are more susceptible to patellar dislocation. Race is a significant factor for this injury, where Hispanics, African-Americans and Caucasians had slightly higher rates of patellar dislocation due to the types of athletic activity involved in: basketball (18.2%), soccer (6.9%), and football (6.9%), according to Brian Waterman.

Lateral Patellar dislocation is common among the child population. Some studies suggest that the annual patellar dislocation rate in children is 43/100,000. The treatment of the skeletally immature is controversial due to the fact that they are so young and are still growing. Surgery is recommended by some experts in order to repair the medial structures early, while others recommend treating it non operatively with physical therapy. If re-dislocation occurs then reconstruction of the medial patellofemoral ligament (MPFL) is the recommended surgical option.

Climbing Injuries

Injuries in rock climbing may occur due to falls, or due to overuse. Injuries due to falls are relatively uncommon; the vast majority of injuries result from overuse, most often occurring in the fingers, elbows, and shoulders. Such injuries are often no worse than torn calluses, cuts, burns and bruises. However, overuse symptoms, if ignored, may lead to permanent damage (esp. to tendons, tendon sheaths, ligaments, and joint capsules).

Risk Groups

The climbers most prone to injuries are intermediate to expert within lead climbing or bouldering.

Overuse Injuries in Climbing

In terms of overuse injuries a British study found that:

- 40 percent occurred in the fingers

- 16 percent in the shoulders

- 12 percent in the elbows

- 5 percent were the knees

- 5 percent back

- 4 percent wrists

One injury that tend to be very common among climbers is Carpal tunnel syndrome. It is found in about 25% of climbers.

Finger Injuries

604 injured rock climbers were prospectively evaluated from January 1998 to December 2001, due to the rapid growth of new complex finger trauma in the mid-1980s. Of the most frequent injuries, three out of four were related to the fingers: pulley injuries accounted for 20%, tendovaginitis for 7%, and joint capsular damage for 6.1%.

Pulleys

Damage to the flexor tendon pulleys that encircle and support the tendons that cross the finger joints is the most common finger injury within the sport. The main culprit for pulley related injuries is the common crimp grip, especially in the closed position. The crimp grip requires a near ninety-degree flexion of the middle finger joint, which produces a tremendous force load on the A2 pulley. Injuries to the A2 pulley can range from microscopic to partial tears and, in the worst case, complete ruptures. Some climbers report hearing a pop, which might be a sign of a significant tear or complete rupture, during an extremely heavy move (e.g. tiny crimp, one- or two-finger pocket). Small partial tears, or inflammation can occur over the course of several sessions.

- Grade I – Sprain of the finger ligaments (collateral ligaments), pain locally at the pulley, pain when squeezing or climbing.

- Grade II – Partial rupture of the pulley tendon. Pain locally at the pulley, pain when squeezing or climbing, possible pain while extending your finger.

- Grade III – Complete rupture of the pulley, causing bowstringing of the tendon. Symptoms can include: Pain locally at the pulley (usually sharp), may feel/hear a 'pop' or 'crack', swelling and possible bruising, pain when squeezing or climbing, pain when extending your finger, pain with resisted flexion of the finger.

Knuckle

- Stress fractures

- Collateral ligament injuries

Shoulder Injuries

Shoulder related injuries include rotator cuff tear, strain or tendinitis, biceps tendinitis and SLAP lesion.

Elbow Injuries

Tennis elbow (Lateral Epicondylitis) is a common elbow injury among climbers, as is Golfer's elbow (Medial Epicondylitis, which is similar, but occurs on the inside of the elbow).

Calluses, Dry Skin

Climbers often develop calluses on their fingers from regular contact with the rock and the rope. When calluses split open they expose a raw layer of skin that can be very painful. This type of injury is commonly referred to as a flapper.

The use of magnesium carbonate (chalk) for better grip dries out the skin and can often lead to cracked and damaged hands

There are a number of skincare products available for climbers that help to treat calluses, moisturise dry hands and reduce recovery time.

Young/Adolescent Climbers

"Any finger injury that is sustained by a young adolescent (12–16) should be seen by a physician and have x-rays performed. These skeletally immature athletes are very susceptible to developing debilitating joint arthritis later in adulthood."

Saddle Sore

A saddle sore in humans is a skin ailment on the buttocks due to, or exacerbated by, horse riding or cycling on a bicycle saddle. It often develops in three stages: skin abrasion, folliculitis (which looks like a small, reddish acne), and finally abscess.

Because it most commonly starts with skin abrasion, it is desirable to reduce the factors which lead to skin abrasion. Some of these factors include:

- Reducing the friction. In equestrian activities, friction is reduced with a proper riding position and using properly fitting clothing and equipment. In cycling, reduce bobbing or swinging motion while pedaling by setting the appropriate saddle height helps reduce friction. Angle and fore/aft position can also play a role, and different cyclists have different needs and preferences in relation to this.

- Selecting an appropriate size and design of horse riding saddle or bicycle saddle.

- Wearing proper clothing. In bicycling, this includes cycling shorts, with chamois padding. For equestrian activity, long, closely fitted pants such as equestrian breeches or jodhpurs minimize chafing. For western riding, closely fitted jeans with no heavy inner seam, sometimes combined with chaps, are preferred. Padded cycling shorts worn under riding pants helps some equestrians, and extra padding, particularly sheepskin, on the seat of the saddle may help in more difficult situations such as long-distance endurance riding.

- Using petroleum jelly, chamois cream or lubricating gel to further reduce friction.

If left untreated over an extended period of time, saddle sores may need to be drained by a physician.

In animals such as horses and other working animals, saddle sores often form on either side of the withers, which is the area where the front of a saddle rests, and also in the girth area behind the animal's elbow, where they are known as a girth gall. Saddle sores can occur over the loin, and occasionally in other locations. These sores are usually caused by ill-fitting gear, dirty gear, lack of proper padding, or unbalanced loads. Reducing friction is also of great help in preventing equine saddle sores. Where there is swelling but not yet open sores, the incidence of sore backs may be reduced by loosening the girth, but not immediately removing the saddle after a long ride, thus allowing normal circulation to return slowly.

Fencing Response

The fencing response is a peculiar position of the arms following a concussion. Immediately after moderate forces have been applied to the brainstem, the forearms are held flexed or extended (typically into the air) for a period lasting up to several seconds after the impact. The fencing response is often observed during athletic competition involving contact, such as American football, hockey, rugby and martial arts. It is used as an overt indicator of injury force magnitude and midbrain localization to aid in injury identification and classification for events including, but not limited to, on-field and/or bystander observations of sports-related head injuries.

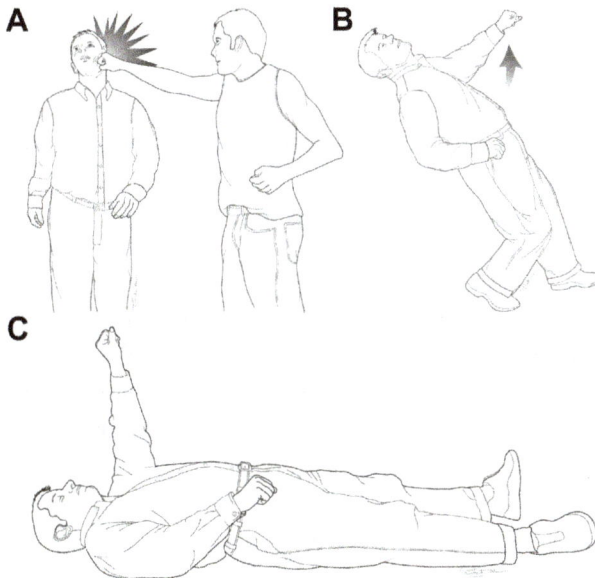

Schematic illustration of the fencing response during a knockout. **A.** The individual receives a punch to the head. **B.** After the traumatic blow to the head, the unconscious individual immediately exhibits arm extension on the same side of the body as the site that received the blow and arm flexion on the opposite side while falling to the ground. **C.** During prostration, the rigidity of the extended and flexed arms is retained for several seconds as flaccidity gradually returns.

Relationship to Fencing Reflex and Posturing

The fencing response designation arises from the similarity to the asymmetrical tonic neck reflex in infants. Like the reflex, a positive fencing response resembles the "en garde" position that initiates a fencing bout, with the extension of one arm and the flexion of the other.

Tonic posturing preceding convulsion has been observed in sports injuries at the moment of impact where extension and flexion of opposite arms occur despite body position or gravity. The fencing response emerges from the separation of tonic posturing from convulsion and refines the tonic posturing phase as an immediate forearm motor response to indicate injury force magnitude and location.

Pathophysiology

The neuromotor manifestation of the fencing response resembles reflexes initiated by vestibular stimuli. Vestibular stimuli activate primitive reflexes in human infants, such as the asymmetric tonic neck reflex, Moro reflex, and parachute reflexes, which are likely mediated by vestibular nuclei in the brainstem. The lateral vestibular nucleus (LVN; Deiter's nucleus) has descending efferent fibers in the vestibulocochlear nerve distributed to the motor nuclei of the anterior column and exerts an excitatory influence on ipsilateral limb extensor motoneurons while suppressing flexor motoneurons. The anatomical location of the LVN, adjacent to the cerebellar peduncles, suggests that mechanical forces to the head may stretch the cerebellar peduncles and activate the LVN. LVN activity would manifest as limb extensor activation and flexor inhibition, defined as a fencing response, while flexion of the contralateral limb is likely mediated by crossed inhibition necessary for pattern generation.

Injury Severity and Sports Applications

In a survey of documented head injuries followed by unconsciousness, most of which involved sporting activities, two thirds of head impacts demonstrated a fencing response, indicating a high incidence of fencing in head injuries leading to unconsciousness, and those pertaining to athletic behavior. Likewise, animal models of diffuse brain injury have illustrated a fencing response upon injury at moderate but not mild levels of severity as well as a correlation between fencing, blood brain barrier disruption, and nuclear shrinkage within the LVN, all of which indicates diagnostic utility of the response. The most challenging aspect to managing sport-related concussion (mild traumatic brain injury, TBI) is recognizing the injury. Consensus conferences have worked toward objective criteria to identify mild TBI in the context of severe TBI. However, few tools are available for distinguishing mild TBI from moderate TBI. As a result, greater emphasis has regularly been placed on the management of concussions in athletes than on the immediate identification and treatment of such an injury. On-field predictors of injury severity can define return-to-play guidelines and urgency of care, but past criteria have either lacked sufficient incidence for effective utility, did not directly address the severity of the injury, or have become cumbersome and fraught with interrater reliability issues. By providing a clear, discernible physiological event immediately upon injury, the fencing response can discern moderate brain injury forces from milder forces, providing an additional criterion by which the identification and classification of concussions can be improved, with immediate application to sport-related on-field diagnoses and decisions affecting return-to-play status for athletes, thereby facilitating the transition from diagnosis to the treatment of any post-concussion symptoms (PCS).

Further Application

The fencing response may also have the potential to indicate traumatic brain injury for soldiers in military settings, specifically with regard to blast injury and subsequent shell shock. There are currently no studies or data to determine the utility of the fencing response in such an arena.

Notable Fencing Displays

Increased awareness of clinical significance on behalf of the bystander is critical to the utility of the fencing response designation. Therefore, notable fencing displays are listed below in order to aid the bystander in identifying the various physical manifestations of the fencing response as well as demonstrating the prevalence of such a response in popular sporting and social events.

Female Athlete Triad

Female athlete triad is a syndrome in which eating disorders (or *low energy availability*), amenorrhoea/*oligomenorrhoea*, and *decreased bone mineral density* (osteoporosis and osteopenia) are present. Also known simply as the Triad, this condition is seen in females participating in sports that emphasize leanness or low body weight. The triad is a serious illness with lifelong health consequences and can potentially be fatal.

Classification

The female athlete triad is a syndrome of three interrelated conditions. Thus, if an athlete is suffering from one element of the Triad, it is likely that she is suffering from the other two components of the triad as well. With the increase in female participation in sports, much of it attributable to Title IX legislation in the United States, the incidence of a triad of disorders particular to women — the female athlete triad—has also increased. Due to this increasing prevalence, the female athlete triad and its relationship with athletics was identified in the 1980s as the symptoms, risk factors, causes and treatments were studied in depth and their relatedness evaluated. The condition is most common in cross country running, gymnastics, and figure skating. Many of those who suffer from the triad are involved in some sort of athletics, in order to promote weight loss and leanness. The competitive sports that promote this physical leanness may result in disordered eating, and be responsible for the origin of the Female Athlete

Triad. For some women, not balancing the needs of their bodies and their sports can have major consequences. In addition, for some competitive female athletes, problems such as low self-esteem, a tendency toward perfectionism, and family stress place them at risk for disordered eating.

Signs and Symptoms

Clinical symptoms of the Triad may include disordered eating, fatigue, hair loss, cold hands and feet, dry skin, noticeable weight loss, increased healing time from injuries, increased incidence of bone fracture and cessation of menses. Affected females may also struggle with low self-esteem and depression.

Upon physical examination, a physician may also note the following symptoms: elevated carotene in the blood, anemia, orthostatic hypotension, electrolyte irregularities, hypoestrogenism, vaginal atrophy, and bradycardia.

An athlete may show signs of restrictive eating, but not meet the clinical criteria for an eating disorder. She may also display subtle menstrual disturbances, such as a change in menstrual cycle length, anovulation, or luteal phase defects, but not yet have developed complete amenorrhea. Likewise, an athlete's bone density may decrease, but may not yet have dropped below her age-matched normal range.

Eating Disorder

Energy availability is defined as energy intake minus energy expended. Energy is taken in through food consumption. Our bodies expend energy through normal functioning as well as through exercise. In the case of female athlete triad, low energy availability may be due to eating disorders, but not necessarily so. Athletes may experience low energy availability by exercising more without a concomitant change in eating habits, or they may increase their energy expenditure while also eating less. Disordered eating is defined among this situation due to the low caloric intake or low energy availability. The disordered eating that accompanies female athlete triad can range from avoiding certain types of food the athlete thinks are "bad" (such as foods containing fat) to serious eating disorders like anorexia nervosa or bulimia nervosa.

While most athletes do not meet the criteria to be diagnosed with an eating disorder such as anorexia nervosa or bulimia nervosa, many will exhibit disordered eating habits. Some examples of disordered eating habits are fasting; binge-eating; purging; and the use of diet-pills, laxatives, diuretics, and enemas. By restricting their diets, athletes worsen the problem of low energy availability.

Having low dietary energy from excessive exercise and/or dietary restrictions leaves too little energy for the body to carry out normal functions such as maintaining a regular menstrual cycle or healthy bone density.

Amenorrhea

Amenorrhea, defined as the cessation of a woman's menstrual cycle for more than three months, is the second disorder in the Triad. Weight fluctuations from dietary restrictions and/or excessive exercise affect the hypothalamus's output of gonadotropic hormones. Gonadotropic hormones "stimulate growth of the gonads and the secretion of sex hormones." (e.g. gonadotropin-releasing hormone, lutenizing hormone and follicle stimulating hormone.) These gonadotropic hormones play a role in stimulating estrogen release from the ovaries. Without estrogen release, the menstrual cycle is disrupted. Exercising intensely and not eating enough calories can lead to decreases in estrogen, the hormone that helps to regulate the menstrual cycle. As a result, a female's periods may become irregular or stop altogether.

There are two types of amenorrhea. A woman who has been having her period and then stops menstruating for ninety days or more is said to have secondary amenorrhea. Primary amenorrhea is characterized by delayed menarche. Menarche is the onset of a girl's first period. Delayed menarche may be associated with delay of the development of secondary sexual characteristics.

Osteoporosis

Osteoporosis is defined by the National Institutes of Health as "a skeletal disorder characterized by compromised bone strength predisposing a person to an increased risk of fracture." Low estrogen levels and poor nutrition, especially low calcium intake, can lead to osteoporosis, the third aspect of the triad. This condition can ruin a female athlete's career because it may lead to stress fractures and other injuries.

Patients with female athlete triad get osteoporosis due to hypoestrogenemia, or low estrogen levels. With estrogen deficiency, the osteoclasts live longer and are therefore able to resorb more bone. In response to the increased bone resorption, there is increased bone formation and a high-turnover state develops which leads to bone loss and perforation of the trabecular plates. As osteoclasts break down bone, patients see a loss of bone mineral density. Low bone mineral density renders bones more brittle and hence susceptible to fracture. Because athletes are active and their bones must endure mechanical stress, the likelihood of experiencing bone fracture is particularly high.

Additionally, because those suffering with female athlete triad are also restricting their diet, they may also not be consuming sufficient amounts vitamins and minerals which contribute to bone density; not getting enough calcium or vitamin D further exacerbates the problem of weak bones.

Bone mass is now thought to peak between the ages of 18-25. Thus, behaviors which result in low bone density in youth could be detrimental to an athlete's bone health throughout her lifetime.

Causes

Gymnastics, figure skating, ballet, diving, swimming, and long distance running are examples of sports which emphasize low body weight. The Triad is seen more often in aesthetic sports such as these versus ball game sports. Women taking part in these sports may be at an increased risk for developing female athlete triad.

Athletes at greatest risk for low energy availability are those who restrict dietary energy intake, who exercise for prolonged periods, who are vegetarian, and who limit the types of food they will eat. Many factors appear to contribute to disordered eating behaviors and clinical eating disorders. Dieting is a common entry point and interest has focused on the contribution of environmental and social factors, psychological predisposition, low self-esteem, family dysfunction, abuse, biological factors, and genetics. Additional factors for athletes include early start of sport-specific training and dieting, injury, and a sudden increase in training volume. Surveys show more negative eating attitude scores in athletic disciplines favoring leanness. Disordered eating behaviors are risk factors for eating disorders.

Treatment

The underlying cause of the female athlete triad is an imbalance between energy taken into the body (through nutrition) and energy used by the body (through exercise). The treatment includes correcting this imbalance by either increasing calories in a diet or by decreasing calories burned by exercise for 12 months or longer. Persons with female athlete triad should get treatment from a multi-disciplinary team that includes a physician, dietitian, and mental health counselor, and seek support from family, friends, and their coach.

Because a symptom of the female athlete triad is menstrual dysfunction, some physicians may recommend oral contraceptives because those pills will regulate the menstrual cycle. However, the underlying cause of the menstrual disorder is an energy imbalance, and using pills to regulate the menstrual cycle without changes in diet and behavior is likely to mask the food deficiency and delay appropriate treatment. A woman taking contraceptives to treat menstrual dysfunction without correcting this energy imbalance will continue to lose bone density.

Less Exercise

Continued participation in training and competition depends on the physical and mental health of the athlete. Athletes who weigh less than 80 percent of their ideal body weight may not be able to safely participate.

Persons with female athlete triad are often asked by health care providers to reduce the amount of time they spend exercising by 10-12 percent.

Eating More

Low energy availability with or without eating disorders, functional hypothalamic amenorrhea, and osteoporosis, alone or in combination, pose significant health risks to physically active girls and women. Prevention, recognition, and treatment of these clinical conditions should be a priority of those who work with female athletes to ensure that they maximize the benefits of regular exercise.

Patients are recommended to work with a dietician who can monitor their nutritional status and help the patient work towards a healthy goal weight. Patients should also meet with a psychiatrist or psychologist to address the psychological aspects of the triad. Therefore, it is important that trainers and coaches are made aware of the athlete's condition and be part of her recovery.

Medicine

Patients are also sometimes treated pharmacologically. To both induce menses and improve bone density, doctors may prescribe cyclic estrogen or progesterone as is used to treat post-menopausal women. Patients may also be put on oral contraceptives to stimulate regular periods. In addition to hormone therapy, nutrition supplements may be recommended. Doctors may prescribe calcium supplements. Vitamin D supplements may be also used because this vitamin aids in calcium absorption. Bisphosphonates and calcitonin, used to treat adults with osteoporosis, may be prescribed, although their effectiveness in adolescents has not yet been established. Finally, if indicated by a psychiatric examination, the affected athlete may be prescribed anti-depressants and in some cases benzodiazepines to help in alleviating severe distress at mealtimes.

Prognosis

Sustained low energy availability, with or without disordered eating, can impair health. Psychological problems associated with eating disorders include low self-esteem, depression, and anxiety disorders. Medical complications involve the cardiovascular, endocrine, reproductive, skeletal, gastrointestinal, renal, and central nervous systems. The prognosis for anorexia nervosa is grave with a six-fold increase in standard mortality rates compared to the general population. In one study, 5.4% of athletes with eating disorders reported suicide attempts. Although 83% of anorexia nervosa patients partially recover, the rate of sustained recovery of weight, menstrual function and eating behavior is only 33%.

Amenorrheic women can be infertile, due to the absence of ovarian follicular development, ovulation, and luteal function. Consequences of hypoestrogenism seen in amenorrheic athletes include impaired endothelium-dependent arterial vasodilation, which reduces the perfusion of working muscle, impaired skeletal muscle oxidative metabolism, elevated low-density lipoprotein cholesterol levels, and vaginal dryness.

Due to low bone mineral density that declines as the number of missed menstrual cycles accumulates, and the loss of BMD may not be fully reversible. Stress fractures occur more commonly in physically active women with menstrual irregularities and/or low BMD with a relative risk for stress fracture two to four times greater in amenorrheic than eumenorrheic athletes. Fractures also occur in the setting of nutritional deficits and low BMD.

Society and Culture

The American Academy of Pediatrics and the AAFP contend that exercise is important and should be promoted in girls for health and enjoyment, however pediatricians should be wary of health problems that may occur in female athlete. The health related issues concerning this topic are grave and can lead to numerous health issues as previously demonstrated. The treatment plan will depend on the severity of the disorder, however some form of treatment has been shown as helpful to produce successful progress towards a better health condition. Clearly, many health problems arise due to disordered eating.

Coaches are discouraged from active participation in the treatment of eating disorders. In addition to conflicts of interest, coaches may be perceived to pressure athletes and potentially perpetuate components of the Female Athlete Triad. For example, in maintaining a place on the team or continued scholarship support, a female athlete may feel compelled to overtrain or restrict eating.

Moving Forward

Coaches, athletic trainers, and healthcare providers should also be educated about the female athlete triad to detect and recognize its components before athletes reach the pathologic end of the spectrum. Awareness levels among athletes, coaches, and healthcare professionals should be assessed to determine where education is needed most. A patient may present with any of the components of the triad; therefore, an awareness of these components among all involved in the care of female athletes is prudent. Athletes should also be taught proper nutrition for athletic performance by their coaches and health providers, because a specific breakdown of macronutrients combined with healthy dietary choices will help these athletes perform the best they possibly can, instead of forcing them to only care about their physique.

Exertional Rhabdomyolysis

Exertional rhabdomyolysis (ER) – sometimes called exercise-induced rhabdomyolysis – is the breakdown of muscle from extreme physical exertion. It is one of many types of rhabdomyolysis that can occur and because of this the exact prevalence and incidence are unclear.

Cause

ER is more likely to occur when strenuous exercise is performed under high temperatures and humidity. Poor hydration levels before, during, and after strenuous bouts of exercise have also been reported to lead to ER. This condition and its signs and symptoms are not well known amongst the sport and fitness community and because of this it is believed that the incidence is greater but highly underreported.

Risks that lead to ER include exercise in hot and humid conditions, improper hydration, inadequate recovery between bouts of exercise, intense physical training, and inadequate fitness levels for beginning high intensity workouts. Dehydration is one of the biggest factors that can give almost immediate feedback from the body by producing very dark colored urine.

Mechanism of Injury

Anatomy

Exertional rhabdomyolysis results from damage to the intercellular proteins inside the sarcolemma. Myosin and actin break down in the sarcomeres when ATP is no longer available due to injury to the sarcoplasmic reticulum. Damage to the sarcolemma and sarcoplasmic reticulum from direct trauma or high force production causes a high influx of calcium into the muscle fibers increasing calcium permeability. Calcium ions build up in the mitochondria, impairing cellular respiration. The mitochondria are unable to produce enough ATP to power the cell properly. Reduction in ATP production impairs the cells ability to extract calcium from the muscle cell.

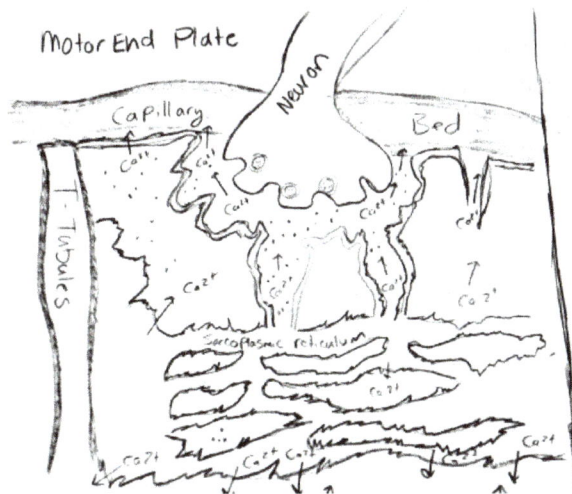

Motor end plate of a person with rhabdomyolysis

The ion imbalance causes calcium-dependent enzymes to activate which break down muscle proteins even further. A high concentration of calcium activates muscle cells, causing the muscle to contract while inhibiting its ability to relax.

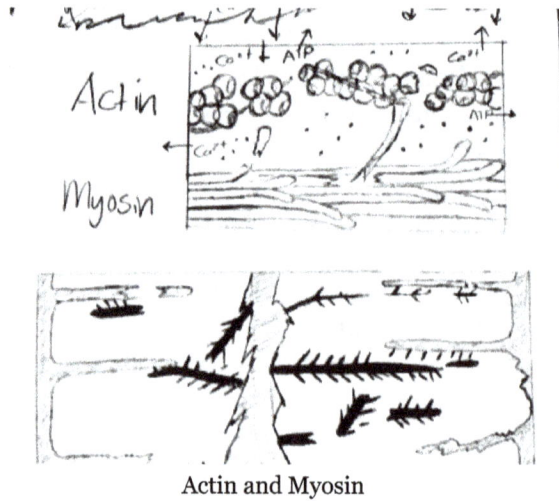

Actin and Myosin

The increase of sustained muscle contraction leads to oxygen and ATP depletion with prolonged exposure to calcium. The muscle cell membrane pump may become damaged allowing free form myoglobin to leak into the bloodstream.

Physiology

Rhabdomyolysis causes the myosin and actin to degenerate into smaller proteins that travel into the circulatory system. The body reacts by increasing intracellular swelling to the injured tissue to send repair cells to the area. This allows creatine kinase and myoglobin to be flushed from the tissue where it travels in the blood until reaching the kidneys. In addition to the proteins released, large quantities of ions such as intracellular potassium, sodium, and chloride find their way into the circulatory system. Intracellular potassium ion has deleterious effects on the heart's ability to generate action potentials leading to cardiac arrhythmias. Consequently, this can affect peripheral and central perfusion that can affect all major organ systems in the body.

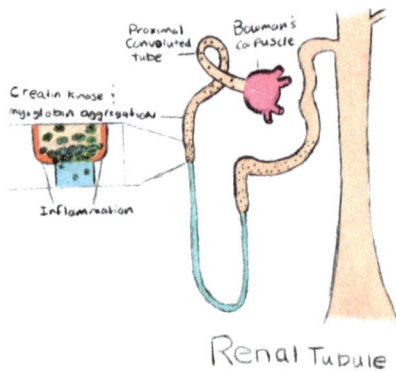

Renal tubules of exertional rhabdomyolysis

When the protein reaches the kidneys it causes a strain on the anatomical structures reducing its effectiveness as a filter for the body. The protein acts like a dam as it forms into tight aggregates when it enters the renal tubules. In addition, the increased intracellular calcium has greater time to bind due to the blockage allowing for renal calculi to form. As a result this causes urine output to decrease allowing for the uric acid to build up inside the organ. The increased acid concentration allows the iron from the aggregate protein to be released into the surrounding renal tissue. Iron then strips away molecular bonds of the surrounding tissue which eventually will lead to renal failure if the tissue damage is too great.

Mechanical Consideration

Muscle degeneration from rhabdomyolysis destroys the myosin and actin filaments in the affected tissue. This initiates the body's natural reaction to increase perfusion to the area allowing for an influx of specialized cells to repair the injury. However, the swelling increases the intracellular pressure beyond normal limits. As the pressure builds in the muscle tissue, the surrounding tissue is crushed against underlying tissue and bone. This is known as compartment syndrome which leads to greater death of the surrounding muscle tissue around the injury. As the muscle dies this will cause pain to radiate from the affected area into the compartmentalized tissue. A loss of range of motion from swelling will also be seen in the affected limb. Along with muscle strength weakness associated with the muscles involved from loss of filament interaction.

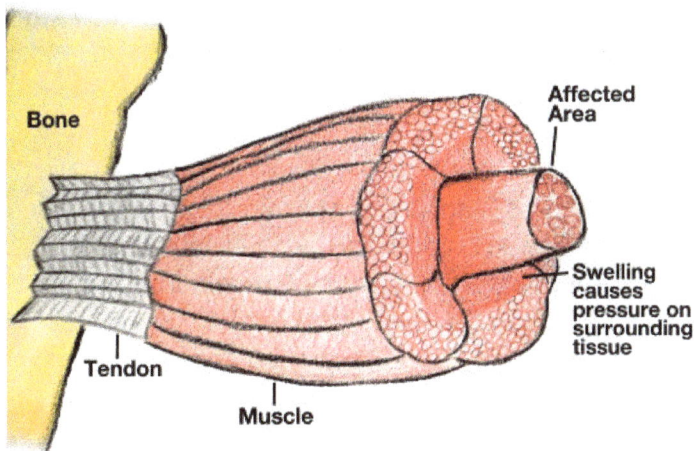

Compartment Syndrome in Muscle

Dehydration is a common risk factor for exertional rhabdomyolsis because it causes a reduction of plasma volume during exertion. This leads to a reduction of blood flow through the vascular system which inhibits blood vessel constriction.

Prevention

Military data suggest lowering the risk of exertional rhabdomyolysis can be obtained by engaging in prolonged lower intensity exercise, as opposed to high intensity exercise over a shorter time period. In all athletic programs, three features should be present; (1)

emphasizing prolonged lower intensity exercise, as opposed to repetitive max intensity exercises. (2) Adequate rest periods and a high carbohydrate diet replenish glycogen stores. (3) Proper hydration will enhance renal clearance of myoglobin. Also, exercise in above average temperature and humidity can increase risk for exertional rhabdomyolysis. Exertional rhabdomyolysis can be avoided by gradually increasing intensity during new exercise regimens, properly hydrating, acclimatization, and avoidance of diuretics during times of strenuous activity.

Supplementation

Sodium bicarbonate supplementation can reduce myoglobin, and prevent exertional rhabdomyolysis.

Diagnosis

Exertional rhabdomyolysis, the exercise-induced muscle breakdown that results in muscle pain/soreness, is commonly diagnosed using the urine myoglobin test accompanied by high levels of creatine kinase (CK). Myoglobin is the protein released into the bloodstream when skeletal muscle is broken down. The urine test simply examines whether myoglobin is present or absent. When results are positive the urine normally obtains a dark, brown color followed by serum CK level evaluation to determine the severity of muscle damage. Elevated levels of serum CK greater than 5,000 U/L that are not caused by myocardial infarction, brain injury, or disease generally indicate serious muscle damage confirming diagnosis of ER.

Treatment

After ER is diagnosed, treatment is applied to 1) avoid renal dysfunction and 2) alleviate symptoms. This should be followed by recommended rehabilitation program, exercise prescription (ExRx). Treatment involves extensive hydration normally done through IV fluid replacement with administration of normal saline until CK levels reduce to a maximum of 1,000 U/L. Proper treatment will ensure hydration and normalize muscle discomfort (pain), flu-like symptoms, CK levels, and myoglobin levels for patient to begin ExRx.

Although sufficient evidence is currently lacking, supplementation with a combination of sodium bicarbonate and mannitol is commonly utilized to prevent renal failure in rhabdomyolysis patients. Sodium bicarbonate alkalizes urine to stop myoglobin from precipitating in renal tubules. Mannitol has several effects including, vasodilatation of renal vasculature, osmotic diuresis, and free radical scavenging.

Recovery

Before initiating any form of physical activity, the individual must demonstrate a normal level of functioning with all previous symptoms absent. Physical activity should be supervised by a health care professional in case of a reoccurrence. However, in some low risk individuals, supervision by a medical professional is not required as long as individual follows up with weekly check ups. Proper hydration prior to performing physical activity and performing exercise in cool, dry environments may reduce the chances of developing a reoccurring episode of ER. Lastly, it is imperative for urine and blood values to be monitored along with careful observation for redevelopment of any signs or symptoms.

The recovery program focuses on progressively conditioning/reconditioning the individual and improving functional mobility. However, special considerations prior to participating in rehabilitation program include the individual's 1) extent of muscle injury, if any 2) level of fitness before incident and 3) weight training experience. These special considerations collectively are a form of assessing the individual's capacity to perform physical activity, which is ultimately used to specify the ExRx design.

Costs

Actual cost for this condition is unknown and also dependent of the level of the condition. In some cases ER can lead to acute renal failure and bring medical costs up due to the need for hemodialysis for recovery/treatment.

Major Trauma

Major trauma is any injury that has the potential to cause prolonged disability or death. There are many causes of major trauma, blunt and penetrating, including falls, motor vehicle collisions, and stabbing and gunshot wounds. Depending on the severity of injury, quick management and transport to an appropriate medical facility (called a trauma center) may be necessary to prevent loss of life or limb. The initial assessment involves a physical evaluation and can also include the use of imaging tools to accurately determine a type of injury and to formulate a course of treatment. Various classification scales exist for use with trauma to determine the severity of injuries, which is used to determine the resources used and for statistical collection. The initial assessment is critical in determining the extent of injuries and what will be needed to manage an injury, and treating immediate life threats.

In 2002, unintentional and intentional injuries were the fifth and seventh leading causes of deaths worldwide, accounting for 6.23% and 2.84% of all deaths. For research purposes the definition is often based on an injury severity score (ISS) of greater than 15.

Classification

Injuries are generally classified by either severity, the location of damage, or a combination of both. Trauma may also be classified by demographic group, such as age or gender. It may also be classified by the type of force applied to the body, such as blunt trauma or penetrating trauma. For research purposes injury may be classified using the Barell matrix, which is based on ICD-9-CM. The purpose of the matrix is to interna-tionally standardize the classification of trauma. Major trauma is sometimes classified by body area; injuries affecting 40% are polytrauma, 30% head injuries, 20% chest trauma, 10%, abdominal trauma and 2%, extremity trauma.

Various scales exist to provide a quantifiable metric to measure the severity of injuries. The value can be used for triaging a patient or for statistical analysis. Injury scales mea-sure damage to anatomical parts, physiological values (blood pressure etc.), comorbidi-ties or a combination of those. The abbreviated injury scale and the Glasgow coma scale are commonly used to quantify injuries for the purpose of triaging and allow a system to monitor or "trend" a patient's condition in a clinical setting. The data can also be used in epidemiological investigations and for research purposes.

About 2% of those who have experienced significant trauma have a spinal cord injury.

Causes

Injuries can be caused by any combination of external forces that act physically against the body. The leading causes of traumatic death are blunt trauma, motor vehicle collisions and falls. Subsets of blunt trauma, are the number one and two causes of traumatic death.

For statistical purposes, injuries are classified as either intentional such as suicide, or unintentional, such as a motor vehicle collision. Intentional injury is a common cause of traumas. Penetrating trauma is caused when a foreign body such as a bullet or a knife enters the body tissue, creating an open wound. In the United States, most deaths caused by penetrating trauma occur in urban areas and 80% of these deaths are caused by firearms. Blast injury is a complex cause of trauma because it commonly includes both blunt and penetrating trauma, and may also be accompanied by a burn injury. Trauma may also be associated with a particular activity, such as an occupational or sports injury.

Pathophysiology

The body responds to traumatic injury both systemically and at the injury site. This response attempts to protect vital organs such as the liver, to allow further cell duplica-tion and to heal the damage. The healing time of an injury depends on various factors including sex, age, and the severity of injury.

The symptoms of injury can manifest in many different ways including:

- Altered mental status
- Fever
- Increased heart rate

- Generalized edema

- Increased cardiac output

- Increased rate of metabolism

Various organ systems respond to injury to restore homeostasis by maintaining perfusion to the heart and brain. Inflammation after injury occurs to protect against further damage and starts the healing process. Prolonged inflammation can cause multiple organ dysfunction syndrome or systemic inflammatory response syndrome. Immediately after injury, the body increases production of glucose through gluconeogenesis and its consumption of fat via lipolysis. Next, the body tries to replenish its energy stores of glucose and protein via anabolism. In this state the body will temporarily increase its maximum expenditure for the purpose of healing injured cells.

Diagnosis

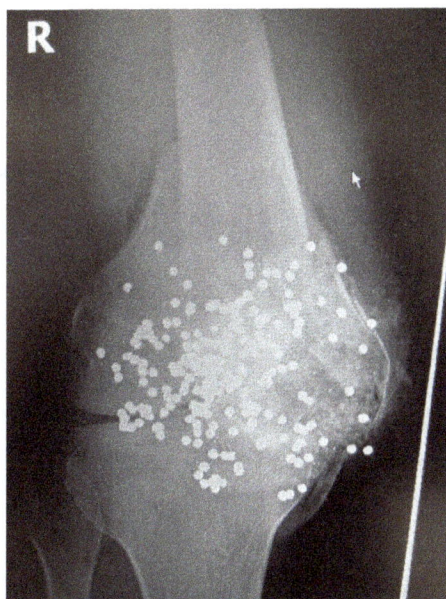

Radiograph of a close-range shotgun blast injury to the knee. Birdshot pellets are visible within and around the shattered patella, distal femur and proximal tibia.

Physical Examination

Primary physical examination is undertaken to identify any life-threatening problems, after which the secondary examination is carried out. This may occur during transportation or upon arrival at the hospital. The secondary examination consists of a systematic assessment of the abdominal, pelvic and thoracic areas, a complete inspection of the body surface to find all injuries, and a neurological examination. Injuries which may manifest themselves later may be missed during the initial assessment, such as when a patient is brought into a hospital's emergency department. Generally the physical examination is performed in a systematic way that first checks for any immediate life threats (primary survey), and then taking a more in depth examination (secondary survey).

Imaging

Persons with major trauma commonly have chest and pelvic X-rays taken, and depending on the mechanism of injury and presentation a focused assessment with sonography for trauma (FAST) exam to check for internal bleeding. For those with relatively stable blood pressure, heart rate, and sufficient oxygenation, CT scans are useful. Full-body CT scans, known as pan-scans, improve the survival rate of those who have suffered major trauma. These scans use intravenous injections for the radiocontrast agent, but not oral administration. There are concerns that intravenous contrast administration in trauma situations without confirming adequate renal function may cause damage to kidneys, but this does not appear to be a significant concern.

In the U.S., CT or MRI scans are performed on 15% of those with trauma in emergency rooms. Where blood pressure is low or the heart rate is increased—likely from bleeding in the abdomen—immediate surgery bypassing a CT scan is recommended. Modern 64-slice CT scans are able to rule out with a high degree of accuracy significant injuries to the neck following blunt trauma.

Surgical Techniques

Surgical techniques, using a tube or catheter to drain fluid from the peritoneum, chest or the pericardium around the heart, are often used in cases of severe blunt trauma to the chest or abdomen, especially when a person is experiencing early signs of shock. In those with low blood-pressure, likely because of bleeding in the abdominal cavity, cutting through the abdominal wall surgically is indicated.

Prevention

By identifying risk factors present within a community and creating solutions to decrease the incidence of injury, trauma referral systems can help to enhance the overall health of a population. Injury prevention strategies are commonly used to prevent injuries in children, who are a high risk population. Injury prevention strategies generally involve educating the general public about specific risk factors and developing strategies to avoid or reduce injuries. Legislation intended to prevent injury typically involves seatbelts, child car-seats, helmets, alcohol control, and increased enforcement of the legislation. Other controllable factors, such as the use of drugs including alcohol or cocaine, increases the risk of trauma by increasing the likelihood of traffic collisions, violence and abuse occurring. Prescription drugs such as benzodiazepines can increase the risk of trauma in elderly people.

The care of acutely injured people in a public health system requires the involvement of bystanders, community members, health care professionals, and health care systems. It encompasses pre-hospital trauma assessment and care by emergency medical services personnel, emergency department assessment, treatment, stabilization, and in-hospital care among all age groups. An established trauma system network is also an important component of community disaster preparedness, facilitating the care of people who have been involved in disasters that cause large numbers of casualties, such as earthquakes.

Management

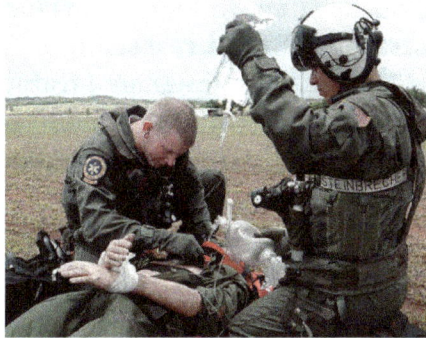

A Navy corpsmen listens for the correct tube placement on an intubated trauma victim during a search and rescue exercise

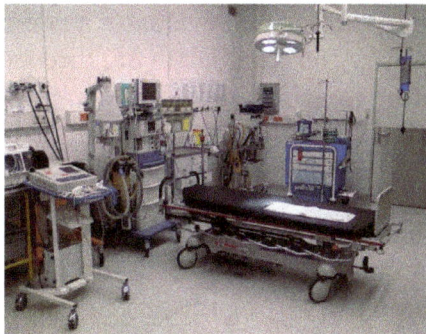

Typical trauma room

Pre-hospital

The pre-hospital use of stabilization techniques improves the chances of a person surviving the journey to the nearest trauma-equipped hospital. Emergency medicine services determines which people need treatment at a trauma center as well as provide primary stabilization by checking and treating airway, breathing, and circulation.

Unnecessary movement of the spine is often minimized by spinal immobilization by securing the neck with a cervical collar and placing the person on a long spine board or scoop stretcher with head supports. This can be accomplished with other medical transport devices such as a Kendrick extrication device, before moving the person. It is important to quickly control severe bleeding with direct pressure to the wound and consider the use of hemostatic agents or tourniquets if the bleeding continues. Conditions like impending airway obstruction, enlargening neck hematoma, or unconsciousness require intubation. It is unclear, however, if this is best done before reaching hospital or in the hospital.

Rapid transportation of severely injured patients improves the outcome in trauma. Helicopter EMS transport reduces mortality compared to ground-based transport in adult trauma patients. Before arrival at the hospital, the availability of advanced life support does not greatly improve the outcome for major trauma when compared to the administration of basic life support. Evidence is inconclusive in determining support for prehospital intravenous fluid resuscitation while some evidence has found it may be harmful. Hospitals with designated trauma centers have improved outcomes when compared to hospitals without them, and outcomes can improve when persons who have experienced trauma are transferred directly to a trauma center.

In-hospital

Management of those with trauma often requires the help of many healthcare specialties including physicians, nurses, respiratory therapists and social workers. Cooperation allows many actions to be completed at once. Generally the first step of managing trauma is to perform a primary survey that evaluates a person's airway, breathing, circulation, and neurologic status. After immediate life threats are controlled a person is either moved into an operating room for immediate surgical correction of the injuries, or a secondary survey is performed which is a more detailed head-to-toe assessment of the person.

Indications for intubation include airway obstruction, inability to protect the airway, and respiratory failure. Examples of these indications include penetrating neck trauma, expanding neck hematoma, and being unconscious among others. In general, the method of intubation used is rapid sequence intubation followed by ventilation. Assessment of circulation in those with trauma includes control of active bleeding. When a person is first brought in, vital signs are checked, an ECG is performed, and, if needed, vascular access is obtained. Other tests should be performed to get a baseline measurement of their current blood chemistry, such as a arterial blood gas or thromboelastography. In those with cardiac arrest due to trauma chest compressions are considered futile but still recommended. Correcting the underlying cause such as a pneumothorax or pericardial tamponade if present may help.

A FAST exam can help assess for internal bleeding. In certain traumas, such as maxillofacial trauma, it can be beneficial to have a highly trained health care provider available to maintain airway, breathing, and circulation.

Intravenous Fluids

Traditionally, high-volume intravenous fluids were given to people who had poor perfusion due to trauma. This is still appropriate in cases with isolated extremity trauma, thermal trauma, or head injuries. However, in general, lots of fluids appear to increase the risk of death. Current evidence supports limiting the use of fluids for penetrating thorax and abdominal injuries, allowing mild hypotension to persist. Targets include a mean arterial pressure of 60 mmHg, a systolic blood pressure of 70–90 mmHg, or the re-establishment of peripheral pulses and adequate ability to think. Hypertonic saline has been studied and found to be of little difference from normal saline.

As no intravenous fluids used for initial resuscitation have been shown to be superior, warmed Lactated Ringer's solution continues to be the solution of choice. If blood products are needed, a greater use of fresh frozen plasma and platelets relative to packed red blood cells has been found to improve survival and lower overall blood product use; a ratio of 1:1:1 is recommended. The success of platelets has been attributed to the fact that they can prevent coagulopathy from developing. Cell salvage and autotransfusion can also be used.

Blood substitutes such as hemoglobin-based oxygen carriers are in development; however, as of 2013 there are none available for commercial use in North America or Europe. These products are only available for general use in South Africa and Russia.

Medications

Tranexamic acid decreases the mortality rate in people who are bleeding due to trauma. However, it only appears to be beneficial if administered within the first three hours after trauma. For severe bleeding, for example from bleeding disorders, recombinant factor VIIa—a protein that assists blood clotting—may be appropriate. While it decreases blood use, it does not appear to decrease the mortality rate. In those without previous factor VII deficiency, its use is not recommended outside trial situations.

Other medications may be used in conjunction with other procedures to stabilize a person who has sustained a significant injury. While positive inotropic medications such as norepinephrine are sometimes used in hemorrhagic shock as a result of trauma, there is a lack of evidence for their use. As of 2012 they have therefore not been recommended. Allowing a low blood pressure may be preferred in some situations.

Surgery

The decision whether to perform surgery is determined by the extent of the damage and the anatomical location of the injury. Bleeding must be controlled before definitive repair can occur. Damage control surgery is used to manage severe trauma in which there is a cycle of metabolic acidosis, hypothermia, and hypotension which can lead to death if not corrected. The main principal of the procedure involves performing the least number of procedures to save life and limb; less critical procedures are left until the victim is more stable.

Prognosis

Trauma deaths occur in immediate, early, or late stages. Immediate deaths are usually due to apnea, severe brain or high spinal cord injury, or rupture of the heart or of large blood vessels. Early deaths occur within minutes to hours and are often due to hemorrhages in the brain's outer meningeal layer, torn arteries, blood around the lungs, air around the lungs, ruptured spleen, liver laceration, or pelvic fracture. Immediate access to care can be crucial to prevent death in persons experiencing major trauma. Late deaths occurs days or weeks after the injury and are often related to infection. Prognosis is better in countries with a dedicated trauma system where injured persons have quick and effective access to proper treatment facilities.

Long-term prognosis is frequently complicated by pain; over half of trauma patients have moderate to severe pain one year after injury. Many also experience a reduced quality of life years after an injury, with 20% of victims sustaining some form of disability. Physical trauma can lead to development of post-traumatic stress disorder (PTSD). One study has found no correlation between the severity of trauma and the development of PTSD.

Epidemiology

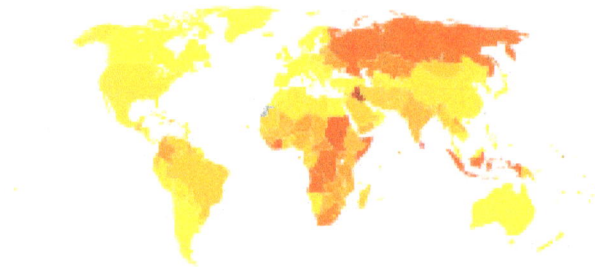

Deaths from injuries per 100,000 inhabitants in 2004

no data	150-175
< 25	175-200
25-50	200-225
50-75	225-250
75-100	250-275
100-125	> 275
125-150	

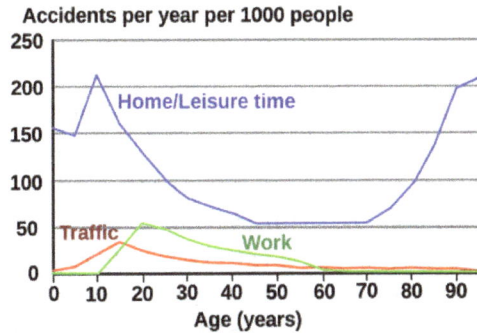

Incidence of accidents by activity in Denmark

Trauma is the sixth leading cause of death worldwide, resulting in five million or 10% of all deaths annually. It is the fifth leading cause of significant disability. About half of trauma deaths are in people aged between 15 and 45 years and is the leading cause of death in this age group. Injury affects more males; 68% of injuries occur in males and death from trauma is twice as common in males as it is in females, this is believed to be because males are much more willing to engage in risk-taking activities. Teenagers and young adults are more likely to need hospitalization from injuries than other age groups. While elderly persons are less likely to be injured, they are more likely to die from injuries sustained due to various physiological differences that make it harder for the body to compensate for the injuries. The primary causes of traumatic death are central nervous system injuries and substantial blood loss.

History

The human remains discovered at the site of Nataruk in Turkana, Kenya, show major trauma blunt and penetrating trauma, and establish the existence of warfare caused by violent trauma to the head, neck, ribs, knees and hands between two groups of hunter-gatherers 10,000 years ago.

Society and Culture

Economics

The financial cost of trauma includes both the amount of money spent on treatment and the loss of potential economic gain through absence from work. The average financial cost for the treatment of traumatic injury in the United States is around US$334,000 per person, making it costlier than the treatment of cancer and cardiovascular diseases. One reason for the high cost of treatment is the increased possibility of complications, which leads to the need for more interventions. Maintaining a trauma center is costly because they are open continuously and maintain a state of readiness to receive patients, even if there are none. In addition to the direct costs of the treatment, there also is a burden on the economy due to lost wages and productivity, which in 2009 accounted for around US$693.5 billion in the United States.

Low and Middle Income Countries

Citizens of low and middle income countries (LMICs) often have higher mortality rates from injury; these countries accounted for 89% of all deaths from injury worldwide. Many of these countries do not have access to sufficient surgical care and many do not have a trauma system in place. In addition, most LMICs do not have a pre-hospital care system to initially treat and transport injured persons to hospital quickly, leading to most casualties being transported by private vehicles. Hospitals lack the appropriate equipment, organizational resources or trained staff. By 2020, the amount of trauma related deaths is expected to decline in high-income countries while in low to middle-income countries it is expected to increase.

Special Populations

Children

Cause	Deaths per year
Traffic collision	260,000
Drowning	175,000
Burns	96,000
Falls	47,000
Toxins	45,000

Due to anatomical and physiological differences, injuries in children need to be approached differently from those in adults. Accidents are the leading cause of death in children between 1 and 14 years old. In the United States, approximately sixteen million children go to an emergency department due to some form of injury every year, with boys being more frequently injured than girls by a ratio of 2:1. The world's five most common unintentional injuries in children as of 2008 are road crashes, drowning, burns, falls and poisoning.

Weight estimation is an important part of managing trauma in children because the accurate dosing of medicine may be critical for resuscitative efforts. A number of methods to estimate weight, including the Broselow tape, Leffler formula and Theron formula exist.

Pregnancy

Trauma occurs in about 5% of all pregnancies, and is the leading cause of maternal death. Pregnant women may additionally experience placental abruption, pre-term labor, and uterine rupture. There are diagnostic issues during pregnancy; ionizing radiation has been shown to cause birth defects, although the doses used for typical exams are generally considered safe. Due to normal physiological changes that occur during pregnancy, shock can be more difficult to diagnose. Where the woman is more than 23 weeks pregnant, it is recommended that the fetus is monitored for at least four hours by cardiotocography.

A number of treatments beyond typical trauma care may be needed when the patient is pregnant. Because the weight of the uterus on the inferior vena cava can decrease blood return to the heart, it can be very beneficial to lay a women in late pregnancy on the left side. Rho(D) immune globulin in those who are rh negative, corticosteroids in those who are 24 to 34 weeks who may need delivery, or a caesarian section in the event of cardiac arrest are also recommended.

Research

Most research on trauma occurs during war and military conflicts as militaries will increase trauma research spending in order to prevent combat related deaths. Some research is being done on patients who were admitted into an intensive care unit or trauma center and received a trauma diagnosis that caused a negative change in their health-related quality of life, with a potential to create anxiety and symptoms of depression. New preserved blood products are also being researched for use in pre-hospital care; it is impractical to use the currently available blood products in a timely fashion in remote, rural settings or in theaters of war.

Strain (Injury)

A strain is an injury to a muscle in which the muscle fibers tear as a result of over-stretching. A strain is also colloquially known as a pulled muscle or torn muscle. The equivalent injury to a ligament is a sprain.

Signs and Symptoms

Typical symptoms of a strain include localized stiffness, discoloration and bruising around the strained muscle.

Causes

Strains are a result of muscular fiber tears due to over stretching; they can range from mild annoyance to very painful. Although strains are not restricted to athletes and can happen while doing everyday tasks, people who play sports are more at risk of developing a strain.

Treatment

The first-line treatment for a muscular strain in the acute phase include five steps commonly known as P.R.I.C.E.

- Protection: Apply soft padding to minimize impact with objects.

- Rest: Rest is necessary to accelerate healing and reduce the potential for reinjury.

- Ice: Apply ice to reduce swelling by reducing blood flow to the injury site. Never ice for more than 20 minutes at a time.

- Compression: Wrap the strained area to reduce swelling with a soft-wrapped bandage.

- Elevation: Keep the strained area as close to the level of the heart as is conveniently possible to keep blood from pooling in the injured area.

The ice and compression (cold compression therapy) will stop the pain and swelling while the injury starts to heal itself. Controlling the inflammation is critical to the healing process, and the icing further restricts fluid leaking into the injured area as well as controlling pain.

Cold compression therapy wraps are a useful way to combine icing and compression to stop swelling and pain.

This immediate treatment is usually accompanied by the use of nonsteroidal anti-inflammatory drugs (e.g., ibuprofen), which both reduce the immediate inflammation and relieve pain. However, NSAIDs, including aspirin and ibuprofen, affect platelet function (this is why they are known as "blood thinners") and should not be taken during the period when tissue is bleeding because they will tend to increase blood flow, inhibit clotting, and thereby increase bleeding and swelling. After the bleeding has stopped, NSAIDs can be used with some effectiveness to reduce inflammation and pain.

It is recommended that the person injured should consult a medical provider if the injury is accompanied by severe pain, if the limb cannot be used, or if there is noticeable tenderness over an isolated spot. These can be signs of a broken or fractured bone, a sprain, or a complete muscle tear.

Surfer's Ear

Surfer's ear is the common name for an exostosis or abnormal bone growth within the ear canal. Surfer's ear is not the same as swimmer's ear, although infection can result as a side effect.

Irritation from cold wind and water exposure causes the bone surrounding the ear canal to develop lumps of new bony growth which constrict the ear canal. Where the ear canal is actually blocked by this condition, water and wax can become trapped and give rise to infection. The condition is so named due to its prevalence among cold water surfers. Warm water surfers are also at risk for exostosis due to the evaporative cooling caused by wind and the presence of water in the ear canal.

Most avid surfers have at least some mild bone growths (exostoses), causing little to no problems. The condition is progressive, making it important to take preventative measures early, preferably whenever surfing. The condition is not limited to surfing and can occur in any activity with cold, wet, windy conditions such as windsurfing, kayaking, sailing, jet skiing, kitesurfing, and diving.

Signs and Symptoms

In general one ear will be somewhat worse than the other due to the prevailing wind direction of the area surfed or the side that most often strikes the wave first.

- Decreased hearing or hearing loss, temporary or ongoing

- Increased prevalence of ear infections, causing ear pain

- Difficulty evacuating debris or water from the ear causing a plugging sensation

-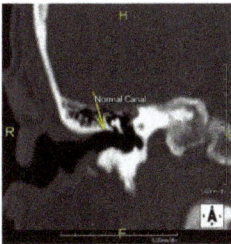

Normal ear canal

Cause

The majority of patients present in their mid-30s to late 40s. This is likely due to a combination of the slow growth of the bone and the decreased participation in activities associated with surfer's ear past the 30's. However surfer's ear is possible at any age and is directly proportional to the amount of time spent in cold, wet, windy weather without adequate protection.

The normal ear canal is approximately 7mm in diameter and has a volume of approximately 0.8 ml (approximately one-sixth of a teaspoon). As the condition progresses the diameter narrows and can even close completely if untreated, although sufferers generally seek help once the passage has constricted to 0.5-2mm due to the noticeable hearing impairment. While not necessarily harmful in and of itself, constriction of the ear canal from these growths can trap debris, leading to painful and difficult to treat infections.

Treatment

Surgery to remove the obstructing ear canal bone is usually performed under general anesthesia in an operating room and aided by the use of a binocular microscope. Most ear surgeons use a drill to remove the bone and may approach the area directly via the ear canal or by making an incision behind the ear and dissecting the ear forward. In using a drilling technique it is important to keep the thin inner ear canal skin away from the drill to preserve the skin and allow optimal skin coverage at the conclusion of the surgery.

Some doctors now prefer to use 1 millimeter chisels to remove the obstructing bone and enter directly through the ear canal. This technique enhances skin preservation. This technique may, in some cases, be performed under sedation with local anesthesia.

During recuperation from surgery it is extremely important not to expose the ear canal to water to minimize the chance of infection or complications.

Depending on the condition of the ear canal and the surgical technique used, the ear canal may require several weeks to several months to heal.

Unprotected exposure of ear canals to cold water and wind after treatment can lead to regrowth of bone and the need for repeated operations on the same ear.

Prevention

The widespread use of wetsuits has allowed people to surf in much colder waters, which has increased the incidence and severity of surfer's ear for people who do not properly protect their ears.

- Avoid activity during extremely cold or windy conditions.

- Keep the ear canal as warm and dry as possible.

  - Ear plugs

  - Neoprene hood

  - Swim cap

References

- Science and Racket Sports Edited by: T. Reilly, M. Hughes and A.Lees. Published by E & FN Spon ISBN 0-419-18500-3.

- *Nilsson Helander, Katarina (April 17, 2009). Acute Achilles tendon rupture; Evaluation of Treatment and Complications (Thesis). University of Gothenburg. ISBN 978-91-628-7720-0. hdl:2077/19390. Lay summary.*

- Graf Ch., e.a.: *Fachlexikon Sportmedizin: Bewegung, Fitness und Ernährung von A-Z*, Deutscher Ärzteverlag, 2008, p. 209, ISBN 3-7691-1223-7, here online

- Reuter P.: *Der grosse Reuter: Springer Universalwörterbuch Medizin, Pharmakologie und Zahnmedizin*, Birkhäuser Verlag, 2005, p. 1300, ISBN 3-540-25104-9, here online

- *Hirata, Isao (1974). The doctor and the athlete (2nd ed.). Philadelphia: J. B. Lippincott. pp. 227–228. ISBN 0-397-50330-X.*

- *Ficat, R. Paul.; Hungerford, David S. (1977). Disorders of the patello-femoral join. Baltimore: Williams Wilkins. ISBN 0-683-03200-3.*

- *Zaffagnini, Stefano.; Dejour, David.; Arendt, Elizabeth A. (Elizabeth Anne) (2010). Patellofemoral pain, instabilty, and arthritis : clinical presentation, imaging, and treatmen. Heidelberg ; New York: Springer. ISBN 978-3-642-05423-5.*

- *Floyd, R. T. (2009). Manual of Structural Kinesiology. Boston: McGraw-Hill Higher Education. ISBN 978-0-07-337643-1.*

- *Saladin, Kenneth S. (2012). Anatomy & physiology : the unity of form and function (6th ed.). New York, NY: McGraw-Hill. p. 268. ISBN 978-0-07-337825-1.*

- *Doran, D. A.; Reay, M. (2000). "Injuries and associated training and performance characteristics in recreational rock climbers". The Science of Rock Climbing and Mountaineering (A collection of scientific articles). Human Kinetics Publishing. ISBN 0-7360-3106-5.*

- *Hörst, Eric J. (2003). Training for Climbing: The Definitive Guide to Improving Your Climbing. Guilford, Connecticut, Helena, Montana: Falcon Publishing. p. 151. ISBN 0-7627-2313-0.*

- *Maki, Allan (28 September 2007). "Darcy Robinson's death brings shock". The Globe and Mail. Retrieved 29 February 2016.*

4

Health Issues in Sports

Health and sports are closely associated. The major health issues in sports are elaborated in the following chapter. It also presents a detailed account on health issues in athletics and youth sports. It will help readers gain a broader perspective on sports medicine.

Health Issues in Athletics

Health issues of athletics concern the health and well-being of athletes who participate in an organized sport. If athletes are physically and mentally underdeveloped, they are susceptible to mental or physical problems. Athletes trying to improve their performance in sports can harm themselves by overtraining, adopting eating habits that damage them physically or psychologically, and using steroids or supplements.

Female Athlete Triad

The Female Athlete Triad is a condition among women that consists of three related health irregularities: disordered eating habits, irregular menstruation, and premature bone loss or osteoporosis. The term was coined in the early 1990s when researchers from the National Institutes of Health noticed unusual health patterns among female athletes. These researchers observed increases in eating habit disorders in young female athletes. Exercising intensely while getting inadequate nutrition can lead to amenorrhea - or irregular menstrual cycles - which in turn can lead to osteoporosis.

Competitive Thinness

Female athletes tend to compare themselves to their competitors, which is another factor for athletes to develop female athlete triad. Competitive thinness is a term used when athletes compare themselves to their rivals who are performing better than them. When athletes begin to compare themselves to their competitors and notice the athletes who are performing better than them are thinner, it can lead to a weight loss mentality. Another risk factor to competitive thinness is related to revealing uniforms. For aesthetic sports, these uniforms are normally very tight, which shows off the athletes' body. These uniforms can cause athletes to develop unhealthy body comparisons.

Over-Training

A female athlete who feels pressured to maintain a certain physique or body weight may exercise excessively and develop eating disorders to restrict calorie intake. Over-exercising increases the need for rest; her overall energy declines, causing her total body fat and estrogen levels to drop - a condition known as amenorrhea. Both male and female athletes may feel the pressure to over-train excessively in order to achieve a certain body image. The human body has a tremendous capacity to adapt to physical stress. "Stress" does not mean only physical damage. It can also refer to activity beneficial to bones, muscles, tendons, and ligaments, making them stronger and more functional. This is also known as "remodeling," and involves both the breakdown and buildup of tissue. However, if breakdown occurs more rapidly than buildup, an overuse injury can result. Nearly half of all injuries encountered in pediatric sports medicine are due to overuse. An overuse injury is traumatic damage to a bone, muscle, or tendon that is subjected to repetitive stress without time to heal naturally, as a result of long and/or high-intensity workouts. Many young athletes participate in sports year-round or on multiple teams at once. Another factor could be parental pressure to compete and succeed. Other risk factors include sleep deprivation, general physical and cognitive immaturity, dietary imbalance and inadequate physical fitness. Among young athletes, a common form of overuse injury is stress fractures, which include injuries of the:

- femoral neck/pubis

- femoral shaft

- tibia

- fibula

- metatarsals

- calcaneus

- cuboid

'Over-training Syndrome' is a term that has been used to describe athletes who, while training for competition, train beyond the body's ability to recover naturally. Common warning signs include tiredness, soreness, drop in performance, headaches, and loss of enthusiasm. Without adequate rest and recovery, training regimens can backfire, eventually harming an athlete's performance. Over-training can also be associated with eating disorders; athletes can turn to excessive exercise in order to lose weight. In cases where athletes are over-training, the most effective treatment is rest and proper nutrition.

Supplements/Steroids

Anabolic steroids are artificially produced hormones called androgens, which are essentially male-type sex hormones in the body. The most powerful of the androgens is testosterone. Another group of steroids are steroidal supplements, a weaker form of androgens. Steroids and supplements are controversial when used for sports because of the health risks associated with them. Some serious and long-term effects on the body are hair loss, dizziness, mood swings, delusions, paranoia, high blood pressure, and increased risk of heart disease, stroke, and even cancer. More recent studies also suggest that steroid users have an increased risk of depression and alcohol use later in life. Doctors call this the 'snowball effect' of steroid-related health problems. Injury patterns suggest that joint ligaments are not able to adapt to steroid-enhanced muscles, leading to injury.

Heat Illness

Heat illness and dehydration are typically brought on by high temperatures and high humidity. These conditions carry increased risk for young athletes, particularly at the beginning of a season, when they are less fit. Other factors that increase vulnerability include: heat-retaining clothing, recent illness, previous experience with heat illness, chronic conditions, and sleep deprivation. Additional precautions should be taken if a child is taking supplements or using cold medication.

Heat illnesses are among the primary causes of sports-related death or disability. They require immediate medical attention. Symptoms to watch for are as follows:

- dry or sticky mouth
- headache
- dizziness
- cramps
- unusual fatigue
- confusion
- loss of consciousness

Injury

Sports injuries are often the result of overuse or trauma to a part of the body. An issue unique to youth athletics is that the participants' bones are still growing, making them especially at risk for injury. Around 8,000 children are rushed to the emergency room daily because of sports injuries. High school athletes suffer approximately 715,000 injuries annually. In American football, for instance, five times as many catastrophic injuries happen in high school as in college-level competition. Injuries include heat illness and dehydration, concussions, and trauma-related deaths. Heat illnesses are a rising concern in youth athletics. These illnesses include heat syncope, muscle cramps, heat exhaustion, heat stroke and exertional hyponatremia. Each year, high school athletes sustain 300,000 head injuries, of which 90% are concussions. By the start of high school, 53% of athletes will have already suffered a concussion, but fewer than 50% of them say anything because they are concerned they will be removed from play. Ice hockey, soccer, lacrosse, wrestling and basketball have a high risk of concussion, with football carrying the most risk. A history of concussion in a football player can contribute to sports-related sudden death.

Prevention

To prevent an injury, proper warm-up is extremely important, because it lets athletes increase their heart rates. Proper warm-up also increases muscle temperature. Warm muscles are less susceptible to injuries because they can contract more forcefully and relax more quickly. As a result, both speed and strength can be enhanced. Also, the probability of over-stretching a muscle and causing injury is much lower. Warm-ups also increase body and blood temperature, which allows more oxygen to reach the muscles, improves muscle elasticity, and reduces the risk of strains and pulls. Other forms of prevention include strengthening muscles, increasing flexibility, taking breaks, weight training, and playing safe. Mental preparation is also important before practice or games. Clearing the mind and visualizing skills and strategy can relax the athlete's muscles and build concentration.

Sports-related Death

Sometimes sports injuries can be so severe that they lead to death. In 2010 48 youths died from sports injuries. The leading causes of death in youth sports are sudden cardiac arrest, concussion, heat illness and external sickling. Cardiac-related deaths are usually due to an undiagnosed cardiovascular disorder. Trauma to the head, neck and spine can also be lethal. Among young American athletes, more than half of trauma-related deaths take place among football players, with track and field, lacrosse, baseball, boxing, and soccer also having relatively high fatality rates.

Health Issues in Youth Sports

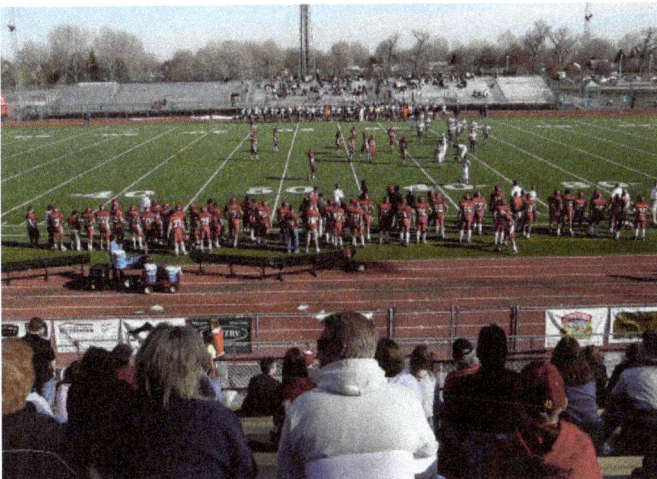

Rocky Mountain High School, football field

The health issues of youth sports are concerns regarding the health and wellbeing of young people between the ages of 6 and 18 who participate in an organized sport. Given that these athletes are physically and mentally underdeveloped, they are particularly susceptible to heat illness, eating disorders and injury; sufficiently severe conditions can result in death.

Heat Illness and Dehydration

Heat illnesses are a recent concern in youth athletics. They include heat syncope, muscle cramps, heat exhaustion, heat stroke and exertional hyponatremia. Heat illness and dehydration are typically brought on by conditions of high temperatures and high humidity. These conditions carry increased risk for young athletes, particularly if at the beginning of a season when they are less fit. Other factors which increase vulnerability include: heat-retaining clothing, recent illness, previous experience with heat illness, chronic conditions, or sleep deprivation. Additional precaution is to be taken if the child is taking supplements or using cold medication.

Heat illnesses are among the primary causes of sports-related death or disability, and as such they require immediate medical attention. Symptoms to watch for are as follows:

- dry or sticky mouth
- headache
- dizziness
- cramps
- unusual fatigue
- confusion
- loss of consciousness

Eating Disorders

Eating disorders are generally not a primary concern amongst youth athletes, however they are unusually prevalent in wrestling and aesthetic sports such as gymnastics. These place heavy emphasis upon weight and body image as ingredients for success in competition. In order to compete, 81% of wrestlers will deliberately lose weight. This involves shedding 3% to 20% of their body weight — most of which being dropped within a short period of time. For rhythmic gymnasts, "success is strongly influenced by visual appeal and body aesthetics. Rhythmic gymnasts are often required to meet certain weight targets to attain and maintain a thin shape." The pressure to please is intense, and correspondingly, 42% of female aesthetic athletes have been diagnosed with eating disorders.

Youth athletes employ a variety of methods to lose weight, including dehydration, fasting, diet pills, laxatives, vomiting, and the use of rubber exercise suits. These practices result in "decreased plasma and blood volume, reduced cardiac outputs, impaired thermoregulatory responses, decreased renal blood flow, and an increase in the amount of electrolytes lost from the body."

Long-term effects

It has been postulated that wrestlers may suffer impaired growth and development due to their fluctuating body weight. However, a study examining high school wrestler growth patterns concluded that participation does not stunt growth. In relation to eating disorders, young female gymnasts may suffer from delayed menarche, menstrual irregularities, low body fat, and delayed maturity. Of these athletes, 11% are at risk for a mental disorder, while 40% risk delayed physical maturation.

Injuries

An issue unique to youth athletics is that the participants' bones are still growing, placing them at highest risk for injury. Around 8,000 children are rushed to the emergency room daily because of sports injuries. High school athletes suffer approximately 715,000 injuries annually. Regarding American football, there are five times more catastrophic injuries in high school than compared to college-level competition.

Overuse injuries

Nearly half of all injuries in pediatric sports medicine are due to overuse. Such injuries can be attributed to inappropriate workout intensity and overlong athletic seasons. Other risk factors include sleep deprivation, general physical and cognitive immaturity, dietary imbalance and inadequate physical fitness. Among young athletes, common overuse injuries are stress fractures, which include injury of the:

- femoral neck/pubis
- femoral shaft
- tibia
- fibula
- metatarsals
- calcaneus
- cuboid

Concussions

Per year, high school athletes sustain 300,000 head injuries, 90% of which being concussions. Though by the beginning of high school, 53% of athletes will have already suffered a concussion. Less than 50% of them say something about it in order to stay in the game. If an athlete returns to competition before being completely healed, they are more susceptible to suffer another concussion. A repeat concussion can have a much slower recovery rate and be accompanied by increased symptoms and long-term effects. The severity of complications from concussion can include brain swelling, blood clots and brain damage. Ice hockey, soccer, wrestling and basketball carry a high risk for concussion, with football at the top.). Concussion causing situations that involve leading with the head, hitting head to head and striking a defenseless athlete have become subject to penalty in order to discourage players and coaches from this type of play. These rule changes have resulted in technique changes at the youngest levels of sports, and youth athletes are now being trained in methods avoiding illegal contact. Youth sport organizations have also made equipment changes to better protect players. A widespread myth is that helmets protect athletes from concussions; they are actually worn to prevent skull fractures. Facts like this have prompted trainings on proper equipment use and not relying on helmets as an implement of contact. A history of concussion in football players can contribute to sports-related sudden death.

Sports-related death

Sometimes sports injuries can be so severe as to result in actual death. Over the past year, 48 youths died from sports injuries. The leading causes of death in youth sports are sudden cardiac arrest, concussion, heat illness and external sickling. Cardiac-related deaths are usually due to an undiagnosed cardiovascular disorder. Trauma to the head, neck and spine can also be lethal. Among young American athletes, more than half of trauma-related deaths are to football players, with track and field, baseball, boxing and soccer also having relatively high fatality rates.

References

- Mayo Clinic staff. "Dehydration and Youth Sports: Curb the Risk." MayoClinic.com. Mayo Clinic,20 Aug. 2011. Web. 7 Oct. 2011. .

- Werkmeister, Joe. "Health and Fitness: Youth Sports Injuries — A Growing Problem." North Shore Sun. TimesReview Newsgroup, 3 Jan. 2011. Web. 7 Oct. 2011.

- Karlin, A M. "Concussion in the Pediatric and Adolescent Population: 'Different Population, Different Concerns.'" PM&R 3.10 Suppl 2 (2011): S369-79. Print.

- Thomas, M, et al. "Epidemiology of Sudden Death in Young, Competitive Athletes Due To Blunt Trauma." Pediatrics 128.1 (2011): e1-8. Print.

- Luke, A, et al. "Sports-Related Injuries in Youth Athletes: Is Overscheduling a Risk Factor?" Clinical Journal of Sport Medicine 21.4 (2011): 307-14. Print.

- Holohan, Ellin. "Youth Sports Injuries Reaching Epidemic Levels, Experts Report." MedicineNet. com. MedicineNet, Inc., 7 Dec. 2010. Web. 7 Oct. 2011.

- Luke, A, et al. "Sports-Related Injuries in Youth Athletes: Is Over scheduling a Risk Factor?" Clinical Journal of Sport Medicine 21.4 (2011): 307-14. Print.

- Brion, R. "Sport-Related Sudden Death and Its Prevention." Bulletin de l'Académie Nationale deMédecine 194.7 (2010): 1237-47. Abstract. Print.

- Biber, Rachel, and Andrew Gregory. "Overuse Injuries in Youth Sports: Is There Such a Thing as Too Much Sports?" Pediatric Annals 39.5 (2010): 286-93. Print.

5

Physical Exercise: An Overview

Physical exercise is an integral part of sports medicine. This chapter will not only provide an overview of physical exercise but it will also comprehensively discuss about the various types of physical exercises like aerobic exercise, strength training, bodyweight exercise and weight training, etc.

Physical Exercise

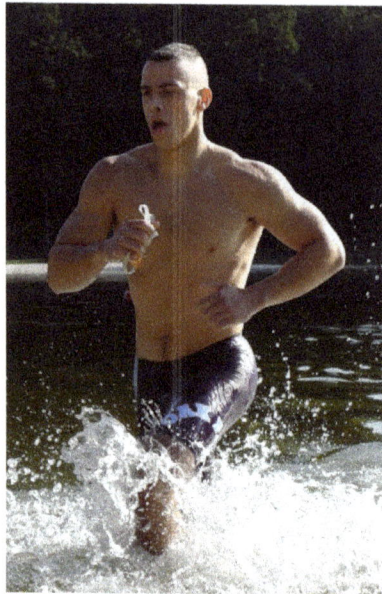

Running in water

Physical exercise is any bodily activity that enhances or maintains physical fitness and overall health and wellness. It is performed for various reasons, including increasing growth and development, preventing aging, strengthening muscles and the cardiovascular system, honing athletic skills, weight loss or maintenance, and merely enjoyment. Frequent and regular physical exercise boosts the immune system and helps prevent "diseases of affluence" such as cardiovascular disease, type 2 diabetes, and obesity. It may also help prevent stress and depression, increase quality of sleep and act as a non-pharmaceutical sleep aid to treat diseases such as insomnia, help promote or maintain positive self-esteem, improve mental health, maintain steady digestion and treat constipation and gas, regulate fertility health, and augment an individual's sex appeal or body image, which has been found to be linked with higher levels of self-esteem. Childhood obesity is a growing global concern, and physical exercise may help decrease some of the effects of childhood and adult obesity. Some care providers call exercise the "miracle" or "wonder" drug—alluding to the wide variety of benefits that it can provide for many individuals.

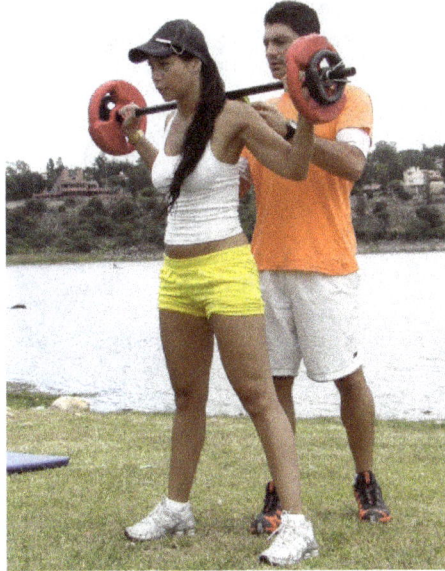

Weight training

In the United Kingdom two to four hours of light activity are recommended during working hours. This includes walking and standing. In the United States, the CDC/ACSM consensus statement and the Surgeon General's report states that every adult should participate in moderate exercise, such as walking, swimming, and household tasks, for a minimum of 30 minutes daily.

Classification

Physical exercises are generally grouped into three types, depending on the overall effect they have on the human body:

- Aerobic exercise is any physical activity that uses large muscle groups and causes the body to use more oxygen than it would while resting. The goal of aerobic exercise is to increase cardiovascular endurance. Examples of aerobic exercise include cycling, swimming, brisk walking, skipping rope, rowing, hiking, playing tennis, continuous training, and long slow distance training.

- Anaerobic exercise, which includes strength and resistance training, can firm, strengthen, and tone muscles, as well as improve bone strength, balance, and coordination. Examples of strength moves are push-ups, pull-ups, lunges, and bicep curls using dumbbells. Anaerobic exercise also include weight training, functional training, eccentric training, Interval training, sprinting, and high-intensity interval training increase short-term muscle strength.

- Flexibility exercises stretch and lengthen muscles. Activities such as stretching help to improve joint flexibility and keep muscles limber. The goal is to improve the range of motion which can reduce the chance of injury.

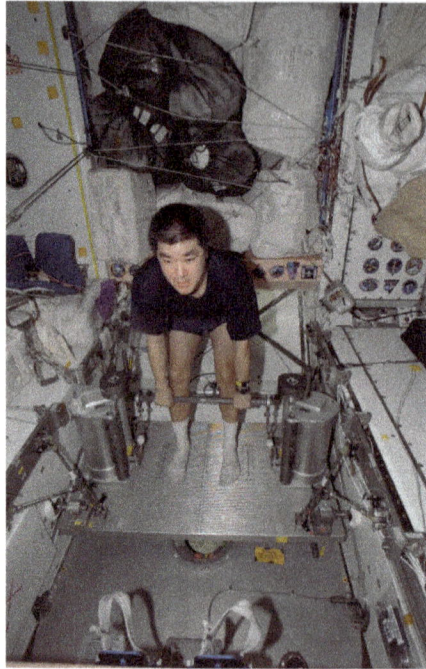

Exercise in space: Astronaut Daniel Tani, Expedition 16 flight engineer, works out at the Unity node of the International Space Station using the short bar of the Interim Resistive Exercise Device (IRED) to perform pull-ups to increase his upper body strength while in a microgravity environment

Physical exercise can also include training that focuses on accuracy, agility, power, and speed.

Sometimes the terms 'dynamic' and 'static' are used. 'Dynamic' exercises such as steady running, tend to produce a lowering of the diastolic blood pressure during exercise, due to the improved blood flow. Conversely, static exercise (such as weight-lifting) can cause the systolic pressure to rise significantly (during the exercise).

Health Effects

Physical exercise is important for maintaining physical fitness and can contribute to maintaining a healthy weight, regulating digestive health, building and maintaining healthy bone density, muscle strength, and joint mobility, promoting physiological well-being, reducing surgical risks, and strengthening the immune system. Some studies indicate that exercise may increase life expectancy and quality of life. People who participate in moderate to high levels of physical exercise have a lower mortality rate compared to individuals who are not physically active. Moderate levels of exercise have been correlated with preventing aging and improving quality of life by reducing inflammatory potential.

The majority of the benefits from exercise are archived with around 3500 MET minutes per week. This means at least 10 minutes of stair climbing, 20 minutes of running, or 25 minutes of biking per day. A lack of physical activity contributes to approximately 17% of heart disease and diabetes, 12% of falls in the elderly, and 10% of breast cancer and colon cancer.

Fitness

There is variation in individual response to training; where most people will see a moderate increase in endurance from aerobic exercise, some individuals will as much as double their oxygen uptake, while others can never augment endurance. However, increase in muscle size from resistance training is primarily determined by diet and testosterone. This genetic variation in improvement from training is one of the key physiological differences between elite athletes and the larger population. Studies have shown that exercising in middle age leads to better physical ability later in life.

Cardiovascular System

The beneficial effect of exercise on the cardiovascular system is well documented. There is a direct correlation between physical inactivity and cardiovascular mortality, and physical inactivity is an independent risk factor for the development of coronary artery disease. Low levels of physical exercise increase the risk of cardiovascular diseases mortality.

Children who participate in physical exercise experience greater loss of body fat and increased cardiovascular fitness. Studies have shown that academic stress in youth increases the risk of cardiovascular disease in later years; however, these risks can be greatly decreased with regular physical exercise. There is a dose-response relation between the amount of exercise performed from approximately 700 to 2000 kcal of energy expenditure per week and all-cause mortality and cardiovascular disease mortality in middle-aged and elderly populations. The greatest potential for reduced mortality is in the sedentary who become moderately active. Studies have shown that since heart disease is the leading cause of death in women, regular exercise in aging women leads to healthier cardiovascular profiles. Most beneficial effects of physical activity on cardiovascular disease mortality can be attained through moderate-intensity activity (40% to 60% of maximal oxygen uptake, depending on age). Persons who modify their behavior after myocardial infarction to include regular exercise have improved rates of survival. Persons who remain sedentary have the highest risk for all-cause and cardiovascular disease mortality. According to the American Heart Association, exercise reduces blood pressure, LDL and total cholesterol, and body weight. It increases HDL cholesterol, insulin sensitivity, and exercise tolerance.

Immune System

Although there have been hundreds of studies on exercise and the immune system, there is little direct evidence on its connection to illness. Epidemiological evidence suggests that moderate exercise has a beneficial effect on the human immune system; an effect which is modeled in a J curve. Moderate exercise has been associated with a 29% decreased incidence of upper respiratory tract infections (URTI), but studies of marathon runners found that their prolonged high-intensity exercise was associated with an increased risk of infection occurrence. However, another study did not find the effect. Immune cell functions are impaired following acute sessions of prolonged, high-intensity exercise, and some studies have found that athletes are at a higher risk for infections. Studies have shown that strenuous stress for long durations, such as training for a marathon, can suppress the immune system by decreasing the concentration of lymphocytes. The immune systems of athletes and nonathletes are generally similar. Athletes may have slightly elevated natural killer cell count and cytolytic action, but these are unlikely to be clinically significant.

Vitamin C supplementation has been associated with lower incidence of URTIs in marathon runners.

Biomarkers of inflammation such as C-reactive protein, which are associated with chronic diseases, are reduced in active individuals relative to sedentary individuals, and the positive effects of exercise may be due to its anti-inflammatory effects. In individuals with heart disease, exercise interventions lower blood levels of fibrinogen and C-reactive protein, an important cardiovascular risk marker. The depression in the immune system following acute bouts of exercise may be one of the mechanisms for this anti-inflammatory effect.

Cancer

A systematic review evaluated 45 studies that examined the relationship between physical activity and cancer survivorship. According to the study results "There was consistent evidence from 27 observational studies that physical activity is associated with reduced all-cause, breast cancer–specific, and colon cancer–specific mortality".

Epigenetic Effects

Physical exercise was correlated with a lower methylation frequency of two tumor suppressor genes, CACNA2D3 and L3MBTL. Hypermethylation of CACNA2D3 is associated with gastric cancer, while hypermethylation of L3MBTL is associated with breast cancer, brain tumors and hematological malignancies. A recent study indicates that exercise results in reduced DNA methylation at CpG sites on genes associated with breast cancer.

Cancer Cachexia

Physical exercise is becoming a widely accepted non-pharmacological intervention for the prevention and attenuation of cancer cachexia. "Cachexia is a multiorganic syndrome associated with cancer, characterized by inflammation, body weight loss (at least 5%) and muscle and adipose tissue wasting". Exercise triggers the activation of the transcriptional coactivator peroxisome proliferator-activated receptor gamma coactivator-1α (PGC-1α), which suppresses FoxO- and NF-κB-dependent gene transcription during muscle atrophy that is induced by fasting or denervation; thus, PGC-1α may be a key intermediate responsible for the beneficial antiatrophic effects of physical exercise on cancer cachexia. The exercise-induced isoform PGC-1α4, which can repress myostatin and induce IGF1 and hypertrophy, is a potential drug target for treatment of cancer cachexia. Other factors, such as JUNB and SIRT1, that maintain skeletal muscle mass and promote hypertrophy are also induced with regular physical exercise.

Neurobiological

The neurobiological effects of physical exercise are numerous and involve a wide range of interrelated effects on brain structure, brain function, and cognition. A large body of research in humans has demonstrated that consistent aerobic exercise (e.g., 30 minutes every day) induces persistent improvements in certain cognitive functions, healthy alterations in gene expression in the brain, and beneficial forms of neuroplasticity and behavioral plasticity; some of these long-term effects include: increased neuron growth, increased neurological activity (e.g., c-Fos and BDNF signaling), improved stress coping, enhanced cognitive control of behavior, improved declarative, spatial, and working memory, and structural and functional improvements in brain structures and pathways associated with cognitive control and memory. The effects of exercise on cognition have important implications for improving academic performance in children and college students, improving adult productivity, preserving cognitive function in old age, preventing or treating certain neurological disorders, and improving overall quality of life.

People who regularly perform aerobic exercise (e.g., running, jogging, brisk walking, swimming, and cycling) have greater scores on neuropsychological function and performance tests that measure certain cognitive functions, such as attentional control, inhibitory control, cognitive flexibility, working memory updating and capacity, declarative memory, spatial memory, and information processing speed. Aerobic exercise is also a potent antidepressant and euphoriant; as a result, consistent exercise produces general improvements in mood and self-esteem.

Regular aerobic exercise improves symptoms associated with a variety of central nervous system disorders and may be used as an adjunct therapy for these disorders. There is clear evidence of exercise treatment efficacy for major depressive disorder and attention deficit hyperactivity disorder. A large body of preclinical evidence and emerging clinical evidence supports the use of exercise therapy for treating and preventing the development of drug addictions. Reviews of clinical evidence also support the use of exercise as an adjunct therapy for certain neurodegenerative disorders, particularly

Alzheimer's disease and Parkinson's disease. Regular exercise is also associated with a lower risk of developing neurodegenerative disorders. Regular exercise has also been proposed as an adjunct therapy for brain cancers.

Depression

Physical exercise has established efficacy as an antidepressant in individuals with depression and current medical evidence supports the use of exercise as both a preventive measure against and an adjunct therapy with antidepressant medication for depressive disorders. A July 2016 meta-analysis concluded that physical exercise improves overall quality of life in individuals with depression relative to controls. One systematic review noted that yoga may be effective in alleviating symptoms of prenatal depression. The biomolecular basis for exercise-induced antidepressant effects is believed to be a result of increased neurotrophic factor signaling, particularly brain-derived neurotrophic factor.

Continuous aerobic exercise can induce a transient state of euphoria, colloquially known as a "runner's high" in distance running or a "rower's high" in crew, through the increased biosynthesis of at least three euphoriant neurochemicals: anandamide (an endocannabinoid), β-endorphin (an endogenous opioid), and phenethylamine (a trace amine and amphetamine analog).

A systematic review noted that, although limited, some evidence suggests that the duration of engagement in a sedentary lifestyle is positively correlated with a risk of developing an anxiety disorder or experiencing anxiety symptoms. It noted that additional research is needed in order to confirm these findings.

Sleep

A 2010 review of published scientific research suggested that exercise generally improves sleep for most people, and helps sleep disorders such as insomnia. The optimum time to exercise *may* be 4 to 8 hours before bedtime, though exercise at any time of day is beneficial, with the possible exception of heavy exercise taken shortly before bedtime, which may disturb sleep. There is, in any case, insufficient evidence to draw detailed conclusions about the relationship between exercise and sleep.

According to a 2005 study, exercise is the most recommended alternative to sleeping pills for resolving insomnia. Sleeping pills are more costly than to make time for a daily routine of staying fit, and may have dangerous side effects in the long run. Exercise can be a healthy, safe and inexpensive way to achieve more and better sleep.

Excessive Exercise

Too much exercise can be harmful. Without proper rest, the chance of stroke or other circulation problems increases, and muscle tissue may develop slowly. Extremely intense, long-term cardiovascular exercise, as can be seen in athletes who train for multiple marathons, has been associated with scarring of the heart and heart rhythm abnormalities. Specifically, high cardiac output has been shown to cause enlargement of the left and right ventricle volumes, increased ventricle wall thickness, and greater cardiac mass. These changes further result in myocardial cell damage in the lining of the heart, leading to scar tissue and thickened walls. During these processes, the protein troponin increases in the bloodstream, indicating cardiac muscle cell death and increased stress on the heart itself.

Inappropriate exercise can do more harm than good, with the definition of "inappropriate" varying according to the individual. For many activities, especially running and cycling, there are significant injuries that occur with poorly regimented exercise schedules. Injuries from accidents also remain a major concern, whereas the effects of increased exposure to air pollution seem only a minor concern.

In extreme instances, over-exercising induces serious performance loss. Unaccustomed overexertion of muscles leads to rhabdomyolysis (damage to muscle) most often seen in new army recruits. Another danger is overtraining, in which the intensity or volume of training exceeds the body's capacity to recover between bouts. One sign of Overtraining Syndrome (OTS) is suppressed immune function, with an increased incidence of upper respiratory tract infection (URTI). An increased incidence of URTIs is also associated with high volume/intensity training, as well as with excessive exercise (EE), such as in a marathon.

Stopping excessive exercise suddenly may create a change in mood. Exercise should be controlled by each body's inherent limitations. While one set of joints and muscles may have the tolerance to withstand multiple marathons, another body may be damaged by 20 minutes of light jogging. This must be determined for each individual.

Too much exercise may cause a woman to miss her periods, a symptom known as amenorrhea. This is a very serious condition which indicates a woman is pushing her body beyond its natural boundaries.

Mechanism of Effects

Skeletal Muscle

Resistance training and subsequent consumption of a protein-rich meal promotes muscle hypertrophy and gains in muscle strength by stimulating myofibrillar muscle protein synthesis (MPS) and inhibiting muscle protein breakdown (MPB). The stimulation of muscle protein synthesis by resistance training occurs via phosphorylation of the mechanistic target of rapamycin (mTOR) and subsequent activation of mTORC1, which leads to protein biosynthesis in the ribosome via phosphorylation of mTORC1's immediate targets (the p70S6 kinase and the translation repressor protein 4EBP1). The suppression of muscle protein breakdown following food consumption occurs primarily via increases in plasma insulin; however, a suppression of MPB of comparable magnitude has also been shown to occur in humans from a sufficient elevation of plasma β-hydroxy β-methylbutyric acid.

Aerobic exercise induces mitochondrial biogenesis and an increased capacity for oxidative phosphorylation in the mitochondria of skeletal muscle, which is one mechanism by which aerobic exercise enhances submaximal endurance performance. These effects occur via an exercise-induced increase in the intracellular AMP:ATP ratio, thereby triggering the activation of AMP-activated protein kinase (AMPK) which subsequently phosphorylates peroxisome proliferator-activated receptor gamma coactivator-1α (PGC-1α), the master regulator of mitochondrial biogenesis.

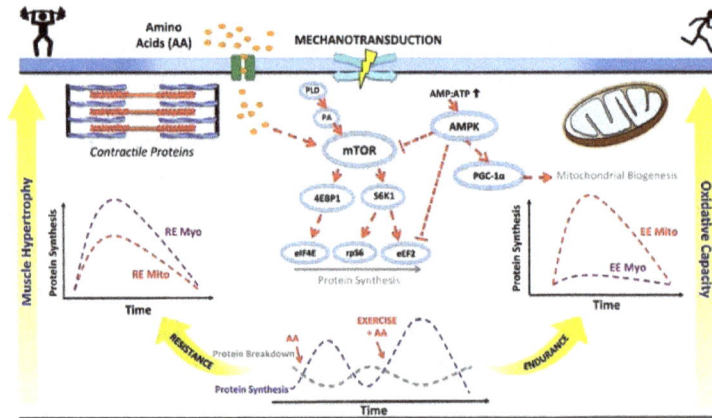

Diagram of the molecular signaling cascades that are involved in myofibrillar muscle protein synthesis and mitochondrial biogenesis in response to physical exercise and specific amino acids or their derivatives (primarily leucine and HMB).

Abbreviations and Representations:

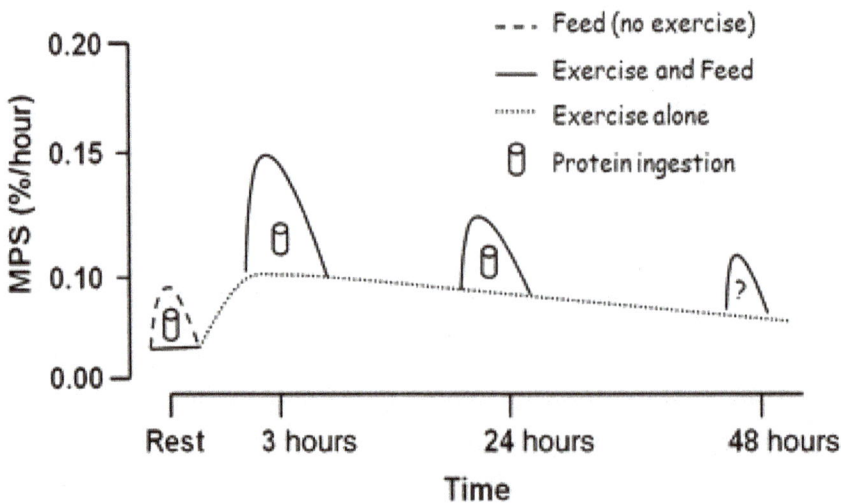

Resistance training stimulates muscle protein synthesis (MPS) for a period of up to 48 hours following exercise (shown by dotted line). Ingestion of a protein-rich meal at any point during this period will augment the exercise-induced increase in muscle protein synthesis (shown by solid lines).

Other Peripheral Organs

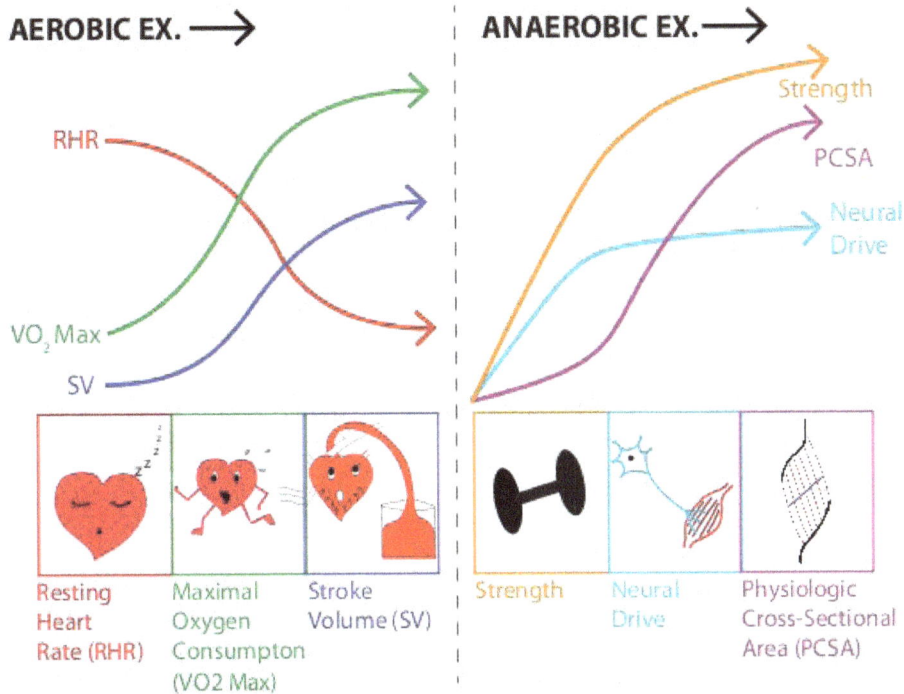

Summary of long-term adaptations to regular aerobic and anaerobic exercise. Aerobic exercise can cause several central cardiovascular adaptations, including an increase in stroke volume (SV) and maximal aerobic capacity (VO_2 max), as well as a decrease in resting heart rate (RHR). Long-term adaptations to resistance training, the most common form of anaerobic exercise, include muscular hypertrophy, an increase in the physiological cross-sectional area (PCSA) of muscle(s), and an increase in neural drive, both of which lead to increased muscular strength. Neural adaptations begin more quickly and plateau prior to the hypertrophic response.

Developing research has demonstrated that many of the benefits of exercise are mediated through the role of skeletal muscle as an endocrine organ. That is, contracting muscles release multiple substances known as myokines which promote the growth of new tissue, tissue repair, and multiple anti-inflammatory functions, which in turn reduce the risk of developing various inflammatory diseases. Exercise reduces levels of cortisol, which causes many health problems, both physical and mental. Endurance exercise before meals lowers blood glucose more than the same exercise after meals. There is evidence that vigorous exercise (90–95% of VO_2 max) induces a greater degree of physiological cardiac hypertrophy than moderate exercise (40 to 70% of VO_2 max), but it is unknown whether this has any effects on overall morbidity and/or mortality. Both aerobic and anaerobic exercise work to increase the mechanical efficiency of the heart by increasing cardiac volume (aerobic exercise), or myocardial thickness (strength training). Ventricular hypertrophy, the thickening of the ventricular walls, is generally beneficial and healthy if it occurs in response to exercise.

Central Nervous System

The persistent long-term neurobiological effects of regular physical exercise are believed to be mediated by transient exercise-induced increases in the concentration of neurotrophic factors (e.g., BDNF, IGF-1, VEGF, and GDNF) and other biomolecules in peripheral blood plasma, which subsequently cross the blood–brain barrier and blood–cerebrospinal fluid barrier and bind to their associated receptors in the brain. Upon binding to their receptors in cerebral vasculature and brain cells (i.e., neurons and glial cells), these biomolecules trigger intracellular signaling cascades that lead to neuroplastic biological responses – such as neurogenesis, synaptogenesis, oligodendrogenesis, and angiogenesis, among others – which ultimately mediate the exercise-induced improvements in cognitive function.

Public Health Measures

Multiple component community-wide campaigns are frequently used in an attempt to increase a population's level of physical activity. A 2015 Cochrane review, however, did not find evidence supporting a benefit. The quality of the underlying evidence was also poor. Survery of brief interventions promoting physical activity found that they are cost-effective, although there are variations between studies.

Environmental approaches appear promising: signs that encourage the use of stairs, as well as community campaigns, may increase exercise levels. The city of Bogotá, Colombia, for example, blocks off 113 kilometers (70 mi) of roads on Sundays and holidays to make it easier for its citizens to get exercise. These pedestrian zones are part of an effort to combat chronic diseases, including obesity.

To identify which public health strategies are effective, a Cochrane overview of reviews is in preparation.

Physical exercise was said to decrease healthcare costs, increase the rate of job attendance, as well as increase the amount of effort women put into their jobs.

Children will mimic the behavior of their parents in relation to physical exercise. Parents can thus promote physical activity and limit the amount of time children spend in front of screens which may decrease the risk of childhood obesity.

Overweight children who participate in physical exercise experience greater loss of body fat and increased cardiovascular fitness. According to the Centers for Disease Control and Prevention in the United States, both children and adults should do 60 minutes or more of physical activity each day. Implementing physical exercise in the school system and ensuring an environment in which children can reduce barriers to maintain a healthy lifestyle is essential.

Exercise Trends

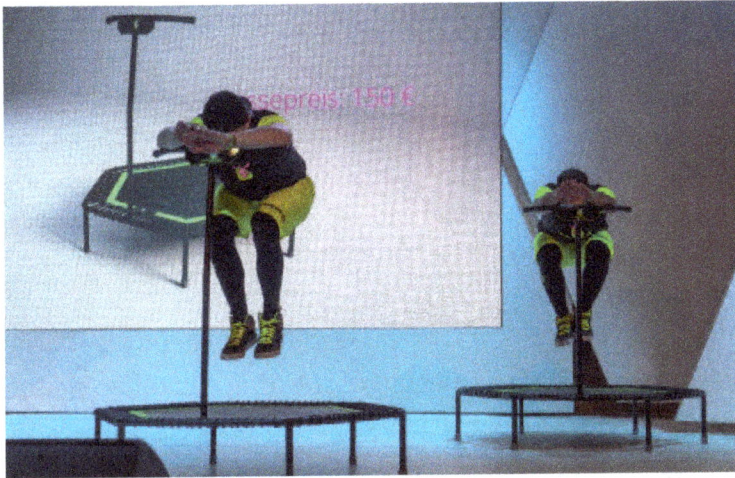

Jumping fitness exercise

Worldwide there has been a large shift towards less physically demanding work. This has been accompanied by increasing use of mechanized transportation, a greater prevalence of labor saving technology in the home, and fewer active recreational pursuits. Personal lifestyle changes however can correct the lack of physical exercise.

Research in 2015 indicates integrating mindfulness to physical exercise interventions increases exercise adherence, self-efficacy and also has positive effects both psychologically and physiologically.

Nutrition and Recovery

Proper nutrition is as important to health as exercise. When exercising, it becomes even more important to have a good diet to ensure that the body has the correct ratio of macronutrients while providing ample micronutrients, in order to aid the body with the recovery process following strenuous exercise.

Active recovery is recommended after participating in physical exercise because it removes lactate from the blood more quickly than inactive recovery. Removing lactate from circulation allows for an easy decline in body temperature, which can also benefit the immune system, as an individual may be vulnerable to minor illnesses if the body temperature drops too abruptly after physical exercise.

History

The benefits of exercise have been known since antiquity. Marcus Cicero, around 65 BCE, stated: "It is exercise alone that supports the spirits, and keeps the mind in vigor."

Several mass exercise movements were started in the early twentieth century to real-ise the benefits of exercise. The first and most significant of these in the UK was the Women's League of Health and Beauty founded in 1930 by Mary Bagot Stack that had 166,000 members in 1937.

However, the link between physical health and exercise (or lack of it) was only discovered in 1949 and reported in 1953 by a team led by Jerry Morris. Dr. Morris noted that men of similar social class and occupation (bus conductors versus bus drivers) had markedly different rates of heart attacks, depending on the level of exercise they got: bus drivers had a sedentary occupation and a higher incidence of heart disease, while bus conductors were forced to move continually and had a lower incidence of heart disease. This link had not previously been noted and was later confirmed by other researchers.

Other Animals

Physical exercise has been shown to benefit a wide range of other mammals, as well as salmon, juvenile crocodiles, and at least one species of bird.

However, several studies have shown that lizards display no benefit from exercise, leading them to be termed "metabolically inflexible". Indeed, damage from overtrain-ing may occur following weeks of forced treadmill exercise in lizards.

A number of studies of both rodents and humans have demonstrated that individual differences in both ability and propensity for exercise (i.e., voluntary exercise) have some genetic basis.

Several studies of rodents have demonstrated that maternal or juvenile access to wheels that allow voluntary exercise can increase the propensity to run as adults. These studies further suggest that physical activity may be more "programmable" than food intake.

- Active living
- Behavioural change theories
- Exercise hypertension
- Exercise-induced nausea
- Exercise intensity
- Exercise intolerance
- Exercise-induced anaphylaxis
- Exercise-induced asthma
- Kinesiology
- Metabolic equivalent
- Supercompensation
- Physical fitness

Types of Physical Exercises

Aerobic Exercise

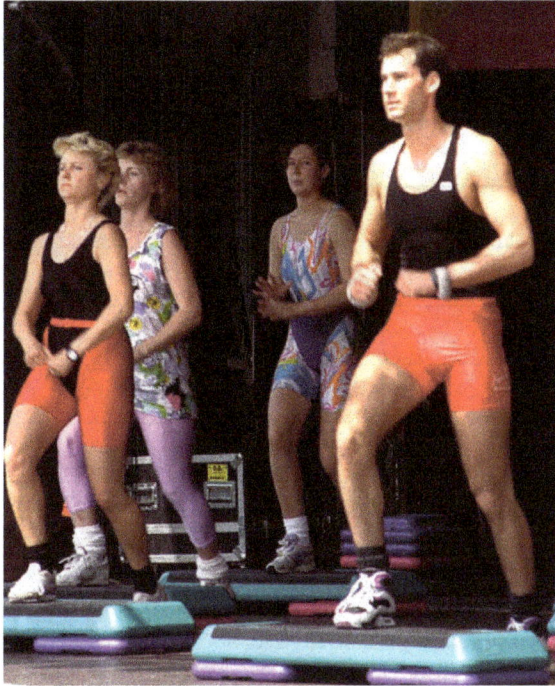

Cardio

Aerobic exercise (also known as cardio) is physical exercise of low to high intensity that depends primarily on the aerobic energy-generating process. Aerobic literally means "relating to, involving, or requiring free oxygen", and refers to the use of oxygen to adequately meet energy demands during exercise via aerobic metabolism. Generally, light-to-moderate intensity activities that are sufficiently supported by aerobic metabolism can be performed for extended periods of time.

When practiced in this way, examples of cardiovascular/aerobic exercise are medium to long distance running/jogging, swimming, cycling, and walking, according to the first extensive research on aerobic exercise, conducted in the 1960s on over 5,000 U.S. Air Force personnel by Dr. Kenneth H. Cooper.

History

Kenneth Cooper was the first person to introduce the concept of aerobic exercise. In the 1960s, Cooper started research into preventive medicine. He became intrigued by the belief that exercise can preserve one's health. In 1970 he created his own institute (the Cooper Institute) for non-profit research and education devoted to preventive medicine. He sparked millions into becoming active and is now known as the "father of aerobics".

Aerobic Versus Anaerobic Exercise

Aerobic exercise and fitness can be contrasted with anaerobic exercise, of which strength training and short-distance running are the most salient examples. The two types of exercise differ by the duration and intensity of muscular contractions involved, as well as by how energy is generated within the muscle.

EXERCISE ZONES										
AGE										
	20	25	30	35	40	45	50	55	65	70
100%	200	195	190	185	180	175	170	165	155	150
VO₂ Max (Maximum effort)										
90%	180	176	171	167	162	158	153	149	140	135
Anaerobic (Hardcore training)										
80%	160	156	152	148	144	140	136	132	124	126
Aerobix (Cardio training / Endurance)										
70%	140	137	133	130	126	123	119	116	109	105
Weight control (Fitness / Fat burn)										
60%	120	117	114	111	108	105	102	99	93	90
Moderate activity (Maintenance / Warm up)										
50%	100	98	95	93	90	88	85	83	78	75

BEATS PER MINUTE

Fox and Haskell formula showing the split between aerobic (light orange) and anaerobic (dark orange) exercise and heart rate

New research on the endocrine functions of contracting muscles has shown that both aerobic and anaerobic exercise promote the secretion of myokines, with attendant benefits including growth of new tissue, tissue repair, and various anti-inflammatory functions, which in turn reduce the risk of developing various inflammatory diseases. Myokine secretion in turn is dependent on the amount of muscle contracted, and the duration and intensity of contraction. As such, both types of exercise produce endocrine benefits.

In almost all conditions, anaerobic exercise is accompanied by aerobic exercises because the less efficient anaerobic metabolism must supplement the aerobic system due to energy demands that exceed the aerobic system's capacity. What is generally called aerobic exercise might be better termed "solely aerobic", because it is designed to be low-intensity enough not to generate lactate via pyruvate fermentation, so that all carbohydrate is aerobically turned into energy.

Initially during increased exertion, muscle glycogen is broken down to produce glucose, which undergoes glycolysis producing pyruvate which then reacts with oxygen (Krebs cycle, Chemiosmosis) to produce carbon dioxide and water and releases energy. If there is a shortage of oxygen (anaerobic exercise, explosive movements), carbohydrate is consumed more rapidly because the pyruvate ferments into lactate. If the intensity of the exercise exceeds the rate with which the cardiovascular system can supply muscles with oxygen, it results in buildup of lactate and quickly makes it impossible to continue the exercise. Unpleasant effects of lactate buildup initially include the burning sensation in the muscles, and may eventually include nausea and even vomiting if the exercise is continued without allowing lactate to clear from the bloodstream.

As glycogen levels in the muscle begin to fall, glucose is released into the bloodstream by the liver, and fat metabolism is increased so that it can fuel the aerobic pathways. Aerobic exercise may be fueled by glycogen reserves, fat reserves, or a combination of both, depending on the intensity. Prolonged moderate-level aerobic exercise at 65% VO2 max (the heart rate of 150 bpm for a 30-year-old human) results in the maximum contribution of fat to the total energy expenditure. At this level, fat may contribute 40% to 60% of total, depending on the duration of the exercise. Vigorous exercise above 75% VO2max (160 bpm) primarily burns glycogen.

Major muscles in a rested, untrained human typically contain enough energy for about 2 hours of vigorous exercise. Exhaustion of glycogen is a major cause of what marathon runners call "hitting the wall". Training, lower intensity levels, and carbohydrate loading may allow postponement of the onset of exhaustion beyond 4 hours.

Aerobic exercise comprises innumerable forms. In general, it is performed at a moderate level of intensity over a relatively long period of time. For example, running a long distance at a moderate pace is an aerobic exercise, but sprinting is not. Playing singles tennis, with near-continuous motion, is generally considered aerobic activity, while golf or two person team tennis, with brief bursts of activity punctuated by more frequent breaks, may not be predominantly aerobic. Some sports are thus inherently "aerobic", while other aerobic exercises, such as fartlek training or aerobic dance classes, are designed specifically to improve aerobic capacity and fitness. It is most common for aerobic exercises to involve the leg muscles, primarily or exclusively. There are some exceptions. For example, rowing to distances of 2,000 m or more is an aerobic sport that exercises several major muscle groups, including those of the legs, abdominals, chest, and arms. Common kettlebell exercises combine aerobic and anaerobic aspects.

Benefits

Among the recognized benefits of doing regular aerobic exercise are:

- Strengthening the muscles involved in respiration, to facilitate the flow of air in and out of the lungs

- Strengthening and enlarging the heart muscle, to improve its pumping efficiency and reduce the resting heart rate, known as aerobic conditioning

- Improving circulation efficiency and reducing blood pressure

- Increasing the total number of red blood cells in the body, facilitating transport of oxygen

- Improved mental health, including reducing stress and lowering the incidence of depression, as well as increased cognitive capacity.

- Reducing the risk for diabetes. One meta-analysis has shown, from multiple conducted studies, that aerobic exercise does help lower Hb A_{1C} levels for type 2 diabetics.

As a result, aerobic exercise can reduce the risk of death due to cardiovascular problems. In addition, high-impact aerobic activities (such as jogging or using a skipping rope) can stimulate bone growth, as well as reduce the risk of osteoporosis for both men and women.

In addition to the health benefits of aerobic exercise, there are numerous performance benefits:

- Increased storage of energy molecules such as fats and carbohydrates within the muscles, allowing for increased endurance

- Neovascularization of the muscle sarcomeres to increase blood flow through the muscles

- Increasing speed at which aerobic metabolism is activated within muscles, allowing a greater portion of energy for intense exercise to be generated aerobically

- Improving the ability of muscles to use fats during exercise, preserving intramuscular glycogen

- Enhancing the speed at which muscles recover from high intensity exercise

- Neurobiological effects: improvements in brain structural connections and increased gray matter density, new neuron growth, improved cognitive function (cognitive control and various forms of memory), and improvement or maintenance of mental health

Some drawbacks of aerobic exercise include:

- Overuse injuries because of repetitive, high-impact exercise such as distance running.

- Is not an effective approach to building muscle.

- Only effective for fat loss when used consistently.

Both the health benefits and the performance benefits, or "training effect", require a minimum duration and frequency of exercise. Most authorities suggest at least twenty minutes performed at least three times per week.

Aerobic Capacity

Aerobic capacity describes the functional capacity of the cardiorespiratory system, (the heart, lungs and blood vessels). Aerobic capacity refers to the maximum amount of oxygen consumed by the body during intense exercises, in a given time frame. It is a function both of cardiorespiratory performance and the maximum ability to remove and utilize oxygen from circulating blood. To measure maximal aerobic capacity, an exercise physiologist or physician will perform a VO_2 max test, in which a subject will undergo progressively more strenuous exercise on a treadmill, from an easy walk through to exhaustion. The individual is typically connected to a respirometer to measure oxygen consumption, and the speed is increased incrementally over a fixed duration of time. The higher the measured cardiorespiratory endurance level, the more oxygen has been transported to and used by exercising muscles, and the higher the level of intensity at which the individual can exercise. More simply put, the higher the aerobic capacity, the higher the level of aerobic fitness. The Cooper and multi-stage fitness tests can also be used to assess functional aerobic capacity for particular jobs or activities.

The degree to which aerobic capacity can be improved by exercise varies very widely in the human population: while the average response to training is an approximately 17% increase in VO_2max, in any population there are "high responders" who may as much as double their capacity, and "low responders" who will see little or no benefit from training. Studies indicate that approximately 10% of otherwise healthy individuals cannot improve their aerobic capacity with exercise at all. The degree of an individual's responsiveness is highly heritable, suggesting that this trait is genetically determined.

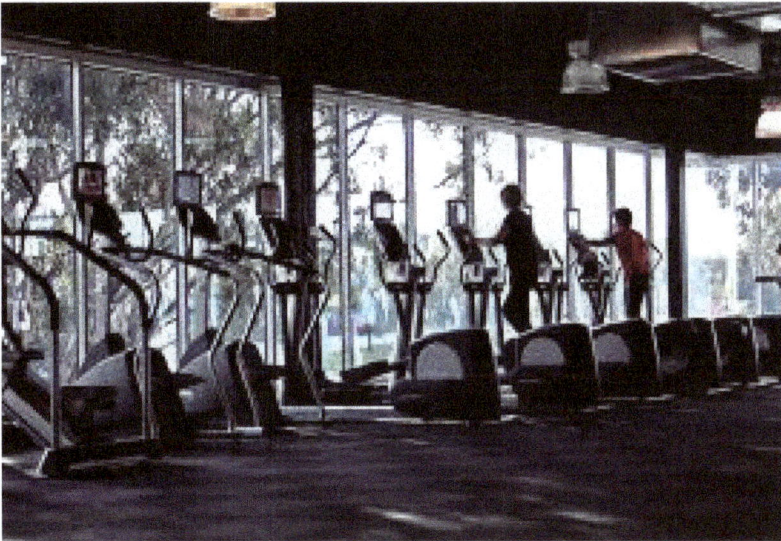

Aerobic workout

Alternatives

Higher intensity exercise, such as High-intensity interval training (HIIT), increases the resting metabolic rate (RMR) in the 24 hours following high intensity exercise, ultimately burning more calories than lower intensity exercise; low intensity exercise burns more calories during the exercise, due to the increased duration, but fewer afterwards.

Commercial Success

Aerobic exercise has long been a popular approach to achieving weight loss and physical fitness, often taking a commercial form.

- In the 1970s Judi Sheppard Missett helped create the market for commercial aerobics with her Jazzercise program

- In the 1980s Richard Simmons hosted an aerobic exercise show on television, and also released a series of exercise videos

- In the 1990s Billy Blanks's Tae Bo helped popularize cardio-boxing workouts that incorporated martial arts movements

Varieties

Indoor

- Stair climbing
- Elliptical trainer
- Indoor rower
- Stairmaster
- Stationary bicycle
- Treadmill

Outdoor

- Walking
- Cycling
- Running
- Cross-country skiing
- Cross-country running
- Nordic walking
- Inline skating
- Rowing

Indoor or outdoor

- Swimming
- Kickboxing
- Skipping rope or jump rope

- Circuit training

- Jumping jacks

- Jogging

- Water aerobics

Strength Training

Strength training is a type of physical exercise specializing in the use of resistance to induce muscular contraction which builds the strength, anaerobic endurance, and size of skeletal muscles.

When properly performed, strength training can provide significant functional benefits and improvement in overall health and well-being, including increased bone, muscle, tendon and ligament strength and toughness, improved joint function, reduced potential for injury, increased bone density, increased metabolism, increased fitness, improved cardiac function, and improved lipoprotein lipid profiles, including elevated HDL ("good") cholesterol. Training commonly uses the technique of progressively increasing the force output of the muscle through incremental weight increases and uses a variety of exercises and types of equipment to target specific muscle groups. Strength training is primarily an anaerobic activity, although some proponents have adapted it to provide the benefits of aerobic exercise through circuit training.

Sports where strength training is central are bodybuilding, weightlifting, powerlifting, strongman, Highland games, shotput, discus throw, and javelin throw. Many other sports use strength training as part of their training regimen, notably American football, wrestling, track and field, rowing, lacrosse, basketball, pole dancing, hockey, professional wrestling, rugby union, rugby league and soccer. Strength training for other sports and physical activities is becoming increasingly popular.

Uses

The benefits of weight training include greater muscular strength, improved muscle tone and appearance, increased endurance and enhanced bone density.

Increased Physical Attractiveness

Many people take up weight training to improve their physical attractiveness. There is evidence that a body type consisting of broad shoulders and a narrow waist, attainable through strength training, is the most physically attractive male attribute according to women participating in the research. Most men can develop substantial muscles; most women lack the testosterone to do it, but they can develop a firm, "toned" physique, and they can increase their strength by the same proportion as that achieved by men (but usually from a significantly lower starting point). An individual's genetic make-up dictates the response to weight training stimuli to a significant extent, training can not exceed a muscle's intrinsic genetically determined qualities, but clearly polymorphic expression of Myosin heavy chains is possible.

Workouts elevate metabolism for up to 14 hours following 45-minutes of vigorous exercise.

Increased General Physical Health

Strength training also provides functional benefits. Stronger muscles improve posture, provide better support for joints, and reduce the risk of injury from everyday activities. Older people who take up weight training can prevent some of the loss of muscle tissue that normally accompanies aging—and even regain some functional strength—and by doing so become less frail. They may be able to avoid some types of physical disability. Weight-bearing exercise also helps to prevent osteoporosis and to improve bone strength in those with osteoporosis. The benefits of weight training for older people have been confirmed by studies of people who began engaging in it even in their 80s and 90s.

Though strength training can stimulate the cardiovascular system, many exercise physiologists, based on their observation of maximal oxygen uptake, argue that aerobics training is a better cardiovascular stimulus. Central catheter monitoring during resistance training reveals increased cardiac output, suggesting that strength training shows potential for cardiovascular exercise. However, a 2007 meta-analysis found that, though aerobic training is an effective therapy for heart failure patients, combined aerobic and strength training is ineffective.

Strength training may be important to metabolic and cardiovascular health. Recent evidence suggests that resistance training may reduce metabolic and cardiovascular disease risk. Overweight individuals with high strength fitness exhibit metabolic/cardiovascular risk profiles similar to normal-weight, fit individuals rather than overweight unfit individuals.

For Rehabilitation or to Address an Impairment

For many people in rehabilitation or with an acquired disability, such as following stroke or orthopaedic surgery, strength training for weak muscles is a key factor to optimise recovery. For people with such a health condition, their strength training is likely to need to be designed by an appropriate health professional, such as a physiotherapist or an occupational therapist.

Increased Sports Performance

Stronger muscles improve performance in a variety of sports. Sport-specific training routines are used by many competitors. These often specify that the speed of muscle contraction during weight training should be the same as that of the particular sport.

For the Pleasure of the Activity

One side effect of any intense exercise is increased levels of dopamine, serotonin, and norepinephrine, which can help to improve mood and counter feelings of depression.

Developing research has demonstrated that many of the benefits of exercise are mediated through the role of skeletal muscle as an endocrine organ. That is, contracting muscles release multiple substances known as myokines which promote the growth of new tissue, tissue repair, and various anti-inflammatory functions, which in turn reduce the risk of developing various inflammatory diseases.

Technique

The basic principles of strength training involve a manipulation of the number of repetitions (reps), sets, tempo, exercises and force to cause desired changes in strength, endurance or size by overloading of a group of muscles. The specific combinations of reps, sets, exercises, resistance and force depend on the purpose of the individual performing the exercise: to gain size and strength multiple (4+) sets with fewer reps must be performed using more force. A wide spectrum of regimens can be adopted to achieve different results, but the classic formula recommended by the American College of Sports Medicine reads as follows:

- 8 to 12 repetitions of a resistance training exercise for each major muscle group at an intensity of 40% to 80% of a one-repetition max (RM) depending on the training level of the participant.

- Two to three minutes of rest is recommended between exercise sets to allow for proper recovery.

- Two to four sets are recommended for each muscle group

Typically failure to use good form during a training set can result in injury or an inability to meet training goals – since the desired muscle group is not challenged sufficiently, the threshold of overload is never reached and the muscle does not gain in strength. There are cases when cheating is beneficial, as is the case where weaker groups become the weak link in the chain and the target muscles are never fully exercised as a result.

The benefits of strength training include increased muscle, tendon and ligament strength, bone density, flexibility, tone, metabolic rate and postural support.

Terminology

Strength training has a variety of specialized terms used to describe parameters of strength training:

- Exercise – different movements which involve rotating joints in specific patterns to challenge muscles in different ways.

- Form – each exercise has a specific form, a topography of movement designed to maximize safety and muscle strength gains.

- Rep – short for repetition, a rep is a single cycle of lifting and lowering a weight in a controlled manner, moving through the form of the exercise.

- Set – a set consists of several repetitions performed one after another with no break between them with the number of reps per set and sets per exercise depending on the goal of the individual. The number of repetitions one can perform at a certain weight is called the Rep Maximum (RM). For example, if one could perform ten reps at 75 lbs, then their RM for that weight would be 10RM. 1RM is therefore the maximum weight that someone can lift in a given exercise – i.e. a weight that they can only lift once without a break.

- Tempo – the speed with which an exercise is performed; the tempo of a movement has implications for the weight that can be moved and the effects on the muscle.

Realization of Training Goals

For developing endurance, gradual increases in volume and gradual decreases in intensity is the most effective program. Sets of thirteen to twenty repetitions develop anaerobic endurance, with some increases to muscle size and limited impact on strength.

It has been shown that for beginners, multiple-set training offers minimal benefits over single-set training with respect to either strength gain or muscle mass increase, but for the experienced athlete multiple-set systems are required for optimal progress. However, one study shows that for leg muscles, three sets are more effective than one set.

Beginning weight-trainers are in the process of training the neurological aspects of strength, the ability of the brain to generate a rate of neuronal action potentials that will produce a muscular contraction that is close to the maximum of the muscle's potential.

Variable	Training goal				
	Strength	Power	Hypertrophy	Endurance	Speed
Load (% of 1RM)	90–80	60–45	80–60	60–40	30
Reps per set	1–5	1–5	6–12	13–60	1–5
Sets per exercise	4–7	3–5	4–8	2–4	3–5

Rest between sets (mins)	2–6	2–6	2–5	1–2	2–5
Duration (seconds per set)	5–10	4–8	20–60	80–150	20–40
Speed per rep (% of max)	60–100	90–100	60–90	60–80	100
Training sessions per week	3–6	3–6	5–7	8–14	3–6
Table reproduced from Siff, 2003					

Weights for each exercise should be chosen so that the desired number of repetitions can just be achieved.

Progressive Overload

In one common method, weight training uses the principle of progressive overload, in which the muscles are overloaded by attempting to lift at least as much weight as they are capable. They respond by growing larger and stronger. This procedure is repeated with progressively heavier weights as the practitioner gains strength and endurance.

However, performing exercises at the absolute limit of one's strength (known as one rep max lifts) is considered too risky for all but the most experienced practitioners. Moreover, most individuals wish to develop a combination of strength, endurance and muscle size. One repetition sets are not well suited to these aims. Practitioners therefore lift lighter (sub-maximal) weights, with more repetitions, to fatigue the muscle and all fibres within that muscle as required by the progressive overload principle.

Commonly, each exercise is continued to the point of momentary muscular failure. Contrary to widespread belief, this is not the point at which the individual thinks they cannot complete any more repetitions, but rather the first repetition that fails due to inadequate muscular strength. Training to failure is a controversial topic with some advocating training to failure on all sets while others believe that this will lead to overtraining, and suggest training to failure only on the last set of an exercise. Some practitioners recommend finishing a set of repetitions just before reaching a personal maximum at a given time. Adrenaline and other hormones may promote additional intensity by stimulating the body to lift additional weight (as well as the neuro-muscular stimulations that happen when in "fight-or-flight" mode, as the body activates more muscle fibres), so getting "psyched up" before a workout can increase the maximum weight lifted.

Weight training can be a very effective form of strength training because exercises can be chosen, and weights precisely adjusted, to safely exhaust each individual muscle group after the specific numbers of sets and repetitions that have been found to be the most effective for the individual. Other strength training exercises lack the flexibility and precision that weights offer.

Split Training

Split training involves working no more than three muscle groups or body parts per day, instead spreading the training of specific body parts throughout a training cycle of several days. It is commonly used by more advanced practitioners due to the logistics involved in training all muscle groups maximally. Training all the muscles in the body individually through their full range of motion in a single day is generally not considered possible due to caloric and time constraints. Split training involves fully exhausting individual muscle groups during a workout, then allowing several days for the muscle to fully recover. Muscles are worked roughly twice per week and allowed roughly 72 hours to recover. Recovery of certain muscle groups is usually achieved on days while training other groups, i.e. a 7-day week can consist of a practitioner training trapezius, side shoulders and upper shoulders to exhaustion on one day, the following day the arms to exhaustion, the day after that the rear, front shoulders and back, the day after that the chest. In this way all mentioned muscle groups are allowed the necessary recovery.

Intensity, Volume, and Frequency

Three important variables of strength training are intensity, volume, and frequency. Intensity refers to the amount of work required to achieve the activity, and is proportional to the mass of the weights being lifted. Volume refers to the number of muscles worked, exercises, sets and reps during a single session. Frequency refers to how many training sessions are performed per week.

These variables are important because they are all mutually conflicting, as the muscle only has so much strength and endurance, and takes time to recover due to microtrauma. Increasing one by any significant amount necessitates the decrease of the other two, e.g. increasing weight means a reduction of reps, and will require more recovery time and therefore fewer workouts per week. Trying to push too much intensity, volume and frequency will result in overtraining, and eventually lead to injury and other health issues such as chronic soreness and general lethargy, illness or even acute trauma such as avulsion fractures. A high-medium-low formula can be used to avoid overtraining, with either intensity, volume, or frequency being high, one of the others being medium, and the other being low. One example of this training strategy can be found in the following chart:

Type	High	Med	Low
Intensity (% of 1RM)	80–100%	50–70%	10–40%
Volume (per muscle)	1 exercise	2 exercises	3+ exercises
Sets	1 set	2–3 sets	4+ sets
Reps	1–6 reps	8–15 reps	20+ reps
Session frequency	1 p/w	2–3 p/w	4+ p/w

A common training strategy is to set the volume and frequency the same each week (e.g. training 3 times per week, with 2 sets of 12 reps each workout), and steadily increase the intensity (weight) on a weekly basis. However, to maximize progress to specific goals, individual programs may require different manipulations, such as decreasing the weight, and increase volume or frequency.

Making program alterations on a daily basis (daily undulating periodization) seems to be more efficient in eliciting strength gains than doing so every 4 weeks (linear periodization), but for beginners there are no differences between different periodization models.

Periodization

There are many complicated definitions for periodization, but the term simply means the division of the overall training program into periods which accomplish different goals.

Periodization is the modulating of volume, intensity, and frequency over time, to both stimulate gains and allow recovery.

In some programs for example; volume is decreased during a training cycle while intensity is increased. In this template, a lifter would begin a training cycle with a higher rep range than he will finish with.

For this example, the lifter has a 1 rep max of 225 lb:

Week	Set 1	Set 2	Set 3	Set 4	Set 5	Volume Lbs.	% Exertion (Last Set)	% of 1 Rep Max(Last Set)
1	125 lb x 8reps	130 lb x 8reps	135 lb x 8reps	140 lb x 8reps	145 lb x 8reps	5,400	78%	64%
2	135 lb x 7reps	140 lb x 7reps	145 lb x 7reps	150 lb x 7reps	155 lb x 7reps	5,075	81%	69%
3	145 lb x 6reps	150 lb x 6reps	155 lb x 6reps	160 lb x 6reps	165 lb x 6reps	4,650	84%	73%
4	155 lb x 5reps	160 lb x 5reps	165 lb x 5reps	170 lb x 5reps	175 lb x 5reps	4,125	87%	78%
5	165 lb x 4reps	170 lb x 4reps	175 lb x 4reps	180 lb x 4reps	185 lb x 4reps	3,500	90%	82%
6	175 lb x 3reps	180 lb x 3reps	185 lb x 3reps	190 lb x 3reps	195 lb x 3reps	2,775	92%	87%

This is an example of periodization where the number of repetitions decreases while the weight increases.

Practice of Weight Training

Methods and Equipment

There are many methods of strength training. Examples include weight training, circuit training, isometric exercise, gymnastics, plyometrics, Parkour, yoga, Pilates, Super Slow.

Strength training may be done with minimal or no equipment, for instance bodyweight exercises. Equipment used for strength training includes barbells and dumbbells, weight machines and other exercise machines, weighted clothing, resistance bands, gymnastics apparatus, Swiss balls, wobble boards, indian clubs, pneumatic exercise equipment, hydraulic exercise equipment.

Aerobic Exercise Versus Anaerobic Exercise

Strength training exercise is primarily anaerobic. Even while training at a lower intensity (training loads of ~20-RM), anaerobic glycolysis is still the major source of power, although aerobic metabolism makes a small contribution. Weight training is commonly perceived as anaerobic exercise, because one of the more common goals is to increase strength by lifting heavy weights. Other goals such as rehabilitation, weight loss, body shaping, and body-building often use lower weights, adding aerobic character to the exercise.

Except in the extremes, a muscle will fire fibres of both the aerobic or anaerobic types on any given exercise, in varying ratio depending on the load on the intensity of the contraction. This is known as the energy system continuum. At higher loads, the muscle will recruit all muscle fibres possible, both anaerobic ("fast-twitch") and aerobic ("slow-twitch"), in order to generate the most force. However, at maximum load, the anaerobic processes contract so forcefully that the aerobic fibers are completely shut out, and all work is done by the anaerobic processes. Because the anaerobic muscle fibre uses its fuel faster than the blood and intracellular restorative cycles can resupply it, the maximum number of repetitions is limited. In the aerobic regime, the blood and intracellular processes can maintain a supply of fuel and oxygen, and continual repetition of the motion will not cause the muscle to fail.

Circuit weight training is a form of exercise that uses a number of weight training exercise sets separated by short intervals. The cardiovascular effort to recover from each set serves a function similar to an aerobic exercise, but this is not the same as saying that a weight training set is itself an aerobic process.

Exercises for Specific Muscle Groups

Weight trainers commonly divide the body's individual muscles into ten major muscle groups. These do not include the hip, neck and forearm muscles, which are rarely trained in isolation. The most common exercises for these muscle groups are listed below.

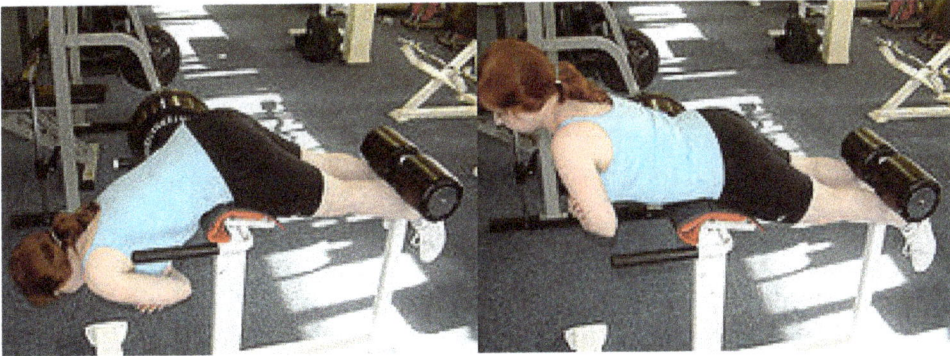

A back extension.

The sequence shown below is one possible way to order the exercises. The large muscles of the lower body are normally trained before the smaller muscles of the upper body, because these first exercises require more mental and physical energy. The core muscles of the torso are trained before the shoulder and arm muscles that assist them. Exercises often alternate between "pushing" and "pulling" movements to allow their specific supporting muscles time to recover. The stabilizing muscles in the waist should be trained last.

Advanced Techniques

A number of techniques have been developed to make weight training exercises more intense, and thereby potentially increase the rate of progress. Many weight lifters use these techniques to bring themselves past a plateau, a duration where a weightlifter may be unable to do more lifting repetitions, sets, or use higher weight resistance.

Set Structure

Drop Sets

Drop sets do not end at the point of momentary muscular failure, but continue with progressively lighter weights.

Pyramid sets

Pyramid sets are weight training sets in which the progression is from lighter weights with a greater number of repetitions in the first set, to heavier weights with fewer repetitions in subsequent sets.

A reverse pyramid is the opposite in which the heavier weights are used at the beginning and progressively lightened.

Burnouts

Burnouts combine pyramids and drop sets, working up to higher weights with low reps and then back down to lower weights and high reps.

Diminishing set

The diminishing set method is where a weight is chosen that can be lifted for 20 reps in one set, and then 70 repetitions are performed in as few sets as possible.

Rest-pause (heavy singles)

Rest-pause heavy singles are performed at or near 1RM, with ten to twenty seconds of rest between each lift. The lift is repeated six to eight times. It is generally recommended to use this method infrequently.

Giant set

The Giant set, is a form of training that targets one muscle group (e.g. the triceps) with four separate exercises performed in quick succession, often to failure and sometimes with the reduction of weight halfway through a set once muscle fatigue sets in. This form of intense training 'shocks' the muscles and as such, is usually performed by experienced trainers and should be used infrequently.

Combined Sets

Supersets

Supersets combine two or more exercises with similar motions to maximize the amount of work of an individual muscle or group of muscles. The exercises are performed with no rest period between the exercises. An example would be doing bench press, which predominantly works the pectoralis and triceps muscles, and then moving to an exercise that works just the triceps such as the triceps extension or the pushdown.

Push-pull supersets

Push-pull supersets are similar to regular supersets, but exercises are chosen which work opposing muscle groups. This is especially popular when applied to arm exercises, for example by combining biceps curls with the triceps pushdown. Other examples include the shoulder press and lat pulldown combination, and the bench press and wide grip row combination.

Pre-exhaustion

Pre-exhaustion combines an isolation exercise with a compound exercise for the same muscle group. The isolation exercise first exhausts the muscle group, and then the compound exercise uses the muscle group's supporting muscles to push it further than would otherwise be possible. For example, the triceps muscles normally help the pectorals perform their function. But in the "bench press" the weaker triceps often fails first, which limits the impact on the pectorals. By preceding the bench press with the pec fly, the pectorals can be pre-exhausted so that both muscles fail at the same time, and both benefit equally from the exercise.

Breakdowns

Breakdowns were developed by Fredrick Hatfield and Mike Quinn to work the different types of muscle fibers for maximum stimulation. Three different exercises that work the same muscle group are selected, and used for a superset. The first exercise uses a heavy weight (~85% of 1 rep max) for around five reps, the second a medium weight (~70% of 1 rep max) for around twelve reps, and finally the third exercise is performed with a light weight (~50% of 1 rep max) for twenty to thirty reps, or even lighter (~40% of 1 rep max) for forty or more reps. (Going to failure is discouraged.) The entire superset is performed three times.

Beyond failure

Forced reps

Forced reps occur after momentary muscular failure. An assistant provides just enough help to get the weight trainer past the sticking point of the exercise, and allow further repetitions to be completed. Weight trainers often do this when they are spotting their exercise partner. With some exercises forced reps can be done without a training partner. For example, with one-arm *biceps curls* the other arm can be used to assist the arm that is being trained.

Cheat reps

Cheating is a deliberate compromise of form to maximize reps. Cheating has the advantage that it can be done without a training partner, but compromises safety. A typical example of cheat reps occurs during biceps curls when, beginning with the load at the waist, the exerciser swings the barbell or dumbbell forward and up during the concentric phase utilizing momentum to assist their bicep muscles in moving the load to a shortened muscle position. Momentum assistance during the concentric phase allows them to move greater loads during the more difficult concentric phase. The objective can be to position greater loads of resistance to the biceps in preparation of performing the eccentric phase than the more difficult concentric phase would otherwise allow. Replacing a typical function of a training partner with a solo exerciser performing cheat reps facilitates forced reps or negative reps when training alone.

Rest-pause (post-failure)

> After a normal set of 6–8 reps (to failure), the weight is re-racked and the trainer takes 10–15 deep breaths, and then performs one more repetition. This process can be repeated for two further repetitions. The twenty-rep squat is another, similar approach, in that it follows a 12–15 rep set of squats with individual rest-pause reps, up to a total of 20 reps.

Weight stripping a.k.a. Number Setting

> Weight stripping is a technique used after failure with a normal resistance in certain exercises, particularly with easily adjustable machines, whereby the weight trainer or a partner gradually reduces the resistance after a full set is taken to failure. With each reduction in resistance, as many possible reps are completed and the resistance is then reduced again. This is continued until the resistance is approximately half the original resistance.

Negative reps

> Negative reps are performed with much heavier weights. Assistants lift the weight, and then the weight trainer attempts to resist its downward progress through an eccentric contraction. Alternatively, an individual can use an exercise machine for negatives by lifting the weight with both arms or legs, and then lowering it with only one. Or they can simply lower weights more slowly than they lift them: for example, by taking two seconds to lift each weight and four seconds to lower it.

Partial reps

> Partial reps, as the name implies, involves movement through only part of the normal path of an exercise. Partial reps can be performed with heavier weights. Usually, only the easiest part of the repetition is attempted.

Burns

> Burns involve mixing partial reps into a set of full range reps in order to increase intensity. The partials can be performed at any part of the exercise movement, depending on what works best for the particular exercise. Also, the partials can either be added after the end of a set or in some alternating fashion with the full range reps. For example, after performing a set of *biceps curls* to failure, an individual would cheat the bar back to the most contracted position, and then perform several partial reps.

Other Techniques

Progressive movement training

Progressive movement training attempts to gradually increase the range of motion throughout a training cycle. The lifter will start with a much heavier weight than they could handle in the full range of motion, only moving through the last 3–5" of the movement. Throughout the training cycle, the lifter will gradually increase the range of motion until the joint moves through the full range of the exercise. This is a style that was made popular by Paul Anderson.

Super slow

Super slow repetitions are performed with lighter weights. The lifting and lowering phases of each repetition take 10 seconds or more.

Timed rests

By strictly controlling the rest periods between reps and sets a trainer can reduce their level of blood oxygenation, which helps to increase the stress on the muscles.

Wrist straps

Wrist straps (lifting straps) are sometimes used to assist in gripping very heavy weights. Wrist straps can be used to isolate muscle groups like in "lat pull-downs", where the trainee would primarily use the latissimus dorsi muscles of the back rather than the biceps. They are particularly useful for the *deadlift*. Some lifters avoid using wrist straps to develop their grip strength, just as some go further by using thick bars. Wrist straps can allow a lifter initially to use more weight than they might be able to handle safely for an entire set, as unlike simply holding a weight, if it is dropped then the lifter must descend with it or be pulled down. Straps place stress on the bones of the wrist which can be potentially harmful if excessive.

Risks and Concerns

Strength training is a safe form of exercise when the movements are controlled, and carefully defined. Or some safety measures can also be taken before the training. However, as with any form of exercise, improper execution and the failure to take appropriate precautions can result in injury. A helmet, boots, gloves, and back belt can aide in injury prevention. Principles of weight training safety apply to strength training.

Bodybuilding

Bodybuilding is a sport in which the goal is to increase muscle size and definition. Bodybuilding increases the endurance of muscles, as well as strength, though not as much as if it were the primary goal. Bodybuilders compete in bodybuilding competitions, and use specific principles and methods of strength training to maximize muscular size and develop extremely low levels of body fat. In contrast, most strength trainers train to improve their strength and endurance while not giving special attention to reducing body fat below normal. Strength trainers tend to focus on compound exercises to build basic strength, whereas bodybuilders often use isolation exercises to visually separate their muscles, and to improve muscular symmetry. Pre-contest training for bodybuilders is different again, in that they attempt to retain as much muscular tissue as possible while undergoing severe dieting. However, the bodybuilding community has been the source of many strength training principles, techniques, vocabulary, and customs.

Nutrition

It is widely accepted that strength training must be matched by changes in diet in order to be effective. Although aerobic exercise has been proven to have an effect on the dietary intake of macronutrients, strength training has not and an increase in dietary protein is generally believed to be required for building skeletal muscle with popular sources advising weight trainers to consume a high-protein diet with from 1.4 to 1.8 g of protein per kg of body weight per day (0.6 to 0.8 g per pound). Protein that is neither needed for cell growth and repair nor consumed for energy is converted into urea mainly through the deamination process and is excreted by the kidneys. It was once thought that a high-protein diet entails risk of kidney damage, but studies have shown that kidney problems only occur in people with previous kidney disease. However failure to properly hydrate can put an increased strain on the kidney's ability to function. An adequate supply of carbohydrates (5–7 g per kg) is also needed as a source of energy and for the body to restore glycogen levels in muscles.

A light, balanced meal prior to the workout (usually one to two hours beforehand) ensures that adequate energy and amino acids are available for the intense bout of exercise. The type of nutrients consumed affects the response of the body, and nutrient timing whereby protein and carbohydrates are consumed prior to and after workout has a beneficial impact on muscle growth. Water is consumed throughout the course of the workout to prevent poor performance due to dehydration. A protein shake is often consumed immediately following the workout, because both protein uptake and protein usage are increased at this time. Glucose (or another simple sugar) is often consumed as well since this quickly replenishes any glycogen lost during the exercise period. To maximise muscle protein anabolism, recovery drink should contain glucose (dextrose), protein (usually whey) hydrosylate containing mainly dipeptides and tripeptides, and leucine. Some weight trainers also take ergogenic aids such as creatine or steroids to aid muscle growth. However, the effectiveness of some products is disputed and others are potentially harmful.

Sex Differences in Mass Gains

Due to the androgenic hormonal differences between males and females, the latter are generally unable to develop large muscles regardless of the training program used. Normally the most that can be achieved is a look similar to that of a fitness model. Muscle is denser than fat, so someone who builds muscle while keeping the same body weight will occupy less volume; if two people weigh the same (and are the same height) but have different lean body mass percentages, the one with more muscle will appear thinner.

In addition, though bodybuilding uses the same principles as strength training, it is with a goal of gaining muscle bulk. Strength trainers with different goals and programs will not gain the same mass as a professional bodybuilder.

Muscle Toning

Some weight trainers perform light, high-repetition exercises in an attempt to "tone" their muscles without increasing their size.

The word tone derives from the Latin "tonus" (meaning "tension"). In anatomy and physiology, as well as medicine, the term "muscle tone" refers to the continuous and passive partial contraction of the muscles, or the muscles' resistance to passive stretching during resting state as determined by a deep tendon reflex. Muscle tonus is dependent on neurological input into the muscle. In medicine, observations of changes in muscle tonus can be used to determine normal or abnormal states which can be indicative of pathology. The common strength training term "tone" is derived from this use.

What muscle builders refer to as a *toned physique* or "muscle firmness" is one that combines reasonable muscular size with moderate levels of body fat, qualities that may result from a combination of diet and exercise.

Muscle tone or firmness is derived from the increase in actin and myosin cross filaments in the sarcomere. When this occurs the same amount of neurological input creates a greater firmness or tone in the resting continuous and passive partial contraction in the muscle.

Exercises of 6–12 reps cause hypertrophy of the sarcoplasm in slow-twitch and high-twitch muscle fibers, contributing to overall increased muscle bulk. Both however can occur to an extent during this rep range. *Even though most are of the opinion that higher repetitions are best for producing the desired effect of muscle firmness or tone, it is not.* Low volume strength training of 5 repetitions or fewer will increase strength by increasing actin and myosin cross filaments thereby increasing muscle firmness or tone. The low volume of this training will inhibit the hypertrophy effect.

Lowered-calorie diets have no positive effect on muscle hypertrophy for muscle of any fiber type. They may, however, decrease the thickness of subcutaneous fat (fat between muscle and skin), through an overall reduction in body fat, thus making muscle striations more visible.

Weight Loss

Exercises like sit-ups, or abdominal crunches, performs less work than whole-body aerobic exercises thereby expending fewer calories during exercise than jogging, for example.

Hypertrophy serves to maintain muscle mass, for an elevated basal metabolic rate, which has the potential to burn more calories in a given period compared to aerobics. This helps to maintain a higher metabolic rate which would otherwise diminish after metabolic adaption to dieting, or upon completion of an aerobic routine.

Weight loss also depends on the type of strength training used. Weight training is generally used for bulking, but the bulking method will more than likely not increase weight because of the diet involved. However, when resistance or circuit training is used, because they are not geared towards bulking, women tend to lose weight more quickly. Lean muscles require calories to maintain themselves at rest, which will help reduce fat through an increase in the basal metabolic rate.

History

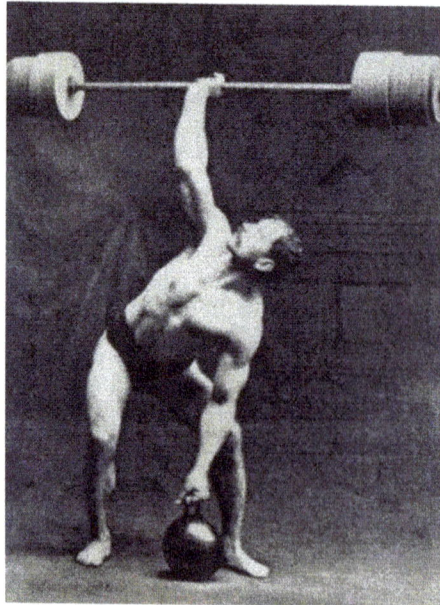

Arthur Saxon performing a Two Hands Anyhow with an early kettlebell and plate-loaded barbell.

Until the 20th century, the history of strength training was very similar to the history of weight training. With the advent of modern technology, materials and knowledge, the methods that can be used for strength training have multiplied significantly.

Hippocrates explained the principle behind strength training when he wrote "that which is used develops, and that which is not used wastes away", referring to muscular hypertrophy and atrophy. Progressive resistance training dates back at least to Ancient Greece, when legend has it that wrestler Milo of Croton trained by carrying a newborn calf on his back every day until it was fully grown. Another Greek, the physician Galen, described strength training exercises using the halteres (an early form of dumbbell) in the 2nd century. Ancient Persians used the *meels*, which became popular during the 19th century as the Indian club, and has recently made a comeback in the form of the clubbell.

The dumbbell was joined by the barbell in the latter half of the 19th century. Early barbells had hollow globes that could be filled with sand or lead shot, but by the end of the century these were replaced by the plate-loading barbell commonly used today.

Strength training with isometric exercise was popularised by Charles Atlas from the 1930s onwards. The 1960s saw the gradual introduction of exercise machines into the still-rare strength training gyms of the time. Strength training became increasingly popular in the 1980s following the release of the bodybuilding movie *Pumping Iron* and the subsequent popularity of Arnold Schwarzenegger.

Special Populations

Safety Concerns Related to Children

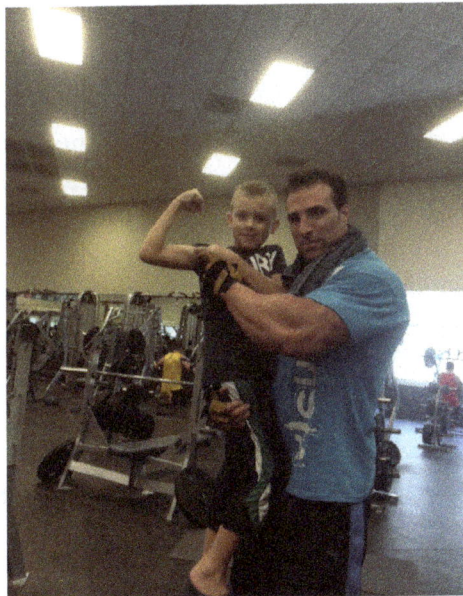

Properly supervised strength training for children.

Orthopaedic specialists used to recommend that children avoid weight training because the growth plates on their bones might be at risk. The very rare reports of growth plate fractures in children who trained with weights occurred as a result of inadequate supervision, improper form or excess weight, and there have been no reports of injuries to growth plates in youth training programs that followed established guidelines. The position of the National Strength and Conditioning Association is that strength training is safe for children if properly designed and supervised.

Younger children are at greater risk of injury than adults if they drop a weight on themselves or perform an exercise incorrectly; further, they may lack understanding of, or ignore the safety precautions around weight training equipment. As a result, supervision of minors is considered vital to ensuring the safety of any youth engaging in strength training.

Australia's Stance on Pre-Adolescence Strength Training

Strength training is the fourth most popular form of fitness in Australia. Due to its popularity amongst all ages, there is great scepticism on what the appropriate age to commence strength training in young athletes is. Some points of the opposing view of strength training in young adolescence are stunted growth, health and bone problems in later stages of life and unhealthy eating habits. Studies by Australian experts that have been recognised by the Australian Institute of Sport (AIS) have debunked these myths. There is no link between any prolonged health risks and strength training in pre-adolescence if the procedures of strength training are followed correctly and under suitable supervision. Strength training for pre-adolescents should focus on skills and techniques. Children should only work on strengthening all the big muscle groups, using free weight and body weight movements with relatively light loads. The benefits of these practices include increased strength performance, injury prevention and learning good training principles.

For Older Adults

Older adults are prone to loss of muscle strength. With more strength older adults have better health, better quality of life, and fewer falls. In cases in which an older person begins strength training, their doctor or health care provider may neglect to emphasize a strength training program which results in muscle gains. Under-dosed strength training programs should be avoided in favor of a program which matches the abilities and goals of the person exercising.

In setting up an exercise program for an older adult, they should go through a baseline fitness assessment to determine their current limits. Any exercise program for older adults should match the intensity, frequency, and duration of exercise that the person can perform. The program should have a goal of increased strength as compared to the baseline measurement.

Recommended training for older adults is three times a week of light strength training exercises. Exercise machines are a commonly used equipment in a gym setting, including treadmills with exercises such as walking or light jogging. Home-based exercises should usually consist of body weight or elastic band exercises that maintain a low level of impact on the muscles. Weights can also be used by older adults if they maintain a lighter weight load with an average amount of repetitions (10–12 REPS) with suitable supervision. It is important for older adults to maintain a light level of strength training with low levels of impact to avoid injuries.

Bodyweight exercise

Bodyweight exercises are strength training exercises that do not require free weights; the individual's own weight provides the resistance for the movement. Movements such as the push-up, the pull-up, and the sit-up are some of the most common bodyweight exercises.

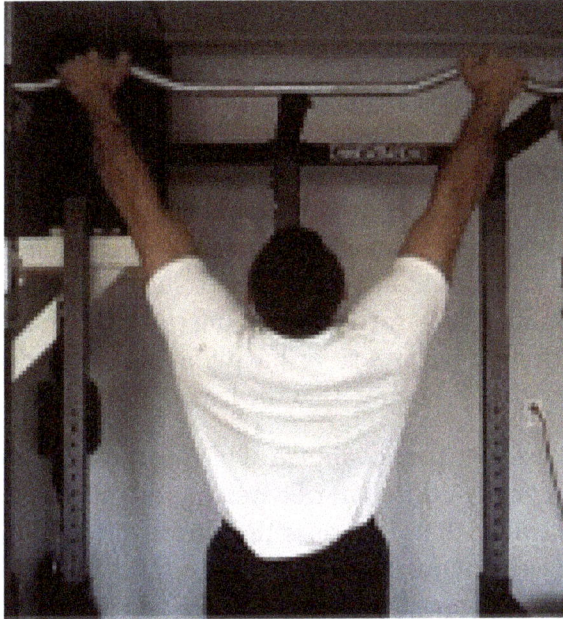

Pull-ups are a common bodyweight exercise.

Advantages

Because they do not require weights, bodyweight exercises are the ideal choice for individuals who are interested in fitness but do not have access to equipment. While some exercises may require some type of equipment, the majority of bodyweight exercises require none. For those exercises that do require equipment, common items found in the household are usually sufficient (such as a bath towel for towel curls), or substitutes can usually be improvised (for example, using a horizontal tree branch to perform pull ups).

Some bodyweight exercises have been shown to benefit not just the young, but the elderly as well.

Most bodyweight exercises can be progressed or regressed to match the individual's abilities. This progression/regression strategy allows people of nearly all levels of fitness to participate. Some basic methods to increase or decrease the difficulty of a bodyweight exercise, without adding extra weight, are: changing the amount of leverage in an exercise (such as elevating the feet for a standard push-up, or performing the push-up with knees on the ground), performing the exercise on an unstable platform (such as performing push-ups on a basketball), modifying the range of motion in an exercise (such as squatting to a 45 degree angle rather than a 90 degree angle), incorporating unilateral movements as opposed to bilateral movements (such as performing a one-armed push-up), and adding isometric pauses during the exercise (such as holding for a few seconds at the bottom of a push-up).

Gymnasts make extensive use of isometrics by doing much of their training with straight arms (such as iron crosses, levers, and planches). When compared to weight lifting, bodyweight exercises often require much more flexibility and balance.

Bodyweight exercises have a far lower risk of injury compared to using free weights and machines due to the absence of an external load that is placing strain on the muscles that they may or may not be able to deal with. However, the lower risk of injury is only provided that the athlete/trainee is progressing through the correct progressions and not immediately skipping to strenuous movements that can place undue and possibly harmful stress on ligaments, tendons, and other tissues. Although falling on the head, chest, buttocks, and falling backwards can occur, these are far less harmful injuries than dropping a weight on a body part, or having a joint extended beyond its natural range of motion due to a weight being used incorrectly.

Bodyweight exercises also give the advantage of having minimal bulking and cutting requirements that are normally utilised in free weight and machines training. This is due to bulking bringing extra fat that decreases the performance of bodyweight exercises, thus bodyweight exercises not only remove the need for a bulking or cutting phase, but it can help a person retain a low body fat percentage all year round.

Bodyweight exercises also work several muscle groups at once, due to the lack of isolation and the need of a large majority of muscles to perform a movement properly. For example, in a pushup, the body must form a rigid straight line, and the elbow joint must move from a straight angle to the smallest angle possible, and thus the core muscles, chest muscles, triceps, and legs are all involved in ensuring proper, strict form.

Disadvantages

As bodyweight exercises use the individual's own weight to provide the resistance for the movement, the weight being lifted is never greater than the weight of one's own body. This can make it difficult to achieve a level of intensity that is near the individual's one rep maximum, which is desirable for strength training.

Bodyweight exercises can be increased in intensity by including additional weights (such as wearing a weighted vest or holding a barbell, kettlebell, sandbell or plate during a sit up), but this deviates from the general premise that bodyweight exercises rely solely on the weight of the individual to provide resistance.

However, difficulty can be added by changing the leverage, which places more emphasis on specific limbs and muscles, e.g. a one legged squat works a leg far stronger than a two legged squat, which not only requires strength but progressing to a one legged squat builds strength along the way. The same can be seen with one arm pushups, pull ups, and many other exercises.

Difficulty can also be added by increasing volume, adding explosiveness to the movements, or slowing down the movement to increase time under tension.

Classes of Exercises

Bodyweight exercises are generally grouped into four rough classes: Push, which requires the individual to use pushing movements to direct the body against gravity; Pull, which requires the practitioner to use pulling to direct the body; Core, which involves contracting movements of the abdominal and back muscles; and Legs/Glutes, which involve movements of the legs and glutes to direct the individual's body against gravity.

Push Exercises

Push bodyweight exercises use a resistive or static pushing motion to work various muscle groups. Most push exercises focus on the pectoral, shoulder, and triceps muscles, but other muscle groups such as the abdominal and back muscles are leveraged to maintain good form during the push exercise.

Bridge

The individual begins in a sit-up position with the hands positioned by the ears, palms down, fingers facing the legs. The individual pushes up with the arms and the back muscles until the body resembles a lowercase 'n'. The spine must be convex and the limbs straight. The difficulty can be increased by entering the bridge from a standing position and bending backwards in a controlled manner into the bridge.

Common variants

>   Inverse Push Ups

Muscle Groups

>   Triceps

>   Trapezius

>   Deltoids

>   Glutes

>   Lower back

4-Count Bodybuilder

From a standing position, the individual drops to a squat with hands on floor (count 1), thrusts the legs back to a pushup position (count 2), returns the legs to the squat position (count 3) and then returns to standing position (count 4). The military 8-Count Bodybuilder adds a full pushup after count 2 (count 3 and 4), and opens and closes the legs while in push-up position (count 5 and 6). The Burpee variation replaces count 4 with a plyometric squat jump before returning to the standing starting position.

Common Variants

> Burpee

> 8-Count Bodybuilders

Muscle Groups

> Legs

> Abdominals

> Shoulders

Dips

The individual begins with the hands placed on two solid surfaces at or around waist height. The knees are then bent to raise the feet from the ground, and the body is lowered as far as possible using the arms, then raised again.

Muscle Groups

> Triceps

> Pectorals

Seated Dip

The individual begins with their feet on the floor, legs out straight, and hands placed on a supporting level surface between knee and waist height. Starting with straight arms with the shoulders above the hands, the body is lowered until the arms are bent at a 90 degrees angle. The body is then raised to the starting position.

The difficulty may be decreased by moving the feet closer to the body. The difficulty may be increased by raising the feet onto a stable surface. The Hanging Dip or Parallel Dip variation requires an apparatus such as a dip bar or two parallel bars (or substitutes such as tree branches or two tables) and the legs are fully raised off the ground, with the individual's bodyweight supported by the arms alone.

Common Variants

> Hanging Dip

Parallel Dip

Muscle Groups

Triceps

Chest

L-sit

The individual sits with the body in an L-position, the upper body perpendicular to the ground and the legs out straight and parallel to the ground. The hands are placed beside the glutes. The hands and arms then push the entire body, including the legs, upwards off the ground with the legs remaining parallel to the ground. This exercise taxes the muscles through isometric tension.

The V-Sit variation increaess the difficulty by holding the legs higher, angled away from the ground, so the individual's body forms a 'V' shape.

Common Variants

V-Sit

Muscle Groups

Obliques

Rectus Abdominis

Triceps

Quadriceps (these are needed to maintain straightness in the legs)

Pectorals

Lunge

The individual stands on flat surface, steps forward with one leg and bends down until the front knee is bent at a 90-degree angle. The back knee bends to almost touch the ground. The front knee should not extend past the front toes in order to maintain good form. The individual then returns to the starting position by pushing back with the front leg and stepping back so both feet are together.

The Back Lunges variation is performed from the same position, but instead the individual steps back with the leg until the front knee is bent at a 90-degree angle and the back knee is almost touching the ground. The Iron Mikes variation starts out in the bottom position of the lunge, whereby the individual performs a plyometric jump and switches leg positions so the landing position is opposite to the starting position. The Walking Lunges variation does not return the front leg to the starting position, but instead the individual steps forward with the back leg to place the feet together.

Common Variants

>Back Lunges

>Iron Mikes

>Walking Lunges

Muscle Groups

>Thigh

>Buttocks

>Hamstrings

Side Lunges

The individual starts with the feet positioned slightly apart and takes a wide step to the side with the left foot, toes pointing slightly outward. As the left foot contacts the ground, the individual shifts their weight to the left so the majority of the individual's bodyweight is supported by the left leg. The individual lowers the hips and slides the hips back until the left thigh is parallel with the ground. The back and the head are kept straight throughout the movement. The individual holds the position for a moment, then raises the body by pushing up with the left leg and moves the feet together again. The exercise is then repeated on the right side.

The difficulty may be increased by performing the Wide Side Lunge variant; the individual starts with the feet in a wide stance instead of together. The individual keeps the feet in the wide stance throughout the exercise and omits the intermediate step of moving the feet together between repetitions.

Common Variants

>Wide Side Lunges

Muscle Groups

>Quadriceps

>Glutes

>Hip flexors

>Hamstrings

Bear Walk

The individual places the hands and the feet on the ground, with the head facing the ground. The individual then proceeds to crawl around by striding with the arms and legs.

Common Variants

Muscle Groups

Shoulders

Chest

Triceps

Trapezius

Core

Rocking Chairs

The individual begins in a fully extended plank or push-up position. The body is then pushed slowly forward about six to ten inches, while the arms are kept straight. The body is then returned to the starting position.

The difficulty of this exercise may be increased by bending the arms and lowering the body until it is close to the floor. The body is then slowly pushed forward and returned to the starting position. The difficulty may be further increased by extending the arms between sets to perform a push-up.

Common Variants

Rocking Chair Press

Muscle Groups

Pectorals

Triceps

Deltoids

Core

Shove Offs

The individual begins by standing in front of an elevated surface with a ledge that will bear the weight of the individual. The body is tilted forward with the hands and arms extended and the back and legs held straight. The body is allowed to continue to fall forward and the individual catches their weight on the elevated surface with their hands in a palm-down position and arms bent. The arms are then forcefully extended to push the body back to the upright position. The waist is not bent at any time during the exercise.

The difficulty of this exercise may be increased by selecting a lower surface which decreases the leverage of the arms and moves the center of gravity forwards towards the hands.

Common Variants

> none

Muscle Groups

> Pectorals

> Shoulders

> Triceps

Mountain Climbers

The individual begins in a push-up position, with the body in a straight line and elbows locked. The left knee is brought to the chest and the left foot placed on the ground, with the right leg remaining outstretched. The individual then performs a small hop and switches the position of the feet so that the right knee is brought to the chest, the right foot placed on the ground and the left leg is extended behind the body. The exercise is then repeated, most commonly at a fast pace for a defined length of time.

Common Variants

> none

Muscle Groups

> Shoulders

> Abdominals

> Core

Pec Crawl

The individual begins in a push-up position on a smooth surface. The body is propelled forward using only the arms which are never bent beyond 90 degrees. The feet are dragged behind the individual, the body held in a straight line. This exercise is best performed on a smooth floor while wearing socks or with a folder towel placed under the feet. If performed on a carpeted surface, sneakers should be worn and the toes pointed backwards while the exercise is performed.

Common Variants

>   none

Muscle Groups

>   Deltoids
>
>   Core
>
>   Pectorals
>
>   Triceps

Dive Bomber

The feet are placed on the ground just a few inches apart, with the legs held straight. The individual bends over at the waist and places their hands on the ground a few feet in front of the toes, forming an inverted 'V' with the body, the hips forming the vertex of the 'V'. The individual swings their chest and shoulders down in an arc, between the hands, so the chest nearly touches the ground. The head and shoulders are curved up in an arc as high as possible, until the back is fully arched, the head is facing forward, and the pelvis is only a few inches off the ground. The motion is then reversed, the chest and shoulders moving through the hands, close to the ground, with the arms pushing the body back to the starting point. The arms should end up straight and in line with the back.

The Half Dive Bomber variant simply stops the movement at the point the chest is between the hands and then reverses the movement to return to the starting position. The Hindu dand variant returns directly to the starting position without bending the arms or arcing the chest and shoulders back through the hands.

The difficulty of the exercise can be decreased by moving the feet further apart, or by elevating the hands on a stable surface. The difficulty can be increased by placing only a single leg on the ground at a time.

Common Variants

>   Half Dive Bomber
>
>   Dand

Muscle Groups

>   Pectorals
>
>   Triceps
>
>   Deltoids
>
>   Core

Pec Flies

The individual starts by lying facedown on a smooth, hard floor. The legs are placed out straight with the toes on the floor, and the arms out to the sides. Two small towels are placed under the palms. With the arms and body kept straight, the palms are slid together in a controlled manner until the hands are under the shoulders. The hands are then slowly slid apart until the chest is barely touching the floor.

Common Variants

Muscle Groups

   Pectorals

   Core

   Shoulders

Side Triceps Extension

The individual starts by lying down on their right side with the body in a straight line. The right hand is placed on the left shoulder, and the left hand is placed palm down on the ground, under the right shoulder, fingers pointing towards the head. The left arm pushes the upper body off the ground until the arm is straight, bending at the waist to keep the lower body on the ground. The body is then lowered to the starting position. The exercise is repeated on the left side to work the right triceps.

Common Variants

Muscle Groups

   Triceps

   Obliques

Crab Walk

The individual starts by sitting on the ground with the knees bent. Both feet and both palms are placed on the floor. The body is lifted off the floor and the individual walks like a crab, both forward and backward.

Common Variants

Muscle Groups

> Triceps

> Core

Hip Raiser

The individual sits on the ground in an L-position with the back perpendicular to the ground and legs out straight. The palms are placed on the ground beside the hips. The soles of the feet are placed on the ground and the pelvis is lifted off the floor until the knees are bent at a 90-degree angle and the body is straight from the head to the knees, with the face pointed straight up. The position is held for a moment and then the body is returned to the starting position.

Common Variants

> none

Muscle Groups

> Triceps

> Shoulders

> Glutes

> Hamstrings

Air Plunges

The individual starts by lying down on the ground flat on the back, with the arms placed palm-down on the ground. The legs are lifted until they are straight in the air, perpendicular to the ground. The arms are used to push the hips off the ground as high as possible, keeping the legs perpendicular to the ground. The hips are then lowered slowly to the starting position. Lie flat on the back, arms to the side, palms on the ground.

The difficulty of the exercise can be increased by holding the hips in the top position for a few seconds before they are lowered to the ground.

Common Variants

> none

Muscle Groups

> Triceps

> Lower abdominals

Surface Triceps Extensions

The individual starts by grasping a stable, waist-level surface such as a couch, railing, table or a horizontal bar. The surface is grasped with an overhand grip, hands shoulder-width apart. The feet are placed back slightly further than a standard push up position. The body is kept straight, while the arms are bent and the body lowered until the head is below the hands. The body is then raised by pushing up with the arms until the arms are locked out straight. The elbows should be kept pointed straight down throughout the movement.

The difficulty of the exercise may be decreased by grasping a higher surface to move the center of gravity closer to the body.

Common Variants

> none

Muscle Groups

> Triceps

> Core

Arm Rotations

The individual starts by standing and placing the arms straight out and perpendicular with the body. The hands and arms are moved in circles, first forward, then backward, for a selected number of rotations.

The targeted muscle groups of this exercise can be modified by repositioning the arm and body: making circles with the arms pointed out straight in front of the individual moves the focus to the front deltoids, while bending over and moving the arms up and down instead of in circles emphasizes the rear deltoids.

Common Variants

> none

Muscle Groups

> Shoulders

The Roof is on Fire

The individual begins in a push up position and performs a single push up. Then the individual will kneel and raise their hands in the air four times as if they are performing an unweighted overhead press. The individual then performs two push ups, then kneels and performs eight unweighted overhead presses. The individual will continue to ladder up in this manner, with the count of unweighted overhead presses equalling four times the number of pushups. When muscle failure is reached, the individual then ladders down with a decreasing number of push ups and a corresponding number of unweighted overhead presses.

Common Variants

> none

Muscle Groups

> Shoulders

> Triceps

> Pectorals

Push-Ups

The bodyweight Push Up is a common marker of an individual's general fitness level; for this reason it is included as one of the "big three" bodyweight exercises in the Navy Seal BUD/S Physical Screening Test. The bodyweight push-up has many distinct variations, many of which are listed below.

Classic Push Up

The individual starts by lying on the ground in the prone position. The feet are placed together and the palms are placed on the ground under the shoulders. The arms then push the body off the ground with the body is kept in a straight line. Once the arms are straight, the body is then lowered until the chest touches the ground.

The difficulty of this exercise may be decreased by elevating the hands onto a stable horizontal surface to move the center of gravity away from the arms. The arms may even be placed on a solid wall or other sturdy vertical surface to make the exercise as easy as possible.

The difficulty of this exercise may be increased by elevating the feet on to a stable horizontal surface to move the center of gravity towards the arms. As well, the exercise may be performed with the hands on an unstable surface such as a medicine ball. The exercise can be further modified by performing the push up on one leg with the other leg held in the air to put more focus on the lower lumbar region. To move the focus to the pectoral muscles, the hands may be moved further apart.

Muscle Groups

> Pectorals

Triceps

Deltoids

Core

Handstand Push Up

The individual starts with the hands about three feet from a wall or other solid vertical surface. The legs are placed on the wall one at a time, then the hands are 'walked' toward the wall, sliding the feet and legs up the wall until the hands are approximately a foot from the wall. The body is lowered in a controlled fashion by bending the arms, until the head nearly touches the ground between the hands.

Muscle Groups

Shoulders

Triceps

Core

Chinese Push Ups

The individual starts with their feet on the ground, heels together. The palms are then placed on the ground five hand lengths away from the toes, forming a diamond with the thumbs and the fingers. The body is bent at the hips to form a 90-degree angle between the torso and legs. The arms are bent at the elbow until the top of the head almost touches the ground between the hands. The arms are then straighted to return to the starting position. The back and legs should be kept as straight as possible throughout the exercise.

The difficulty of the exercise may be decreased by placing the hands on an elevated surface, while placing the feet on the elevated surface will cause the exercise to become more difficult.

Muscle Groups

Triceps

Deltoids

Get in Line

The individual starts in a push up position, but places one hand directly under the forehead while the other hand is placed under the sternum. The arms are bent and the body lowered to the floor as in a normal pu`sh up, the elbows kept as close to the body as possible. The hands may be alternated with every repetition or with every set.

Muscle Groups

Triceps

Deltoids

Close Grip Push Ups

This exercise is performed just as a classic push up, but the hands are moved closer together to approximately one or two hand widths apart. As with the classic push up, the hands may be elevated to decrease the difficulty, or the feet raised to increase the difficulty.

Muscle Groups

Triceps

Pectorals

Shoulders

Core

Military Press

The Military Press is performed in a similar manner to the Chinese Push Up, but the hands are placed shoulder-width apart.

Muscle Groups

Triceps

Pectorals

Shoulders

Core

Shoulder Drop Push Ups

The Shoulder Drop is performed in a similar manner to the Classic Push Up, but one shoulder is lowered to the ground as the opposite shoulder is raised high in the air.

Muscle Groups

Pectorals

Triceps

Deltoids

Core

Deep Push Ups

Deep Push Ups are performed as a Classic Push-up, with each hand placed on a raised surface so the body can be lowered between the hands at the bottom of the movement. This modification places more emphasis on the pectorals and deltoids.

Muscle Groups

Pectorals

Triceps

Deltoids

Core

Staggered Hands Push Up

Performed like a Classic Push Up, except one hand is placed forward of the normal starting position and one hand is placed slightly behind.

Muscle Groups

Pectorals

Triceps

Deltoids

Core

Bouncing Push Ups

Performed as a Classic Push Up, but the body is propelled upwards with a plyometric movement so the hands leave the floor for a moment. The individual then lands gently on the fingers and palms of the hand and lowers the body again to the floor.

Muscle Groups

Pectorals

Triceps

Deltoids

Core

Semi-Planche Push Up

The individual begins in a prone position, with the hands palm-down on the ground with the fingers pointed toward the feet. The arms are then extended to raise the entire body off the ground so that only the palms of the hands and the toes are touching the ground. The body is then returned to the starting position.

Muscle Groups

>Pectorals

>Triceps

>Deltoids

>Core

Planche Push Up

Performed as a Semi-Planche Push Up, but the toes are also raised off the ground and the entire body is balanced on the hands which remain stationary on the ground.

Muscle Groups

>Pectorals

>Triceps

>Deltoids

>Core

One-Arm Push Up

Performed in the form of a Classic Push Up, but one arm is placed behind the back, with the elbow of the other arm held tightly against the ribs. The feet are spread apart to provide balance, and the body is lowered and raised using only a single arm.

Muscle Groups

>Pectorals

>Triceps

>Deltoids

>Core

>Abdominals

>Obliques

Lower back

Spidermans

The individual begins in a prone position on the ground, the balls of the feet on the ground and the hands placed on the ground above the head, fingers splayed. The body is then raised in the air, keeping the midsection as straight as possible, until only the fingers and balls of the feet touch the ground. The body is then lowered to the starting position.

Muscle Groups

>   Core

>   Back

>   Pectorals

Pull

Pull bodyweight exercises use a resistive or static pulling motion to work various muscle groups.

Human Flag

The individual starts by grabbing a vertical object such as a pole or tree trunk, with both hands palms pronated. The body is then lifted into a horizontal position using the abdominal muscles, with the arms remaining as straight as possible.

Common Variants

>   none

Muscle Groups

>   Abdominals (mainly obliques)

>   Shoulders

>   Triceps (this is for the pushing down by the lower arm)

>   Biceps (this is done by the pulling of the upper arm)

Muscle Up

The individual starts with an aggressive standard Pull Up with an overhand grip to chest level, at which point the wrists are rotated forward to permit the elbows and arms to swing above the bar. The arms then push the body up until the arms are straight and the waist is at the level of the bar. The motion is then reversed so the body can be lowered back to the starting position. The transition between the high pull up and the low dip is the most difficult part and emphasizes the trapezius.

Common Variants

Muscle Groups

Deltoids

Trapezius

Erector spinae

Latissimus dorsi

Biceps

Brachialis

Pull Up

The bodyweight Pull Up is another common indicator of an individual's general fitness level and is also included as one of the "big three" bodyweight exercises in the Navy Seal BUD/S Physical Screening Test.

The individual starts by hanging from a bar with the arms extended and the palms facing away from the exerciser. The body is then pulled up using the arms until the elbows are bent and the head is higher than the hands. If the hands are moved closer, more emphasis is placed on the biceps and elbow flexors.

Common Variants

Muscle Groups

Deltoids

Trapezius

Erector spinae

Latissimus dorsi

Biceps

Brachialis

Abdominals

Let Me Ins

The individual starts by facing the outer edge of an open door that has a standard doorknob set. The feet are placed on either side of the door and the door pressed between the feet, the heels directly below the doorknob. The individual then leans back until the arms are straight and bends the knees so a 90-degree angle is formed between the thighs and back. The body is then pulled toward the door until the chest touches the edge of the door. The thighs and back should remain locked into a 90-degree angle throughout the exercise. The body is then lowered to the starting point.

The exercise can be performed with either a side grip or over-handed grip, which places emphasis on the extensors on the outside of the forearm, or an under-handed grip, which shifts the focus to the flexors on the inside of the forearms.

The difficulty can be modified by moving the feet; moving them forward increases the difficulty while moving the feet back decreases the difficulty. The exercise can also be performed with unilateral movements (one-handed) to increase the difficulty.

The Towel Grip variation works to increase grip strength. A small towel or rope is hooked around the doorknob and the individual grasps one end of the towel in each hand to perform the exercise. In lieu of a door, the same exercise can be performed with a tree trunk, railing, or any vertical stable pole.

Common Variants

> Towel Grip Let Me In
>
> One-Handed Let Me In

Muscle Groups

> Latissimus dorsi
>
> Biceps
>
> Forearms
>
> Deltoids

Let Me Ups

The individual starts by lying on the ground in the supine position, and grasps a bar mounted at arm's length above the chest. The arms are bent to pull the body up to the bar, while the body remains as straight as possible from the ankles to the shoulders. The body is then lowered until the arms are straight.

The exercise may be made less difficult by moving the feet closer to the bar and bending the knees. The exercise may be increased in difficulty by raising the feet onto a raised surface. Performing the exercise with an overhand grip focuses on the extensors on the outside of the forearm, while an underhand grip changes the focus to the flexors on the inside of the forearm.

Common Variants

> none

Muscle Groups

> Latissimus dorsi
>
> Biceps
>
> Forearms
>
> Deltoids

Towel Curls

The individual starts in a standing position with the back against a wall. The ends of a bath-sized towel are grasped in each hand, and the towel is looped under the foot of one leg. The towel is pulled upwards with the arms, the elbows locked against the side of the body, while pushing down with the foot to provide resistance. The arms are then lowered slowly as the foot continues to provide resistance until the arms are at the starting position.

The difficulty of the exercise may be modified by providing more or less resistance with the foot; the exercise may be made even more difficult by performing it with one hand.

The Ledge Curl variant uses a fixed ledge between waist and chest height to provide resistance. The hands are balled into fists and placed under the ledge. The individual then bends over slowly while pressing up against the bottom of the ledge, then returns slowly to the starting position, maintaining the same level of resistance along the way.

The Isometric Curl variant uses one hand placed on the wrist of the other hand to provide resistance to the curling motion; the curling arm does not move in this case but instead benefits from the isometric tension of the exercise.

Common Variants

> Ledge Curls
>
> Isometric Curls

Muscle Groups

> Biceps
>
> Forearms

The Claw

The individual places the arms in front of the body, and opens and closes the hands and fingers as tightly and as quickly as possible. This exercise is usually performed for a large number of repetitions.

Common Variants

>   none

Muscle Groups

>   Hands

>   Forearms

Core

Core exercises primarily involve dynamic and static contraction of the back and abdominal muscles. Core exercises can aid with improved balance and overall stability.

Crunch

The Curl-Up, or Crunch, is another measure of a person's fitness level and is the third of the "big three" bodyweight exercises in the Navy Seal BUD/S Physical Screening Test.

The individual starts in a supine position on the ground. The shoulders are curled towards the pelvis while the lower back remains flat against the floor. The focus is placed on contracting the abdominal muscles.

The Crunch It Up variant places the feet under a stationary object such as a low bed or couch. The arms are crossed over the stomach and the knees bent. Using the abdominal muscles, the torse is brought up just until the arms touch the thighs. The torso is then lowered to the starting position.

The V-Ups variant starts with the individual in a supine position with arms straight out on the ground and parallel to the body. The body is bent at the hips, the torso is raised off the ground and the legs brought to the chest with knees bent. The legs and torso are then lowered until they are just a few inches off the ground, but not touching it.

The Side-V variant starts with the individual on the ground, lying on one side of the body, with the arm closest to the ground stretched out perpendicular to the body. The other arm is bent and the hand placed behind the head. The torso is raised and the legs, kept straight, are raised until the legs form a 90-degree angle with the torso. The legs and torso are then lowered until they are just a few inches off the ground, but not touching it.

The Jack-Knife variant starts with the individual on the ground, legs stretched out straight and the arms on the ground extended straight up over the head. The chest and legs are simultaneously brought up until the hands touch the feet. The legs and torso are then lowered until they are just a few inches off the ground, but not touching it.

The Bicycle variant starts with the individual on the ground, the hands behind the head. The knee is pulled in toward the chest while the upper body curls up to touch the opposite elbow to the knee. The leg is then straightened and the exercise performed on the other side. The legs should be suspended off the ground during the exercise.

Common Variants

>	Crunch It Ups

>	V-Ups

>	Side V-Ups

>	Jack Knives

>	Bicycle

Muscle Groups

>	Abdominals

Hyperextension

The individual starts in a prone position on the ground with the arms straight out in front of the body. The arms, legs and upper chest are lifted off the ground, and then slowly lowered back to the ground. This exercise is also known as "Supermans".

The Thumbs-Up variant starts in the same position, but the individual forms two fists with the thumbs pointed straight up, then lifts the head, shoulders and chest off the ground as high as possible.

The Swimmers variation raises and lowers the opposite leg and arm and alternates sides.

The Pillow Humpers variant places a towel under the hips and the feet under a stationary object like a low bed or couch. The hands are placed behind the head and the torso is raised off the ground as far as possible.

Common Variants

>	Thumbs Up

>	Swimmers

    Supermans

    Pillow Humpers

Muscle Groups

    Lower back

    Erector spinae

Planche

The individual starts on the ground in a prone position, with the hands at the side of the body by the hips, palm down. The body is held straight while the arms push the body off the floor until the arms are straight. The entire weight of the individual is balanced on the arms. The body is then lowered to the ground.

Common Variants

    none

Muscle Groups

    Full Body [explain]

Plank

The individual places the toes and the forearms on the ground, with the elbows underneath the shoulders and the arm bent at a 90-degree angle. This position is maintained for as long as possible.

The Static Push Up variant simply holds the starting position of a Classic Push Up for as long as possible.

The S&M Push Up variant builds on the Static Push Up variant, but opposite legs and arms are lifted from the ground. The position is held as long as possible before switching sides.

Common Variants

    Front Plank

    Side Plank

    Reverse Plank

    Static Push Up

    S&M Push Ups

Muscle Groups

>   Core

>   Abdominals

>   Back

>   Shoulders

Russian Twist

The individual starts by sitting upright on the ground, with arms crossed and knees bent. The feet are lifted off the ground while the torso is twisted so the left elbow can touch the right knee, then twisted in the opposite direction so the right elbow can touch the left knee. The movement is repeated as long as possible.

Common Variants

>   none

Muscle Groups

>   Abdominals

>   Intercostals

>   Obliques

Standing Knee Raises

The individual starts by standing upright, with arms raised out in front of the body. The left knee is brought up as high as possible, held up for a few moments, then lowered to the ground. The right knee is then raised as high as possible, held, then lowered to the ground.

Common Variants

>   none

Muscle Groups

>   Abdominals

Leg Raises

The individual starts in a supine position on the floor, palms on the floor under the lower back or buttocks. The legs are slowly raised to a 45-degree angle with the ground, then slowly lowered to the ground.

The exercise can be increased in difficulty by raising the legs to a 90-degree angle, and not allowing the legs to return fully to the floor between repetitions.

The Flutter Kicks variation raises both legs off the ground by several inches, then alternates lifting each leg to the 45-degree position and returning it to its starting position.

The Hello Darlings variant raises both legs off the ground by several inches, then opens and closes the legs with a horizontal movement.

The Hanging Leg Lift variant starts with the individual hanging from a horizontal bar by their hands. The knees are brought slowly up to the chest and then returned to the starting position. The difficulty can be increased by keeping the legs straight as they are raised as high as possible.

Common Variants

> Flutter Kicks
>
> Hello Darlings
>
> Hanging Leg Lifts

Muscle Groups

> Abdominals
>
> Hip flexors

Beach Scissors

The individual begins by lying on the side, one hand propping up the head, both legs kept straight. The upper leg is raised as high as possible, held in the air for a moment, then lowered to the starting position. The difficulty may be increased by propping up the body on one elbow.

Common Variants

> none

Muscle Groups

> Hip flexors
>
> Obliques

Hip Ups

The individual begins by lying on the ground, propped up on one elbow, hip and feet touching the ground. The hips are then raised until the body is in a straight line. The hips are then lowered to the starting position.

Common Variants

    none

Muscle Groups

    Obliques

    Intercostals

Supine Windshield Wipers

The individual begins by lying on the ground in a supine position, legs raised in the air at 90 degrees, arms stretched out the sides. The legs are then lowered to the right side by rotating the hips, then brought back to the starting position. The legs are then lowered to the left side, then returned to the starting position.

Common Variants

    Half Windshield Wipers

    Full Windshield Wipers

Muscle Groups

    Abdominals

    Obliques

    Intercostals

Yes, No, Maybes

The individual begins in a supine position on a raised surface, with the head and neck extending off the edge. The head is then moved up and down in a "yes" fashion. The head is then turned from side to side in a "no" fashion. Finally, the head is moved from side to side, bringing each ear to the nearest shoulder in a "maybe" fashion. The exercise may also be performed in a prone position, with the hands placed on the back of the head to provide extra resistance.

Common Variants

    none

Muscle Groups

Neck

Legs/Glutes

Bodyweight exercises that work the thigh, calf and glute muscles are generally performed in the upright, seated, and all-fours positions. Increasing the difficulty of exercises in this class is usually accomplished through unilateral modifications (performed on one leg) or providing additional weight over and above the individual's own bodyweight.

Calf Raises

The individual starts with both feet on the edge of a raised surface, with the toes on the surface and the heels lower than the toes. The heels are raised as high as possible, then returned to the starting position.

The difficulty may be increased by performing the exercise on one leg.

The Cliffhanger variant requires one foot only to be placed on the surface and the position held as long as possible in isometric tension.

The Donkey Calf Raises variant requires that the individual bend at the waist to about 90 degrees and rest the arms on a chair or other stable surface.

The Little Piggies variant is performed by placing the heels on the surface, and moves the toes instead.

Common Variants

> The Cliffhanger

> Donkey Calf Raises

> Little Piggies

Muscle Groups

> Calves

Squat

The individual starts in a standing position with feet shoulder width apart. The legs are bent at the nees and hips, and the torso is lowered between the legs. The knees should remain behind the toes at all times. The body is then raised to the starting position.

The Invisible Chair variant is performed with the back against the wall, knees bent at 90 degrees, and the body is held in this position for as long as possible.

The Wall Squat variant is performed with the back against the wall and the feet one step forward from the wall. The back slides down the wall as the knees are bent to a 90-degree angle.

The Sumo Squat variant is performed with a wide stance, and the body is lowered until the thighs are parallel to the ground.

The One-Legged Squat is performed with one leg held out straight in front of the body while the other leg bears the full weight of the individual during the squat.

The Pistol Squat variant builds on the One-Legged Squat and brings the buttocks all the way down to the heel of the foot on the ground. This variety of squats is made to challenge your balance.

The Bulgarian Split Squat. Put the rear leg on a bench, drop straight down, and make sure that the front heel always stays in contact with the ground to avoid any excess stress on the knees. Retain a tall posture throughout the whole exercise. These can work the abs, quads and glutes, as well as the ability to stabilize. Moreover, 3 sets of 6-10 reps do the job to satisfaction.

The Sissy Squat variant uses a pole or other support to hold with one hand, while the body leans backward through the squat until the buttocks are resting on the heels.

Common Variants

     Invisible Chair

     Wall Squat

     Sumo Squat

     One-Legged Squats

     Pistol Squat

     Bulgarian Split Squat

     Sissy Squats

Muscle Groups

     Legs

Good Mornings

The individual starts in a standing position, hands behind the head. The body is bent at the waist and the back is kept straight until the legs and torso form a 90-degree angle.

The torso is returned slowly to the starting position.

Common Variants

Muscle Groups

Glutes

Hamstrings

Lower back

Dirty Dogs

The individual starts in an all-fours position, then lifts one knee off the ground and swings the knee out to the side as far as possible, maintaining the bent knee at a 90-degree angle. The leg is then returned to the starting position and the exercise is then performed with the other leg.

The Mule Kick variant is performed by straightening the leg as it is lifted away from the body as high as possible.

Common Variants

Mule Kick

Muscle Groups

Glutes

Lower back

Hip flexors

Standing Side Leg Lift

The individual stands with their feet hip-width apart. The leg is lifted to the side in a slow, controlled manner until it forms a 45-degree angle with the stationary leg. The leg is then returned to the starting position and the exercise performed on the other side. One hand may be rested on a chair or other stable surface for support.

Common Variants

Muscle Groups

Glutes

Hip flexors

Lower back

Standing Leg Curls

The individual starts with the feet shoulder-width apart. The leg is lifted from the ground, with the knee bent, and the foot curled in toward the buttocks. The leg is returned to the starting position and the exercise performed on the other side. One or two hands may be rested on a chair or other stable surface for support.

Common Variants

    none

Muscle Groups

    Glutes

    Hamstrings

One-Legged Romanian Dead Lifts

The individual starts in a standing position with the feet together. Bending at the waist, one leg is raised in the air while the hand reaches for the floor. The leg is lowered to the starting position and the body returned to the upright position. The leg and back should stay straight at all times during the exercise.

Common Variants

    none

Muscle Groups

    Hamstrings

    Lower back

    Core

Hip Extensions

The individual starts with the back resting on the ground, and the legs bent at 90 degrees with the feet resting on an elevated surface such as a chair. Using only the legs, the hips are pushed up as high as possible, held in contraction for a moment, then lowered to the starting position.

Common Variants

Muscle Groups

> Glutes
>
> Hamstrings
>
> Lower back

King of the Klutz

The individual stands on one leg, body held vertically, closes the eyes, then holds the position for as long as possible. The difficulty may be increased by performing the exercise on a soft or unstable surface.

Common Variants

> none

Muscle Groups

> Calves
>
> Quadriceps
>
> Hamstrings
>
> Hip flexors

Bam Bams

The individual lies in a prone position on a raised, horizontal surface so the legs may project freely beyond the edge of the surface and the toes rest on the ground. The legs are then spread as wide as possible, then raised slowly and brought together until the heels touch. The feet are then returned to the ground. The legs are held as straight as possible throughout the exericse.

Common Variants

> none

Muscle Groups

> Glutes

Ham Sandwich

The individual kneels on the ground, with the feet anchored under a solid surface, or held to the ground by another person. The body is then lowered until the chest is touching the ground. The individual then uses a plyometric movement with the arms to return to the starting position.

Common Variants

Muscle Groups

    Hamstrings

    Pectorals

    Shoulders

Beat Your Boots

The feet are placed together on the ground and the individual bends at the waist to grab the ankles, with the legs kept straight. The knees are then bent until the buttocks touch the ankles. The body is then returned to the starting position.

Common Variants

Muscle Groups

    Hamstrings

    Quadriceps

The Arabesque

The arabesque is a technique that is borrowed from the ballet moves. It works excellently for the butt muscles, and does not even make the use of free weights. However, if you want to add cuffs or ankle weights, you need to follow the following procedure. Place your hands on the back of the chair or on a railing, and lift one leg behind you as high as possible, while holding your glutes and squeezing them for a count of about 4 or 5. Make sure to maintain an upright position so that you do not stress your lower back instead of the glutes.

Common Variants

Muscle Groups

    Hamstrings

    Glutes

The Duck Walk

Duck walks are really good exercises to help shape your butt. The procedure to do this exercise is to assume and hold a squatting position while walking forward for the repetitions and then walk backwards in the same positions for the repetitions. This position might not be very "diva" looking, but is highly effective all the same.

Common Variants

> none

Muscle Groups

> Quadriceps

> Hamstrings

> Glutes

Weight Training

Weight training is a common type of strength training for developing the strength and size of skeletal muscles. It utilizes the force of gravity in the form of weighted bars, dumbbells or weight stacks in order to oppose the force generated by muscle through concentric or eccentric contraction. Weight training uses a variety of specialized equipment to target specific muscle groups and types of movement.

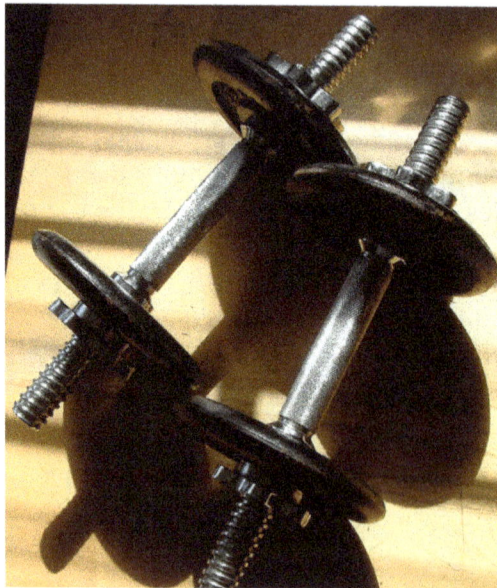

A complete weight training workout can be performed with a pair of adjustable dumbbells and a set of weight disks (plates).

Sports where strength training is central are bodybuilding, weightlifting, powerlifting, and strongman, Highland games, shotput, discus throw, and javelin throw. Many other sports use strength training as part of their training regimen, notably; mixed martial arts, American football, wrestling, rugby football, track and field, rowing, lacrosse, basketball, baseball and hockey. Strength training for other sports and physical activities is becoming increasingly popular.

Weight Training Versus Other Types of Exercise

Strength training is an inclusive term that describes all exercises devoted toward increasing physical strength. Weight training is a type of strength training that uses weights, Eccentric Training or muscular resistance to increase strength. Endurance training is associated with aerobic exercise while flexibility training is associated with stretching exercise like yoga or pilates. *Weight training* is often used as a synonym for strength training, but is actually a specific type within the more inclusive category. Contrary to popular belief, weight training can be beneficial for both men and women.

History

The genealogy of lifting can be traced back to the beginning of history where humanity's fascination with physical abilities can be found among numerous ancient writings. Progressive resistance training dates back at least to Ancient Greece, when legend has it that wrestler Milo of Croton trained by carrying a newborn calf on his back every day until it was fully grown. Another Greek, the physician Galen, described strength training exercises using the halteres (an early form of dumbbell) in the 2nd century.

Ancient Greek sculptures also depict lifting feats. The weights were generally stones, but later gave way to dumbbells. The dumbbell was joined by the barbell in the later half of the 19th century. Early barbells had hollow globes that could be filled with sand or lead shot, but by the end of the century these were replaced by the plate-loading barbell commonly used today.

Another early device was the Indian club, which came from ancient Persia where it was called the "meels". It subsequently became popular during the 19th century, and has recently made a comeback in the form of the clubbell.

The 1960s saw the gradual introduction of exercise machines into the still-rare strength training gyms of the time. Weight training became increasingly popular in the 1970s, following the release of the bodybuilding movie *Pumping Iron,* and the subsequent popularity of Arnold Schwarzenegger. Since the late 1990s increasing numbers of women have taken up weight training, influenced by programs like Body for Life; currently nearly one in five U.S. women engage in weight training on a regular basis.

Basic Principles

The basic principles of weight training are essentially identical to those of strength training, and involve a manipulation of the number of repetitions (reps), sets, tempo, exercise types, and weight moved to cause desired increases in strength, endurance, and size. The specific combinations of reps, sets, exercises, and weights depends on the aims of the individual performing the exercise. Sets with fewer reps can be performed with heavier weights contributing to an increase in lean muscle mass and sets with higher reps can be performed with lighter weights contributing to increased muscular endurance.

In addition to the basic principles of *strength training*, a further consideration added by weight training is the equipment used. Types of equipment include barbells, dumbbells, pulleys and stacks in the form of weight machines, and the body's own weight in the case of chin-ups and push-ups. Different types of weights will give different types of resistance, and often the same absolute weight can have different relative weights depending on the type of equipment used. For example, lifting 10 kilograms using a dumbbell sometimes requires more force than moving 10 kilograms on a weight stack if certain pulley arrangements are used. In other cases, the weight stack may require more force than the equivalent dumbbell weight due to additional torque or resistance in the machine. Additionally, although they may display the same weight stack, different machines may be heavier or lighter depending on the number of pulleys and their arrangements.

Weight training also requires the use of 'good form', performing the movements with the appropriate muscle group, and not transferring the weight to different body parts in order to move greater weight (called 'cheating'). Failure to use good form during a training set can result in injury or a failure to meet training goals; since the desired muscle group is not challenged sufficiently, the threshold of overload is never reached and the muscle does not gain in strength. At a particularly advanced level; however, "cheating" can be used to break through strength plateaus and encourage neurological and muscular adaptation.

Comparison to Other Types of Strength Training

The benefits of weight training overall are comparable to most other types of strength training: increased muscle, tendon and ligament strength, bone density, flexibility, tone, metabolic rate, and postural support. There are benefits and limitations to weight training as compared to other types of strength training. Jumping and rotation with a barbell on shoulders, shown on the right animation, is one of the illustrations.

Weight Training Versus Isometric Training

Isometric exercise provides a maximum amount of resistance based on the force output of the muscle, or muscles pitted against one another. This maximum force maximally strengthens the muscles over all of the joint angles at which the isometric exercise occurs. By comparison, weight training also strengthens the muscle throughout the range of motion the joint is trained in, but only maximally at one angle, causing a lesser increase in physical strength at other angles from the initial through terminating joint angle as compared with isometric exercise. In addition, the risk of injury from weights used in weight training is greater than with isometric exercise (no weights), and the risk of asymmetric training is also greater than with isometric exercise of identical opposing muscles.

Weight Training and Bodybuilding

Although weight training is similar to bodybuilding, they have different objectives. Bodybuilders use weight training to develop their muscles for size, shape, and symmetry regardless of any increase in strength for competition in bodybuilding contests; they train to maximize their muscular size and develop extremely low levels of body fat. In contrast, many weight trainers train to improve their strength and anaerobic endurance while not giving special attention to reducing body fat far below normal.

The bodybuilding community has been the source of many of weight training's principles, techniques, vocabulary, and customs. Weight training does allow tremendous flexibility in exercises and weights which can allow bodybuilders to target specific muscles and muscle groups, as well as attain specific goals. Not all bodybuilding is undertaken to compete in bodybuilding contests and, in fact, the vast majority of bodybuilders never compete, but bodybuild for their own personal reasons.

Safety

Weight training is a safe form of exercise when the movements are controlled and carefully defined. However, as with any form of exercise, improper execution and the failure to take appropriate precautions can result in injury.

Maintaining Proper Form

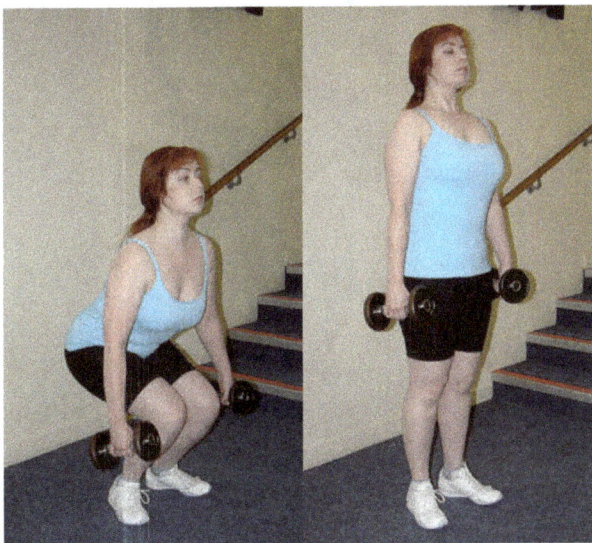

A dumbbell half-squat.

Maintaining proper form is one of the many steps in order to perfectly perform a certain technique. Correct form in weight training improves strength, muscle tone, and maintaining a healthy weight. Proper form will prevent any strains or fractures. When the exercise becomes difficult towards the end of a set, there is a temptation to cheat, i.e., to use poor form to recruit other muscle groups to assist the effort. Avoid heavy weight and keep the number of repetitions to a minimum. This may shift the effort to weaker muscles that cannot handle the weight. For example, the *squat* and the *deadlift* are used to exercise the largest muscles in the body—the leg and buttock muscles—so they require substantial weight. Beginners are tempted to round their back while performing these exercises. The relaxation of the spinal erectors which allows the lower back to round can cause shearing in the vertebrae of the lumbar spine, potentially damaging the spinal discs.

Stretching and Warm-Up

Weight trainers commonly spend 5 to 20 minutes warming up their muscles before starting a workout. It is common to stretch the entire body to increase overall flexibility; however, many people stretch just the area being worked that day. The main reason for warming up is injury prevention. Warming up increases blood flow and flexibility, which lessens the chance of a muscle pull or joint pain.

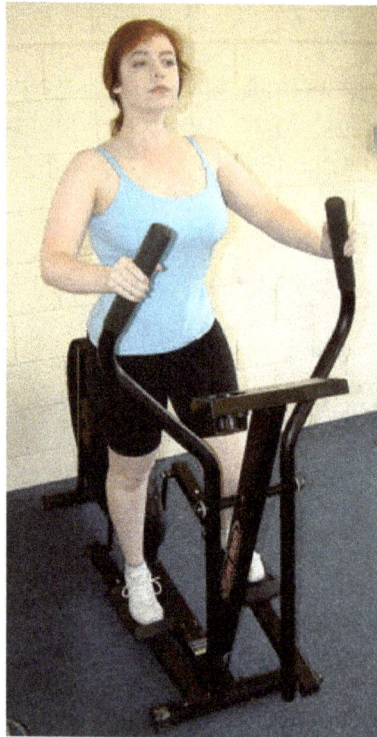

The cross trainer can be used to warm up muscles in both the upper and lower body.

Warm up sets are also important. For example, the same lifter working on his chest would also be advised to complete at least two warm up sets prior to hitting his "core tonnage." Core tonnage refers to the heavier lifts that actually strain your muscles. For example, if the lifter's main sets were at 205 lbs, 225 lbs and 235 lbs on the bench, then a warmup of 5 reps of 135 and 5 reps of 185 would be advisable. When properly warmed up the lifter will then have more strength and stamina since the blood has begun to flow to the muscle groups.

Breathing

Breathing shallowly or holding one's breath while working out limits the oxygen supply to the muscles and the brain, decreasing performance and, under extreme stress, risking a black-out or a stroke by aneurysm. Most trainers advise weight trainees to consciously "exhale on effort" and to inhale when lowering the weight. This technique ensures that the trainee breathes through the most difficult part of the exercise, where one would reflexively hold one's breath.

However, biomechanics and kinesiology expert Stuart McGill indicates that spine stabilization is assured by "the ability to cocontract the abdominal wall (abdominal brace) independently of any lung ventilation patterns. Good stabilizers maintain the critical symmetrical muscle stiffness...Poor stabilizers allow abdominal contraction levels to cycle with breathing at critical moments when stability is required. Grooving muscular activation patterns so that a particular direction in lung air flow is entrained to a particular part of any exertion is not helpful. This would be of little carryover value to other activities; in fact it would be counterproductive."

Other coaches advise trainees to perform the valsalva maneuver during exercises which place a load on the spine, since the risk of a stroke by aneurysm is astronomically lower than the risk of an orthopedic injury caused by inadequate rigidity of the torso. Stuart McGill adds that the mechanism of building "high levels of intra-abdominal pressure (IAP)...produced by breath holding using the Valsava maneuver", to "ensure spine stiffness and stability during these extraordinary demands", "should be considered only for extreme weight-lifting challenges — not for rehabilitation exercise".

Hydration

As with other sports, weight trainers should avoid dehydration throughout the workout by drinking sufficient water. This is particularly true in hot environments, or for those older than 65.

Some athletic trainers advise athletes to drink about 7 imperial fluid ounces (200 mL) every 15 minutes while exercising, and about 80 imperial fluid ounces (2.3 L) throughout the day.

However, a much more accurate determination of how much fluid is necessary can be made by performing appropriate weight measurements before and after a typical exercise session, to determine how much fluid is lost during the workout. The greatest source of fluid loss during exercise is through perspiration, but as long as your fluid intake is roughly equivalent to your rate of perspiration, hydration levels will be maintained.

Under most circumstances, sports drinks do not offer a physiological benefit over water during weight training. However, high-intensity exercise for a continuous duration of at least one hour may require the replenishment of electrolytes which a sports drink may provide. Some may maintain that energy drinks, such as Red Bull that contain caffeine, improve performance in weight training and other physical exercise, but in fact, these energy drinks can cause dehydration, tremors, heat stroke, and heart attack when consumed in excess. 'Sports drinks' that contain simple carbohydrates & water do not cause ill effects, but are most likely unnecessary for the average trainee.

Insufficient hydration may cause lethargy, soreness or muscle cramps. The urine of well-hydrated persons should be nearly colorless, while an intense yellow color is normally a sign of insufficient hydration.

Avoiding Pain

An exercise should be halted if marked or sudden pain is felt, to prevent further injury. However, not all discomfort indicates injury. Weight training exercises are brief but very intense, and many people are unaccustomed to this level of effort. The expression "no pain, no gain" refers to working through the discomfort expected from such vigorous effort, rather than to willfully ignore extreme pain, which may indicate serious soft tissue injuries.

Discomfort can arise from other factors. Individuals who perform large numbers of repetitions, sets, and exercises for each muscle group may experience a burning sensation in their muscles. These individuals may also experience a swelling sensation in their muscles from increased blood flow (the "pump"). True muscle fatigue is experienced as a marked and uncontrollable loss of strength in a muscle, arising from the nervous system (motor unit) rather than from the muscle fibers themselves. Extreme neural fatigue can be experienced as temporary muscle failure. Some weight training programs, such as Metabolic Resistance Training, actively seek temporary muscle failure; evidence to support this type of training is mixed at best. Irrespective of their program, however, most athletes engaged in high-intensity weight training will experience muscle failure during their regimens.

Beginners are advised to build up slowly to a weight training program. Untrained individuals may have some muscles that are comparatively stronger than others. An injury can result if, in a particular exercise, the primary muscle is stronger than its stabilising muscles. Building up slowly allows muscles time to develop appropriate strengths relative to each other. This can also help to minimize delayed onset muscle soreness. A sudden start to an intense program can cause significant muscular soreness. Unexercised muscles contain cross-linkages that are torn during intense exercise.

Other Precautions

Anyone beginning an intensive physical training program is typically advised to consult a physician, because of possible undetected heart or other conditions for which such activity is contraindicated.

Exercises like the bench press or the squat in which a failed lift can potentially result in the lifter becoming trapped under the weight are normally performed inside a power rack or in the presence of one or more spotters, who can safely re-rack the barbell if the weight trainer is unable to do so.

Equipment

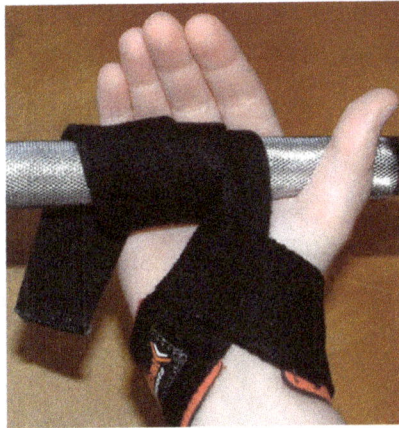

A lifting strap.

Weight training usually requires different types of equipment, most commonly dumbbells, barbells, and weight machines. Various combinations of specific exercises, machines, dumbbells, and barbells allow trainees to exercise body parts in numerous ways.

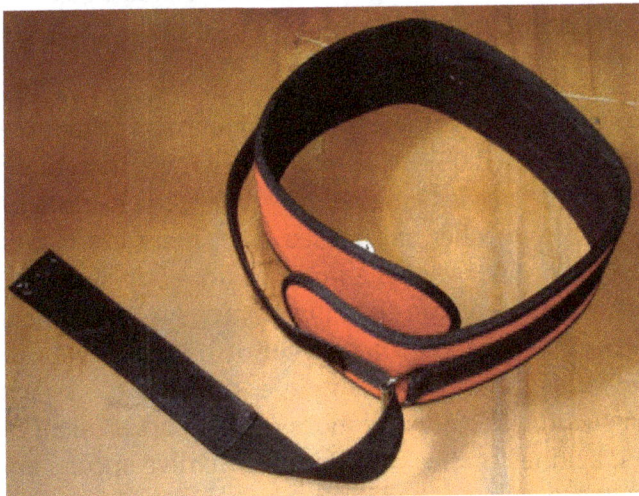

A lifting belt.

Other types of equipment include:

- Lifting straps, which allow more weight to be lifted by transferring the load to the wrists and avoiding limitations in forearm muscles and grip strength

- Weightlifting belts, which are meant to brace the core through intra-abdominal pressure. Controversy exists regarding the safety of these devices and their proper use is often misunderstood.

- Weighted clothing, bags of sand, lead shot, or other materials that are strapped to wrists, ankles, torso or other body parts to increase the amount of work required by muscles

- Gloves can improve grip, prevent the formation of calluses on the hands, relieve pressure on the wrists, and provide support.

- Chalk, which dries out sweaty hands, improving grip

- Wrist and knee wraps

- Shoes, which have a flat, rigid sole to provide a sturdy base of support, and may feature a raised heel of varying height (usually 0.5" or 0.75") to accommodate a lifter's biomechanics for more efficient squats, deadlifts, overhead presses, and Olympic lifts.

Types of Exercises

Isotonic and Plyometric Exercises

These terms combine the prefix "iso" (meaning "same") with "tonic" (strength) and "plio" (more) with "metric" (distance). In "isotonic" exercises the force applied to the muscle does not change (while the length of the muscle decreases or increases) while in "plyometric" exercises the length of the muscle stretches and contracts rapidly to increase the power output of a muscle.

Weight training is primarily an isotonic form of exercise, as the force produced by the muscle to push or pull weighted objects should not change (though in practice the force produced does decrease as muscles fatigue). Any object can be used for weight training, but dumbbells, barbells, and other specialised equipment are normally used because they can be adjusted to specific weights and are easily gripped. Many exercises are not strictly isotonic because the force on the muscle varies as the joint moves through its range of motion. Movements can become easier or harder depending on the angle of muscular force relative to gravity; for example, a standard biceps curl becomes easier as the hand approaches the shoulder as more of the load is taken by the structure of the elbow. Certain machines such as the Nautilus involve special adaptations to keep resistance constant irrespective of the joint angle.

Plyometrics exploit the stretch-shortening cycle of muscles to enhance the myotatic (stretch) reflex. This involves rapid alternation of lengthening and shortening of muscle fibers against resistance. The resistance involved is often a weighted object such as a medicine ball or sandbag, but can also be the body itself as in jumping exercises or the body with a weight vest that allows movement with resistance. Plyometrics is used to develop explosive speed, and focuses on maximal power instead of maximal strength by compressing the force of muscular contraction into as short a period as possible, and may be used to improve the effectiveness of a boxer's punch, or to increase the vertical jumping ability of a basketball player. Care must be taken when performing plyometric exercises because they inflict greater stress upon the involved joints and tendons than other forms of exercise.

Isolation Exercises Versus Compound Exercises

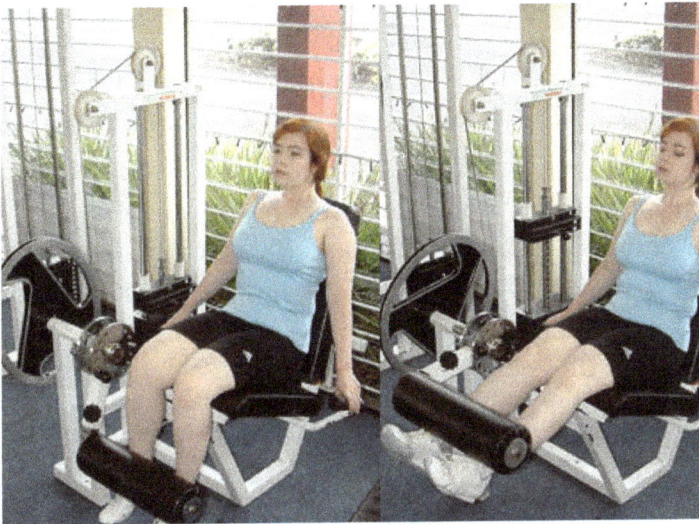

The *leg extension* is an isolation exercise.

An isolation exercise is one where the movement is restricted to one joint only. For example, the *leg extension* is an isolation exercise for the quadriceps. Specialized types of equipment are used to ensure that other muscle groups are only minimally involved—they just help the individual maintain a stable posture—and movement occurs only around the knee joint. Most isolation exercises involve machines rather than dumbbells and barbells (free weights), though free weights can be used when combined with special positions and joint bracing.

Compound exercises work several muscle groups at once, and include movement around two or more joints. For example, in the leg press, movement occurs around the hip, knee and ankle joints. This exercise is primarily used to develop the quadriceps, but it also involves the hamstrings, glutes and calves. Compound exercises are generally similar to the ways that people naturally push, pull and lift objects, whereas isolation exercises often feel a little unnatural.

Each type of exercise has its uses. Compound exercises build the basic strength that is needed to perform everyday pushing, pulling and lifting activities. Isolation exercises are useful for "rounding out" a routine, by directly exercising muscle groups that cannot be fully exercised in the compound exercises. Compound exercises are also very useful in promoting the production of testosterone.

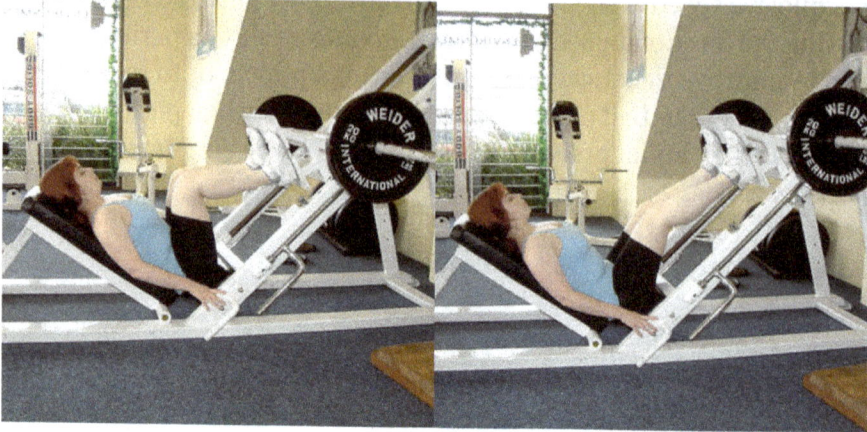

The leg press is a compound exercise.

The type of exercise performed also depends on the individual's goals. Those who seek to increase their performance in sports would focus mostly on compound exercises, with isolation exercises being used to strengthen just those muscles that are holding the athlete back. Similarly, a powerlifter would focus on the specific compound exercises that are performed at powerlifting competitions. However, those who seek to improve the look of their body without necessarily maximizing their strength gains (including bodybuilders) would put more of an emphasis on isolation exercises. Both types of athletes, however, generally make use of both compound and isolation exercises.

Free Weights Versus Weight Machines

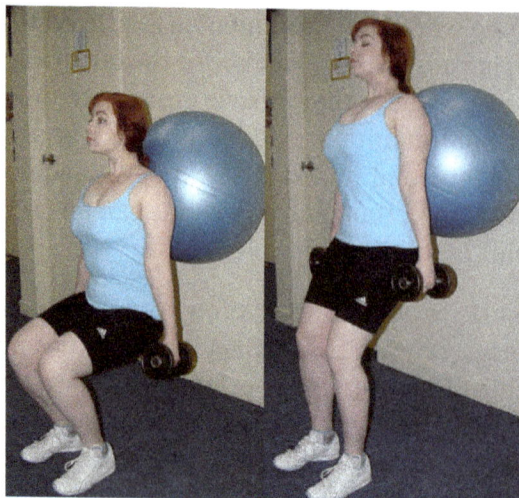

Exercise balls allow a wider range of free weight exercises to be performed. They are also known as Swiss balls, stability balls, fitness balls, gym balls, sports balls, therapy balls or body balls. They are sometimes confused with medicine balls

Free weights include dumbbells, barbells, medicine balls, sandbells, and kettlebells. Unlike weight machines, they do not constrain users to specific, fixed movements, and therefore require more effort from the individual's stabilizer muscles. It is often argued that free weight exercises are superior for precisely this reason. For example, they are recommended for golf players, since golf is a unilateral exercise that can break body balances, requiring exercises to keep the balance in muscles.

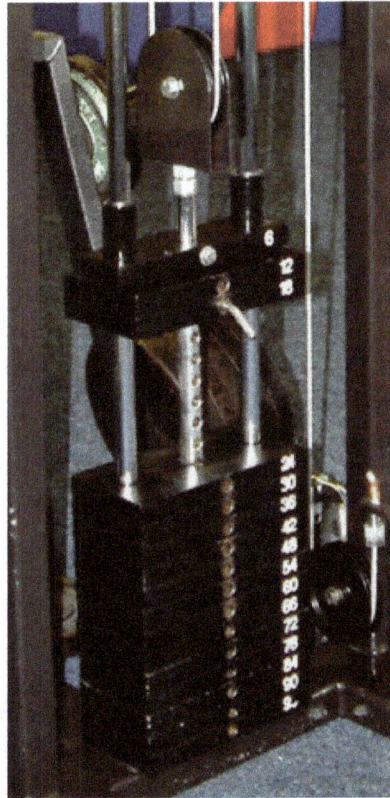

The weight stack from a Cable machine.

Some free weight exercises can be performed while sitting or lying on an exercise ball. This makes it extremely difficult to maintain proper form, thus preventing the use of heavier weight, severely limiting any long-term gains in strength.

There are a number of weight machines that are commonly found in neighborhood gyms. The Smith machine is a barbell that is constrained to vertical movement. The cable machine consists of two weight stacks separated by 2.5 metres, with cables running through adjustable pulleys (that can be fixed at any height) to various types of handles. There are also exercise-specific weight machines such as the leg press. A multigym includes a variety of exercise-specific mechanisms in one apparatus.

One limitation of many free weight exercises and exercise machines is that the muscle is working maximally against gravity during only a small portion of the lift. Some exercise-specific machines feature an oval cam (first introduced by Nautilus) which varies the resistance, so that the resistance, and the muscle force required, remains constant throughout the full range of motion of the exercise.

Push-Pull Workout

A push–pull workout is a method of arranging a weight training routine so that exercises alternate between push motions and pull motions. A push–pull superset is two complementary segments (one pull/one push) done back-to-back. An example is bench press (push) / bent-over row (pull). Another push–pull technique is to arrange workout routines so that one day involves only push (usually chest, shoulders and triceps) exercises, and an alternate day only pull (usually back and biceps) exercises.

Health Benefits

Benefits of weight training include increased strength, muscle mass, endurance, bone and bone mineral density, insulin sensitivity, GLUT 4 density, HDL cholesterol, improved cardiovascular health and appearance, and decreased body fat, blood pressure, LDL cholesterol and triglycerides.

The body's basal metabolic rate increases with increases in muscle mass, which promotes long-term fat loss and helps dieters avoid yo-yo dieting. Moreover, intense workouts elevate metabolism for several hours following the workout, which also promotes fat loss.

Weight training also provides functional benefits. Stronger muscles improve posture, provide better support for joints, and reduce the risk of injury from everyday activities. Older people who take up weight training can prevent some of the loss of muscle tissue that normally accompanies aging—and even regain some functional strength—and by doing so become less frail. They may be able to avoid some types of physical disability. Weight-bearing exercise also helps to prevent osteoporosis. The benefits of weight training for older people have been confirmed by studies of people who began engaging in it even in their 80s and 90s.

For many people in rehabilitation or with an acquired disability, such as following stroke or orthopaedic surgery, strength training for weak muscles is a key factor to optimise recovery. For people with such a health condition, their strength training is likely to need to be designed by an appropriate health professional, such as a physiotherapist.

Stronger muscles improve performance in a variety of sports. Sport-specific training routines are used by many competitors. These often specify that the speed of muscle contraction during weight training should be the same as that of the particular sport.

Sport-specific training routines also often include variations to both free weight and machine movements that may not be common for traditional weightlifting.

Though weight training can stimulate the cardiovascular system, many exercise physiologists, based on their observation of maximal oxygen uptake, argue that aerobics training is a better cardiovascular stimulus. Central catheter monitoring during resistance training reveals increased cardiac output, suggesting that strength training shows potential for cardiovascular exercise. However, a 2007 meta-analysis found that, though aerobic training is an effective therapy for heart failure patients, combined aerobic and strength training is ineffective; "the favorable antiremodeling role of aerobic exercise was not confirmed when this mode of exercise was combined with strength training".

One side-effect of any intense exercise is increased levels of dopamine, serotonin and norepinephrine, which can help to improve mood and counter feelings of depression.

Weight training has also been shown to benefit dieters as it inhibits lean body mass loss (as opposed to fat loss) when under a caloric deficit. Weight training also strengthens bones, helping to prevent bone loss and osteoporosis. By increasing muscular strength and improving balance, weight training can also reduce falls by elderly persons.

Anaerobic Exercise

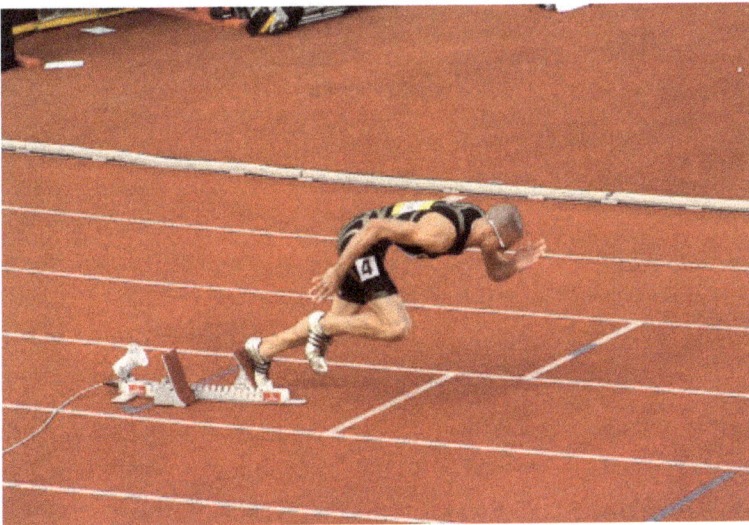

Anaerobic exercise

Anaerobic exercise is a physical exercise intense enough to cause lactate to form. It is used by athletes in non-endurance sports to promote strength, speed and power and by body builders to build muscle mass. Muscle energy systems trained using anaerobic exercise develop differently compared to aerobic exercise, leading to greater performance in short duration, high intensity activities, which last from mere seconds to up to about 2 minutes. Any activity lasting longer than about two minutes has a large aerobic metabolic component.

Metabolism

Anaerobic metabolism, or anaerobic energy expenditure, is a natural part of whole-body metabolic energy expenditure. Fast twitch muscle (as compared to slow twitch muscle) operates using anaerobic metabolic systems, such that any recruitment of fast twitch muscle fibers leads to increased anaerobic energy expenditure. Intense exercise lasting upwards of about four minutes (e.g., a mile race) may still have a considerable anaerobic energy expenditure component. High-intensity interval training, although based on aerobic exercises like running, cycling and rowing, effectively becomes anaerobic when performed in excess of 90% maximum heart rate. Anaerobic energy expenditure is difficult to accurately quantify, although several reasonable methods to estimate the anaerobic component to exercise are available.

EXERCISE ZONES										
	AGE									
BEATS PER MINUTE	20	25	30	35	40	45	50	55	65	70
100%	200	195	190	185	180	175	170	165	155	150
90% VO₂ Max (Maximum effort)	180	176	171	167	162	158	153	149	140	135
80% Anaerobic (Hardcore training)	160	156	152	148	144	140	136	132	124	126
70% Aerobix (Cardio training / Endurance)	140	137	133	130	126	123	119	116	109	105
60% Weight control (Fitness / Fat burn)	120	117	114	111	108	105	102	99	93	90
50% Moderate activity (Maintenance / Warm up)	100	98	95	93	90	88	85	83	78	75

Fox and Haskell formula

In contrast, aerobic exercise includes lower intensity activities performed for longer periods of time. Activities such as walking, long slow runs, rowing, and cycling require a great deal of oxygen to generate the energy needed for prolonged exercise (i.e., aerobic energy expenditure). In sports which require repeated short bursts of exercise however, the anaerobic system enables muscles to recover for the next burst. Therefore training for many sports demands that both energy producing systems be developed.

The two types of anaerobic energy systems are: 1) high energy phosphates, adenosine triphosphate and creatine phosphate; and 2) anaerobic glycolysis. The former is called *alactic anaerobic* and the latter *lactic anaerobic* system. High energy phosphates are stored in limited quantities within muscle cells. Anaerobic glycolysis exclusively uses glucose (and glycogen) as a fuel in the absence of oxygen, or more specifically when ATP is needed at rates that exceed those provided by aerobic metabolism. The consequence of such rapid glucose breakdown is the formation of lactic acid (or more appropriately, its conjugate base lactate at biological pH levels). Physical activities that last up to about thirty seconds rely primarily on the former, ATP-CP phosphagen system. Beyond this time both aerobic and anaerobic glycolysis-based metabolic systems begin to predominate.

The by-product of anaerobic glycolysis, lactate, has traditionally been thought to be detrimental to muscle function. However, this appears likely only when lactate levels are very high. Elevated lactate levels are only one of many changes that occur within and around muscle cells during intense exercise that can lead to fatigue. Fatigue, that is muscle failure, is a complex subject. Elevated muscle and blood lactate concentrations are a natural consequence of any physical exertion. The effectiveness of anaerobic activity can be improved through training.

Physical Fitness

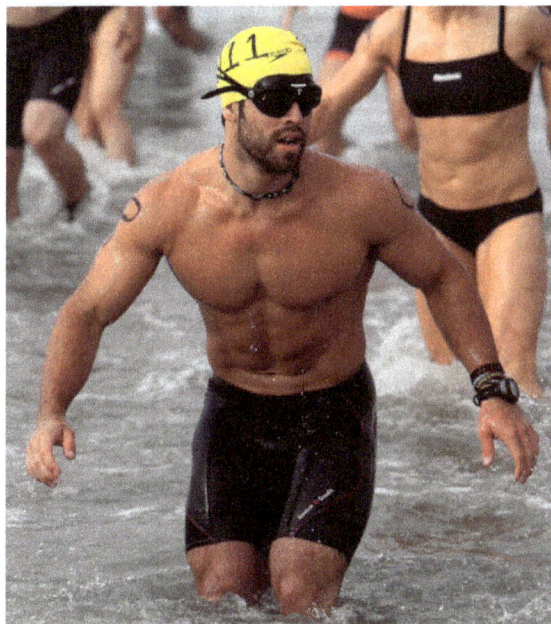

Physical fitness can be achieved through exercise.
Photo shows Rich Froning Jr. – four-time winner of "Fittest Man on Earth" title.

Physical fitness is a general state of health and well-being and, more specifically, the ability to perform aspects of sports, occupations and daily activities. Physical fitness is generally achieved through proper nutrition, moderate-vigorous physical exercise, and sufficient rest.

Before the industrial revolution, *fitness* was defined as the capacity to carry out the day's activities without undue fatigue. However, with automation and changes in lifestyles *physical fitness* is now considered a measure of the body's ability to function efficiently and effectively in work and leisure activities, to be healthy, to resist hypokinetic diseases, and to meet emergency situations.

Fitness

Fitness is defined as the quality or state of being fit. Around 1950, perhaps consistent with the Industrial Revolution and the treatise of World War II, the term "fitness" increased in western vernacular by a factor of ten. Modern definition of fitness describe either a person or machine's ability to perform a specific function or a holistic definition of human adaptability to cope with various situations. This has led to an interrelation of human fitness and attractiveness which has mobilized global fitness and fitness equipment industries. Regarding specific function, fitness is attributed to personnel who possess significant aerobic or anaerobic ability, i.e. strength or endurance. A holistic definition of fitness is described by Greg Glassman in the CrossFit journal as an increased work capacity across broad times and modal domains; mastery of several attributes of fitness including strength, endurance, power, speed, balance and coordination and being able to improve the amount of work done in a given time with any of these domains. A well rounded fitness program will improve a person in all aspects of fitness, rather than one, such as only cardio/respiratory endurance or only weight training.

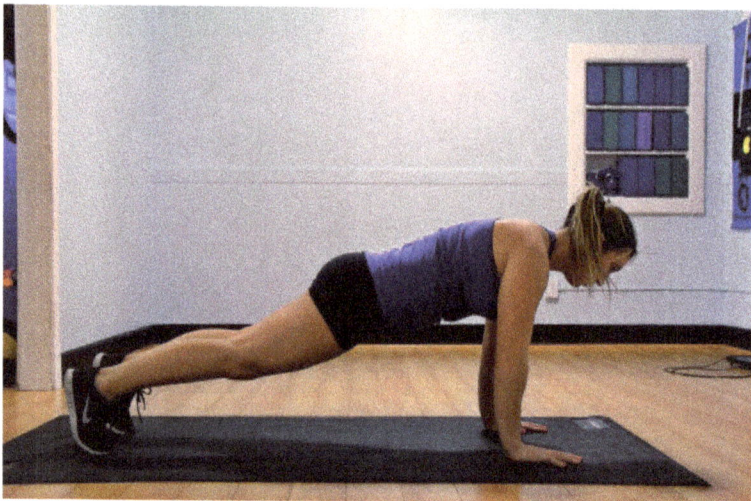

A woman performs plank exercise for strengthening of muscles

A comprehensive fitness program tailored to an individual typically focuses on one or more specific skills, and on age- or health-related needs such as bone health. Many sources also cite mental, social and emotional health as an important part of overall fitness. This is often presented in textbooks as a triangle made up of three points, which represent physical, emotional, and mental fitness. Physical fitness can also prevent or treat many chronic health conditions brought on by unhealthy lifestyle or aging. Working out can also help some people sleep better and possibly alleviate some mood disorders in certain individuals.

Developing research has demonstrated that many of the benefits of exercise are mediated through the role of skeletal muscle as an endocrine organ. That is, contracting muscles release multiple substances known as myokines which promote the growth of new tissue, tissue repair, and various anti-inflammatory functions, which in turn reduce the risk of developing various inflammatory diseases.

Activity Guidelines

The Physical Activity Guidelines for Americans was created by the Office of Disease Prevention and Health Promotion. This publication suggests that all adults should avoid inactivity to promote good health mentally and physically. For substantial health benefits, adults should participate in at least 150 minutes (two hours and 30 minutes) a week of moderate-intensity, or 75 minutes (1 hour and 15 minutes) a week of vigorous-intensity aerobic physical activity, or an equivalent combination of moderate- and vigorous-intensity aerobic activity. Aerobic activity should be performed in episodes of at least 10 minutes, and preferably, it should be spread throughout the week. For additional and more extensive health benefits, adults should increase their aerobic physical activity to 300 minutes (5 hours) a week of moderate-intensity, or 150 minutes a week of vigorous-intensity aerobic physical activity, or an equivalent combination of moderate- and vigorous-intensity activity. Additional health benefits are gained by engaging in physical activity beyond this amount. Adults should also do muscle-strengthening activities that are moderate or high intensity and involve all major muscle groups on 2 or more days a week, as these activities provide additional health benefits.

Training

Specific or task-oriented fitness is a person's ability to perform in a specific activity with a reasonable efficiency: for example, sports or military service. Specific training prepares athletes to perform well in their sports.

Examples are:

- 100 m sprint: in a sprint the athlete must be trained to work anaerobically throughout the race, an example of how to do this would be interval training.

- Middle distance running: athletes require both speed and endurance to gain benefit out of this training. The hard working muscles are at their peak for a longer period of time as they are being used at that level for longer period of time.

- Marathon: in this case the athlete must be trained to work aerobically and their endurance must be built-up to a maximum.

- Many fire fighters and police officers undergo regular fitness testing to determine if they are capable of the physically demanding tasks required of the job.

- Members of armed forces will often be required to pass a formal fitness test – for example soldiers of the US Army must be able to pass the Army Physical Fitness Test (APFT).

- Hill sprints: requires a level of fitness to begin with, the exercise is particularly good for the leg muscles. The army often trains doing mountain climbing and races.

- Plyometric and Isometric Exercises: An excellent way to build strength and increase muscular endurance.

- Sand running creates less strain on leg muscles than running on grass or concrete. This is because sand collapses beneath the foot softening the landing. Sand training is an effective way to lose weight and become fit as its proven you need more effort (one and a half times more) to run on the soft sand than on a hard surface.

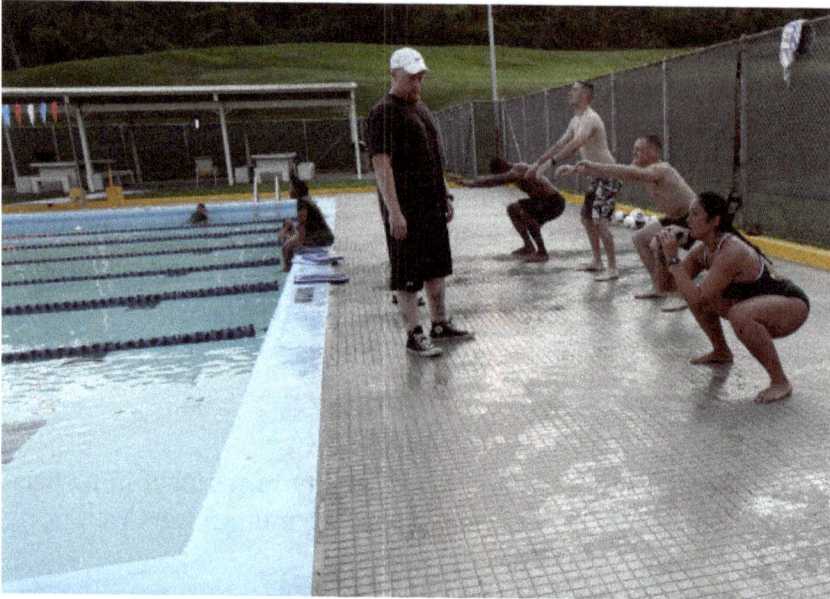

Swimmers perform squats prior to entering the pool in a U.S. military base, 2011

- Aquajogging is a form of exercise that decreases strain on joints and bones. The water supplies minimal impact to muscles and bones which is good for those recovering from injury. Furthermore, the resistance of the water as one jogs through it provides an enhanced effect of exercise (the deeper you are the greater the force needed to pull your leg through).

- Swimming: Squatting exercise helps in enhancing a swimmer's start.

In order for physical fitness to benefit the health of an individual, an unknown response in the person called a stimulus will be triggered by the exertion. When exercise is performed with the correct amount of intensity, duration and frequency, a significant amount of improvement can occur. The person may overall feel better but the physical effects on the human body take weeks or months to notice and possibly years for full development. For training purposes, exercise must provide a stress or demand on either a function or tissue. To continue improvements, this demand must eventually increase little over an extended period of time. This sort of exercise training has three basic principles: overload, specificity, and progression. These principles are related to health but also enhancement of physical working capacity.

High Intensity Interval Training (HIIT)

High Intensity Interval Training consists of repeated, short bursts of exercise, completed at a high level of intensity. These sets of intense activity are followed by a predetermined time of rest or low intensity activity. Studies have shown that exercising at a higher intensity has increased cardiac benefits for humans, compared to when exercising at a low or moderate level. When your workout consists of an HIIT session, your body has to work harder to replace the oxygen it lost. Research into the benefits of HIIT have revealed that it can be very successful for reducing fat, especially around the abdominal region. Furthermore, when compared to continuous moderate exercise, HIIT proves to burn more calories and increase the amount of fat burned post- HIIT session. Lack of time is one of the main reasons stated for not exercising; HIIT is a great alternative for those people because the duration of an HIIT session can be as short as 10 minutes, making it much quicker than conventional workouts.

Aerobic Exercise

Cardiorespiratory fitness can be measured using VO2 max, a measure of the amount of oxygen the body can uptake and utilize. Aerobic exercise, which improves cardiorespiratory fitness, involves movement that increases the heart rate to improve the body's oxygen consumption. This form of exercise is an important part of all training regiments ranging from professional athletes to the everyday person. Also, it helps increase stamina.

Examples are:

- Jogging – Running at a steady and gentle pace. This form of exercise is great for maintaining weight.

- Elliptical Training – This is a stationary exercise machine used to perform walking, or running without causing excessive stress on the joints. This form of exercise is perfect for people with achy hips, knees and ankles.

- Walking – Moving at a fairly regular pace for a short, medium or long distance.

- Treadmill training – Many treadmills have programs set up that offers a numerous amount of different workout plans. One effective cardiovascular activity would be to switch between running and walking. Typically warm up first by walking and then switch off between walking for three minutes and running for three minutes.

- Swimming – Using the arms and legs to keep oneself afloat and moving either forwards or backwards. This is a good full body exercise for those who are looking to strengthen their core while improving cardiovascular endurance.

- Cycling – Riding a bicycle typically involves longer distances than walking or jogging. This is another low stress exercise on the joints and is great for improving leg strength.

Effects

Controlling Blood Pressure

Physical fitness has proven to result in positive effects on the body's blood pressure because staying active and exercising regularly builds up a stronger heart. The heart is the main organ in charge of systolic blood pressure and diastolic blood pressure. Engaging in a physical activity will create a rise in blood pressure, once the activity is stopped, however, the individual's blood pressure will return to normal. The more physical activity that one engages in, the easier this process becomes, resulting in a more 'fit' individual. Through regular physical fitness, the heart does not have to work as hard to create a rise in blood pressure, which lowers the force on the arteries, and lowers the over all blood pressure.

Cancer Prevention

Centers for disease control and prevention provide lifestyle guidelines of maintaining a balanced diet and engaging in physical activity to reduce the risk of disease. The WCRF/ American Institute for Cancer Research (AICR) published a list of recommendations that reflect the evidence they have found through consistency in fitness and dietary factors that directly relate to Cancer prevention.

The WCRF/AICR recommendations include the following:

- "Be as lean as possible without becoming underweight

- Each week, adults should engage in at least 150 minutes of moderate intensity physical activity or 75 minutes of vigorous intensity physical activity

- Children should engage in at least one hour of moderate or vigorous physical activity each week

- Be physically active for at least thirty minutes every day

- Avoid sugar, limit the consumption of energy packed foods

- Balance your diet with a variety of vegetables, grains, fruits, legumes, etc.

- Limit sodium intake, the consumption of red meats and the consumption of processed meats

- Limit alcoholic drinks to two for men and one for women a day"

These recommendations are also widely supported by the American Cancer Society. The guidelines have been evaluated and individuals that have higher guideline adherence scores substantially reduce cancer risk as well as help towards control with a multitude of chronic health problems. Regular physical activity is a factor that helps reduce an individual's blood pressure and improves cholesterol levels, two key components that correlate with heart disease and Type 2 Diabetes. The American Cancer Society encourages the public to "adopt a physically active lifestyle" by meeting the criteria in a variety of physical activities such as hiking, swimming, circuit training, resistance raining, lifting, etc. It is understood that cancer is not a disease that can be cured by physical fitness alone, however because it is a multifactorial disease, physical fitness is a controllable prevention. The large associations tied with being physically fit and reduced cancer risk are enough to provide a strategy to reduce cancer risk. The American Cancer Society assorts different levels of activity ranging from moderate to vigorous to clarify the recommended time spent on a physical activity. These classifications of physical activity consider the intentional exercise and basic activities done on a daily basis and give the public a greater understanding by what fitness levels suffice as future disease prevention.

Inflammation

Studies have shown an association between increased physical activity and reduced inflammation. It produces both a short-term inflammatory response and a long-term anti-inflammatory effect. Physical activity reduces inflammation in conjunction with or independent of changes in body weight. However, the mechanisms linking physical activity to inflammation are unknown.

Immune System

Physical activity boosts the immune system. This is dependent on the concentration of endogenous factors (such as sex hormones, metabolic hormones and growth hormones), body temperature, blood flow, hydration status and body position. Physical activity has shown to increase the levels of natural killer (NK) cells, NK T cells, macrophages, neutrophils and eosinophils, complements, cytokines, antibodies and T cytotoxic cells. However, the mechanism linking physical activity to immune system is not fully understood.

Cardiovascular Disease Prevention

Physical activity affects one's blood pressure, cholesterol levels, blood lipid levels, blood clotting factors and the strength of blood vessels. All factors that directly correlate to cardiovascular disease. It also improves the body's use of insulin. People who are at risk for diabetes, Type 2 (insulin resistant) especially, benefit greatly from physical activity because it activates a better usage of insulin and protects the heart. Those who develop diabetes have an increased risk of developing cardiovascular disease. In a study where a sample of around ten thousand adults from the Third National Health and Nutrition Examination Survey, physical activity and metabolic risk factors such as insulin resistance, inflammation, dyslipidemia were assessed. The study adjusted basic confounders with moderate/vigorous physical activity and the relation with CVD mortality. The results displayed physical activity being associated with a lower risk of CVD mortality that was independent of traditional metabolic risk factors.

The American Heart Association recommendations include the same findings as provided in the WCRF/ AICR recommendations list for people who are healthy. In regards to people with lower blood pressure or cholesterol, the association recommends that these individuals aim for around forty minutes of moderate to vigorous physical activity around three or four times a week.

Weight Control

Achieving resilience through physical fitness promotes a vast and complex range of health related benefits. Individuals who keep up physical fitness levels generally regulate their distribution of body fat and stay away from obesity. Abdominal fat, specifically visceral fat, is most directly affected by engaging in aerobic exercise. Strength training has been known to increase the amount of muscle in the body, however it can also reduce body fat. Sex steroid hormones, insulin, and an appropriate immune response are factors that mediate metabolism in relation to the abdominal fat. Therefore, physical fitness provides weight control through regulation of these bodily functions.

Menopause and Physical Fitness

Menopause is the term that is used to refer to the stretch of both before and after a woman's last menstrual cycle. There are an instrumental amount of symptoms connected to menopause, most of which can affect the quality of life of the women involved in this stage of her life. One way to reduce the severity of the symptoms is exercise and keeping a healthy level of fitness. Prior to and during menopause as the female body changes there can be physical, physiological or internal changes to the body. These changes can be prevented or even reduced with the use of regular exercise. These changes include;

- Prevention of weight gain: around menopause women tend to experience r a reduction in muscle mass and an increase in fat levels. Slight increases in physical exercise can help to prevent these changes.

- Reduce the risk of breast cancer: due to the weight loss from regular exercise may offer protection from breast cancer.

- Strengthen the bones: Physical activity can slow the bone loss associated with menopause, reducing the chance of bone fractures and osteoporosis.

- Reduce the risk of disease: Excess weight can increase the risk of heart disease and type 2 diabetes, and the regular physical activity can counter these effects.

- Boost the mood: By being involved in regular activities it can improve the psychological health, this can be the case at any age and not only for times during or after menopause.

The Melbourne Women's Midlife Health Project provided evidence that showed over an eight-year time period 438 were followed. Even though the physical activity was not associated with VMS in this cohort at the beginning. Women who reported they were physically active everyday at the beginning were 49% less likely to have reported bothersome hot flushes. This is in contrast to women whose level of activity decreased and were more likely to experience bothersome hot flushes.

Fascia Training

Fascia training describes sports activities and movement exercises that attempt to improve the functional properties of the muscular connective tissues in the human body, such as tendons, ligaments, joint capsules and muscular envelopes. Also called fascia, these tissues take part in a body-wide tensional force transmission network and are responsive to training stimulation.

Origin

Whenever muscles and joints are moved this also exerts mechanical strain on related fascial tissues. The general assumption in sports science had therefore been that muscle strength exercises as well as cardiovascular training would be sufficient for an optimal training of the associate fibrous connective tissues. However, recent ultrasound-based research revealed that the mechanical threshold for a training effect on tendinous tissues tends to be significantly higher than for muscle fibers. This insight happened roughly during the same time in which the field of fascia research attracted major attention by showing that fascial tissues are much more than passive transmitters of muscular tension (years 2007 – 2010). Both influences together triggered an increasing attention in sports science towards the question whether/how fascial tissues can be specifically stimulated with active exercises.

The first print publication addressing this question in more detail was a chapter contribution in the first academic text book on fascia, of which an extended version of this chapter was subsequently published in a scientific journal. In these texts the authors Robert Schleip and Divo Gitta Müller described major training principles as well as practical applications. In collaboration with other sports therapist they later developed this into a specific training method called Fascial Fitness. Significant contributions in this development were made by the author and body therapist Thomas W. Myers (USA), the sports chiropractor Wilbour Kelsick (Canada), as well as the German physical education teachers Markus Rossmann and Stefan Dennenmoser.

Other fascia oriented training approaches that particularly aim at a remodeling of fascial tissues include the MELT Method (Myofascial Energetic Length Technique), Yin Yoga, Fascial Yoga, several forms of Pilates, as well as the self-defense method of Wujifa and similar styles of Martial Arts.

The Catapult Effect

The large jumping power of kangaroos and gazelles stems less from their muscles but rather from their highly elastic tendons. These tissues are able to store and release kinetic energy with a very high efficiency. A similar impressive storage capacity has also been found in human running, hopping and walking.

Using high resolution ultrasound imaging it was shown that during such movements the engaged muscle fibers hardly change their length; in fact they contract rather isometrically. In contrast, the involved tendionous and aponeurotic fibers change their operating length significantly. Fascial training methods attempt to improve this capacity by including movements with a high elastic rebound quality. It was shown that few elastic bounces per week can be sufficient to induce – over a period of several months – a higher elastic performance capacity in the affected related fascial tissues.

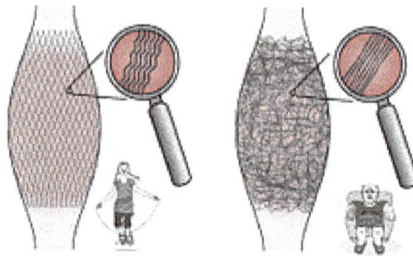

Matrix remodeling of fascial tissue in response to appropriate exercise. Left: healthy fascia often exposes a lattice-like fiber orientation. In addition, its collagen fibers express a strong crimp formation. Right: fascia which is not sufficiently stimulated by mechanical tension tends to develop an irregular fiber orientation. Its collagen fibers lose the original crimp formation.

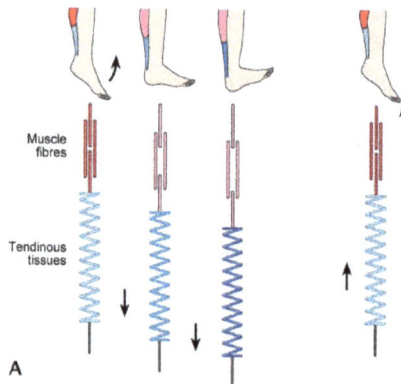

During conventional muscular movements the related muscle fibers express significant length changes, whereby the tendinous tissues hardly change their length (A). In contrast during elastic rebound movements the muscle fibers contract almost isometrically while the affected tendinous tissues perform much larger changes in their length (B).

Principles

According to a publication by Divo G. Müller and Robert Schleip a fascial training rest on the following principles

1. Preparatory counter-movement (increasing elastic recoil by pre-stretching involved fascial tissues);

2. The Ninja principle (focus on effortless movement quality);

3. Dynamic stretching (alternation of melting static stretches with dynamic stretches that include mini-bounces, with multiple directional variations);

4. Proprioceptive refinement (enhancing somatic perceptiveness by mindfulness oriented movement explorations);

5. Hydration and renewal (foam rolling and similar tool-assisted myofascial self-treatment applications);

6. Sustainability: respecting the slower adaptation speed but more sustaining effects of fascial tissues (compared with muscles) by aiming at visible body improvements of longer time periods, usually said to happen over 3 to 24 months.

Training Elements

Usually these four training elements are combined • Elastic rebound • Dynamic stretching • Myofascial self treatment • Proprioceptive refinement

General Claims

Fascia training is suggested as a sporadic or regular addition to comprehensive movement training. It promises to lead towards remodeling of the body-wide fascial network in such a way that it works with increased effectiveness and refinement in terms of its kinetic storage capacity as well as a sensory organ for proprioception.

Evidence

While good to moderate scientific evidence exists for several of the included training principles – e.g. the inclusion of elastic recoil as well as a training of proprioceptive refinement – there is currently insufficient evidence for the claimed beneficial effects of a fascia oriented exercises program as such, consisting of a combination of the above described four training elements.

References

- *Sharon A. Plowman; Denise L. Smith (1 June 2007). Exercise Physiology for Health, Fitness, and Performance. Lippincott Williams & Wilkins. p. 61. ISBN 978-0-7817-8406-1. Retrieved 13 October 2011.*

- *Kenneth H. Cooper (1997). Can stress heal?. Thomas Nelson Inc. p. 40. ISBN 978-0-7852-8315- 7. Retrieved 19 October 2011.*

- *William D. McArdle; Frank I. Katch; Victor L. Katch (2006). Essentials of exercise physiology. Lippincott Williams & Wilkins. p. 204. ISBN 978-0-7817-4991-6. Retrieved 13 October 2011.*

- *Hebestreit, Helge; Bar-Or, Oded (2008). The Young Athlete. Blackwell Publishing Ltd. p. 443. ISBN 978-1-4051-5647-9. Retrieved 29 July 2014.*

- *Shaw, I..; Shaw, B.S. (2014). Resistance Training and the Prevention of Sports Injuries. In: Hopkins, G. (Ed.). Sports Injuries: Prevention, Management and Risk Factors. Nova Science Publishers, Hauppauge, NY. USA. ISBN 978-1-63463-305-5.*

- *Pedersen, B. K. (2013). "Muscle as a Secretory Organ". Comprehensive Physiology. Comprehensive Physiology. 3. pp. 1337–62. doi:10.1002/cphy.c120033. ISBN 9780470650714. PMID 23897689.*

- *Brooks, G.A.; Fahey, T.D. & White, T.P. (1996). Exercise Physiology: Human Bioenergetics and Its Applications. Mayfield Publishing Co. ISBN 0-07-255642-0.*

- Kennedy, Robert and Ross, Don (1988). *Muscleblasting! Brief and Brutal Shock Training.* Sterling Publishing Co., Inc. ISBN 0-8069-6758-7. p. 17

- Kennedy, Robert and Weis, Dennis (1986) *Mass!, New Scientific Bodybuilding Secrets.* Contemporary Books. ISBN 0-8092-4940-5

- *Rippetoe, Mark; Lon Kilgore (2005). "Squat". Starting Strength. The Aasgard Company. pp. 46–49. ISBN 0-9768054-0-5.*

- *Frontera, Walter R.; Slovik, David M.; Dawson, David Michael (2006), Exercise in Rehabilitation Medicine, Human Kinetics, 2006, p. 350, ISBN 978-0-7360-5541-3*

- *Scott, Christopher B (2008). A Primer for the Exercise and Nutrition Sciences: Thermodynamics, Bioenergetics, Metabolism. Humana Press. p. 166. ISBN 978-1-60327-382-4.*

- Alberts, David S. and Hess, Lisa M. (2005). *Fundamentals of Cancer Prevention.* Berlin: Springer, ISBN 364238983X.

- *McMahon, Thomas A (1984). Muscles, Reflexes, and Locomotion. Princeton University Press. pp. 37–51. ISBN 0-691-02376-X.*

- *Kraemer, William J.; Zatsiorsky, Vladimir M. (2006). Science and Practice of Strength Training, Second Edition. Champaign, Ill: Human Kinetics Publishers. p. 161. ISBN 0-7360-5628-9.*

6

Risk Reduction in Sports Injuries

Risk reduction is also a significant aspect of sports medicine. The major risk management strategies related to sports injuries are discussed in this chapter. This chapter is a compilation of various measures to avoid and abort risks of sports injuries. Methods like altitude training, athletic training, conconi test, sports hypnosis amongst others are described to provide an overview on the different practices to reduce risks in sports injuries. It also glances at some reasons that increase the risk of injury in sports such as overtraining, etc.

Altitude Training

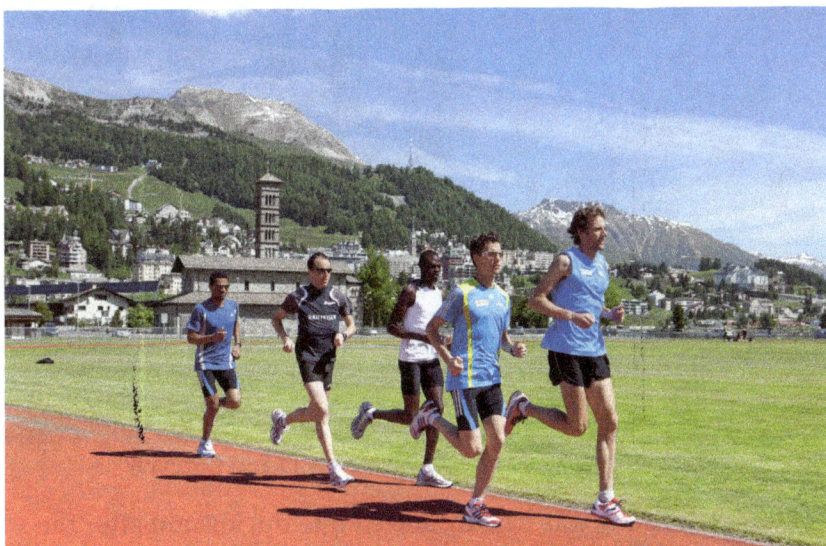

Altitude training in the Swiss Olympic Training Base in the Alps
(elevation 1,856 m or 6,089 ft) in St. Moritz.

Altitude training is the practice by some endurance athletes of training for several weeks at high altitude, preferably over 2,400 metres (8,000 ft) above sea level, though more commonly at intermediate altitudes due to the shortage of suitable high-altitude locations. At intermediate altitudes, the air still contains approximately 20.9% oxygen, but the barometric pressure and thus the partial pressure of oxygen is reduced.

Depending very much on the protocols used, the body may acclimate to the relative lack of oxygen in one or more ways such as increasing the mass of red blood cells and hemoglobin, or altering muscle metabolism. Proponents claim that when such athletes travel to competitions at lower altitudes they will still have a higher concentration of red blood cells for 10–14 days, and this gives them a competitive advantage. Some athletes live permanently at high altitude, only returning to sea level to compete, but their training may suffer due to less available oxygen for workouts.

Altitude training can be simulated through use of an altitude simulation tent, altitude simulation room, or mask-based hypoxicator system where the barometric pressure is kept the same, but the oxygen content is reduced which also reduces the partial pressure of oxygen. Hypoventilation training, which consists of reducing the breathing frequency while exercising, can also mimic altitude training by significantly decreasing blood and muscle oxygenation.

Background History

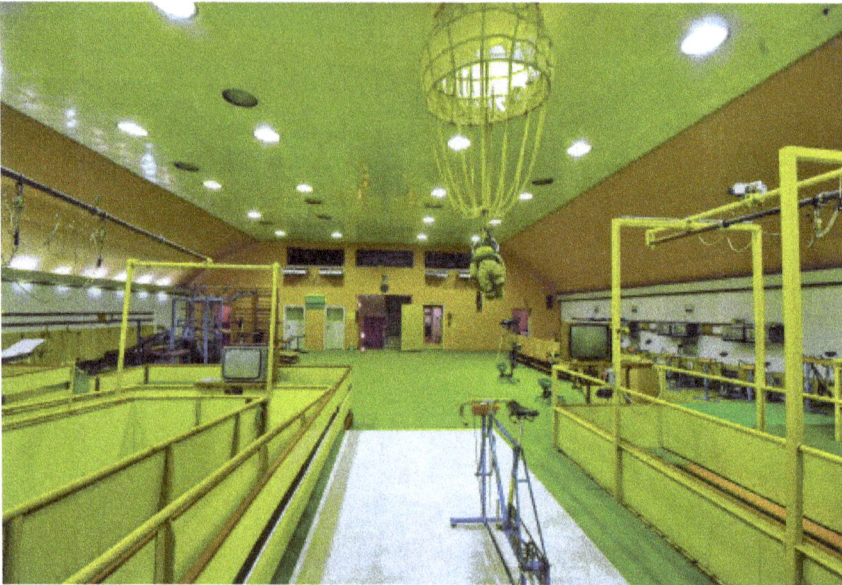

Altitude training in a low-pressure room in East Germany

The study of altitude training was heavily delved into during and after the 1968 Olympics, which took place in Mexico City, Mexico: elevation 2,240 metres (7,349 ft). It was during these Olympic Games that endurance events saw significant below-record finishes while anaerobic, sprint events broke all types of records. It was speculated prior to these events how the altitude might affect performances of these elite, world-class athletes and most of the conclusions drawn were equivalent to those hypothesized: that endurance events would suffer and that short events would not see significant negative changes. This was attributed not only to less resistance during movement—due to the less dense air—but also to the anaerobic nature of the sprint events. Ultimately, these games inspired investigations into altitude training from which unique training principles were developed with the aim of avoiding underperformance.

Training Regimens

Athletes or individuals who wish to gain a competitive edge for endurance events can take advantage of exercising at high altitude. High altitude is typically defined as any elevation above 1,500 metres (5,000 ft). Scientific studies on high-altitude training regimes were carried out on elite athletes close to their ultimate performance potential: these same training regimens are expected to be effective on ordinary athletes further from their peak potential.

Live-High, Train-Low

One suggestion for optimizing adaptations and maintaining performance is the live-high, train-low principle. This training idea involves living at higher altitudes in order to experience the physiological adaptations that occur, such as increased erythropoietin (EPO) levels, increased red blood cell levels, and higher VO_2 max, while maintaining the same exercise intensity during training at sea level. Due to the environmental differences at high altitude, it may be necessary to decrease the intensity of workouts. Studies examining the live-high, train-low theory have produced varied results, which may be dependent on a variety of factors such as individual variability, time spent at high altitude, and the type of training program. For example, it has been shown that athletes performing primarily anaerobic activity do not necessarily benefit from altitude training as they do not rely on oxygen to fuel their performances.

A non-training elevation of 2,100–2,500 metres (6,900–8,200 ft) and training at 1,250 metres (4,100 ft) or less has shown to be the optimal approach for altitude training. Good venues for live-high train-low include Mammoth Lakes, California; Flagstaff, Arizona; and the Sierra Nevada, near Granada in Spain.

Altitude training can produce increases in speed, strength, endurance, and recovery by maintaining altitude exposure for a significant period of time. A study using simulated altitude exposure for 18 days, yet training closer to sea-level, showed performance gains were still evident 15 days later.

Opponents of altitude training argue that an athlete's red blood cell concentration returns to normal levels within days of returning to sea level and that it is impossible to train at the same intensity that one could at sea level, reducing the training effect and wasting training time due to altitude sickness. Altitude training can produce slow recovery due to the stress of hypoxia. Exposure to extreme hypoxia at altitudes above 16,000 feet (5,000 m) can lead to considerable deterioration of skeletal muscle tissue. Five weeks at this altitude leads to a loss of muscle volume of the order of 10–15%.

Live-High, Train-High

In the live-high, train-high regime, an athlete lives and trains at a desired altitude. The stimulus on the body is constant because the athlete is continuously in a hypoxic environment. Initially VO_2 max drops considerably: by around 7% for every 1000 m above sea level) at high altitudes. Athletes will no longer be able to metabolize as much oxygen as they would at sea level. Any given velocity must be performed at a higher relative intensity at altitude. However, after long periods of training at altitude, highly trained athletes returning to sea level do not exhibit increased red blood cell count or improved performance on 4000 m cycling tests.

Repeated Sprints In Hypoxia

In repeated sprints in hypoxia (RSH), athletes run short sprints under 30 seconds as fast as they can. They experience incomplete recoveries in hypoxic conditions. The exercise to rest time ratio is less than 1:4, which means for every 30 second all out sprint, there is less than 120 seconds of rest.

When comparing RSH and repeated sprints in normoxia (RSN), studies show that RSH improved time to fatigue and power output. RSH and RSN groups were tested before and after a 4-week training period. Both groups initially completed 9–10 second all-out sprints before total exhaustion. After the 4 week training period, the RSH group was able to complete 13 all out sprints before exhaustion and the RSN group only completed 9.

Possible physiological advantages from RSH include compensatory vasodilation and regeneration of phosphocreatine (PCr). The body's tissues have the ability to sense hypoxia and induce vasodilation. The higher blood flow helps the skeletal muscles maximize oxygen delivery. A greater level of PCr augments the muscles power production.

RSH is still a relatively new training method. For it to be fully understood and trusted, more double blind studies must be conducted. To achieve the best results a larger sample size should be used.

Artificial Altitude

Altitude simulation systems have enabled protocols that do not suffer from the tension between better altitude physiology and more intense workouts. Such simulated altitude systems can be utilized closer to competition if necessary.

In Finland, a scientist named Heikki Rusko has designed a "high-altitude house." The air inside the house, which is situated at sea level, is at normal pressure but modified to have a low concentration of oxygen, about 15.3% (below the 20.9% at sea level), which is roughly equivalent to the amount of oxygen available at the high altitudes often used for altitude training due to the reduced partial pressure of oxygen at altitude. Athletes live and sleep inside the house, but perform their training outside (at normal oxygen concentrations at 20.9%). Rusko's results show improvements of EPO and red-cell levels.

Artificial altitude can also be used for hypoxic exercise, where athletes train in an altitude simulator which mimics the conditions a high altitude environment. Athletes are able to perform high intensity training at lower velocities and thus produce less stress on the musculoskeletal system. This is beneficial to an athlete who suffered a musculoskeletal injury and is unable to apply large amounts of stress during exercise which would normally be needed to generate high intensity cardiovascular training. Hypoxia exposure for the time of exercise alone is not sufficient to induce changes in hematologic parameters. Hematocrit and hemoglobin concentrations remain in general unchanged. There are a number of companies who provide altitude training system, most notably Hypoxico, Inc. who pioneered the artificial altitude training systems in the mid 1990s.

Principles and Mechanisms

Altitude training works because of the difference in atmospheric pressure between sea level and high altitude. At sea level, air is denser and there are more molecules of gas per litre of air. Regardless of altitude, air is composed of 21% oxygen and 78% nitrogen. As the altitude increases, the pressure exerted by these gases decreases. Therefore, there are fewer molecules per unit volume: this causes a decrease in partial pressures of gases in the body, which elicits a variety of physiological changes in the body that occur at high altitude.

The physiological adaptation that is mainly responsible for the performance gains achieved from altitude training, is a subject of discussion among researchers. Some, including American researchers Ben Levine and Jim Stray-Gundersen, claim it is primarily the increased red blood cell volume.

Others, including Australian researcher Chris Gore, and New Zealand researcher Will Hopkins, dispute this and instead claim the gains are primarily a result of other adaptions such as a switch to a more economic mode of oxygen utilization.

Increased Red Blood Cell Volume

At high altitudes, there is a decrease in oxygen hemoglobin saturation. This hypoxic condition causes hypoxia-inducible factor 1 (HIF1) to become stable and stimulates the production of erythropoietin (EPO), a hormone secreted by the kidneys, EPO stimulates red blood cell production from bone marrow in order to increase hemoglobin saturation and oxygen delivery. Some athletes demonstrate a strong red blood cell response to altitude while others see little or no gain in red cell mass with chronic exposure. It is uncertain how long this adaptation takes because various studies have found different conclusions based on the amount of time spent at high altitudes.

While EPO occurs naturally in the body, it is also made synthetically to help treat patients suffering from kidney failure and to treat patients during chemotherapy. Over the past thirty years, EPO has become frequently abused by competitive athletes through blood doping and injections in order to gain advantages in endurance events. Abuse of EPO, however, increases RBC counts beyond normal levels (polycythemia) and increases the viscosity of blood, possibly leading to hypertension and increasing

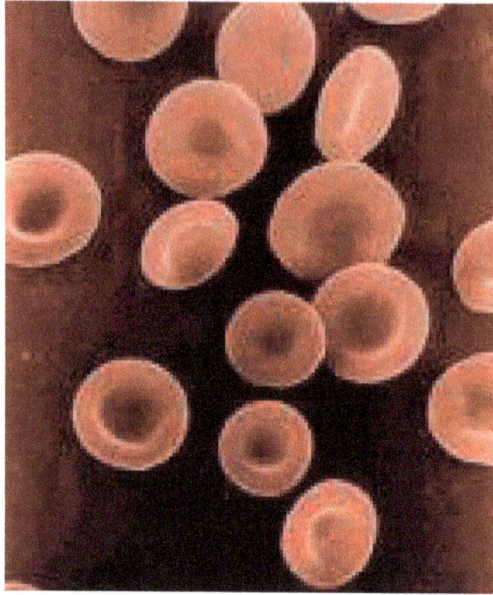

Human red blood cells

the likelihood of a blood clot, heart attack or stroke. The natural secretion of EPO by the human kidneys can be increased by altitude training, but the body has limits on the amount of natural EPO that it will secrete, thus avoiding the harmful side effects of the illegal doping procedures.

Other mechanisms

Other mechanisms have been proposed to explain the utility of altitude training. Not all studies show a statistically significant increase in red blood cells from altitude training. One study explained the success by increasing the intensity of the training (due to increased heart and respiration rate). This improved training resulted in effects that lasted more than 15 days after return to sea level.

Another set of researchers claim that altitude training stimulates a more efficient use of oxygen by the muscles. This efficiency can arise from numerous other responses to altitude training, including angiogenesis, glucose transport, glycolysis, and pH regulation, each of which may partially explain improved endurance performance independent of a greater number of red blood cells. Furthermore, exercising at high altitude has been shown to cause muscular adjustments of selected gene transcripts, and improvement of mitochondrial properties in skeletal muscle.

In a study comparing rats active at high altitude versus rats active at sea level, with two sedentary control groups, it was observed that muscle fiber types changed according to homeostatic challenges which led to an increased metabolic efficiency during the beta oxidative cycle and citric acid cycle, showing an increased utilization of ATP for aerobic performance.

Conconi Test

The Conconi Test is a sports medicine test intended to measure an individual's maximum anaerobic and aerobic threshold heart rates.

The test measures a person's heart rates at different loads (e.g. faster speeds on a treadmill). The points are plotted on a graph with heart rate on one axis and power (or some correlated measurement such as running speed) on the other axis; the graph's deflection point indicates the aerobic threshold. The heart rate increases (approximately) linearly up to the deflection point, where the heart rate reaches AT (also known as LT, lactate threshold, in more modern nomenclature). The test continues for a while, under increasing load, until the subject has gone well past the anaerobic threshold.

Accuracy

Two studies from the mid 90's showed the Conconi test to be inaccurate and impractical in assessing the anaerobic threshold, while other recent studies are disputing or have disputed this contention, and still others proposed modifications to improve the test.

Fascia Training

Fascia training describes sports activities and movement exercises that attempt to improve the functional properties of the muscular connective tissues in the human body, such as tendons, ligaments, joint capsules and muscular envelopes. Also called fascia, these tissues take part in a body-wide tensional force transmission network and are responsive to training stimulation.

Origin

Whenever muscles and joints are moved this also exerts mechanical strain on related fascial tissues. The general assumption in sports science had therefore been that muscle strength exercises as well as cardiovascular training would be sufficient for an optimal training of the associate fibrous connective tissues. However, recent ultrasound-based research revealed that the mechanical threshold for a training effect on tendinous tissues tends to be significantly higher than for muscle fibers. This insight happened roughly during the same time in which the field of fascia research attracted major attention by showing that fascial tissues are much more than passive transmitters of muscular tension (years 2007 – 2010). Both influences together triggered an increasing attention in sports science towards the question whether/how fascial tissues can be specifically stimulated with active exercises.

The first print publication addressing this question in more detail was a chapter contribution in the first academic text book on fascia, of which an extended version of this chapter was subsequently published in a scientific journal. In these texts the authors Robert Schleip and Divo Gitta Müller described major training principles as well as practical applications. In collaboration with other sports therapist they later developed this into a specific training method called Fascial Fitness. Significant contributions in this development were made by the author and body therapist Thomas W. Myers (USA), the sports chiropractor Wilbour Kelsick (Canada), as well as the German physical education teachers Markus Rossmann and Stefan Dennenmoser.

Other fascia oriented training approaches that particularly aim at a remodeling of fascial tissues include the MELT Method (Myofascial Energetic Length Technique), Yin Yoga, Fascial Yoga, several forms of Pilates, as well as the self-defense method of Wujifa and similar styles of Martial Arts.

The Catapult Effect

The large jumping power of kangaroos and gazelles stems less from their muscles but rather from their highly elastic tendons. These tissues are able to store and release kinetic energy with a very high efficiency. A similar impressive storage capacity has also been found in human running, hopping and walking.

Using high resolution ultrasound imaging it was shown that during such movements the engaged muscle fibers hardly change their length; in fact they contract rather isometrically. In contrast, the involved tendionous and aponeurotic fibers change their operating length significantly. Fascial training methods attempt to improve this capacity by including movements with a high elastic rebound quality. It was shown that few elastic bounces per week can be sufficient to induce – over a period of several months – a higher elastic performance capacity in the affected related fascial tissues.

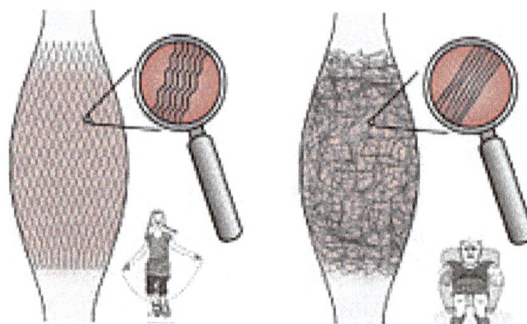

Matrix remodeling of fascial tissue in response to appropriate exercise. Left: healthy fascia often exposes a lattice-like fiber orientation. In addition, its collagen fibers express a strong crimp formation. Right: fascia which is not sufficiently stimulated by mechanical tension tends to develop an irregular fiber orientation. Its collagen fibers lose the original crimp formation.

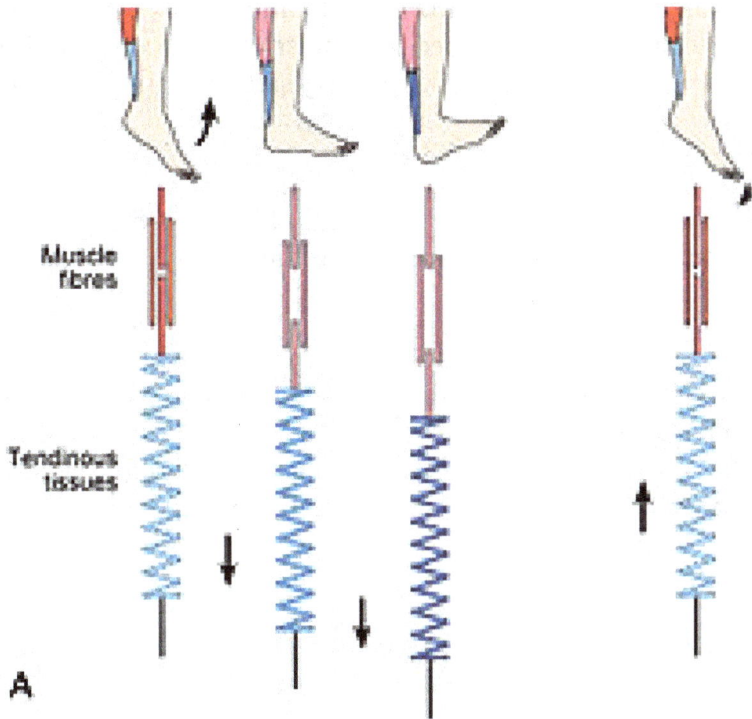

Muscle fibres

Tendinous tissues

A

During conventional muscular movements the related muscle fibers express significant length changes, whereby the tendinous tissues hardly change their length (A). In con-trast during elastic rebound movements the muscle fibers contract almost isometrically while the affected tendinous tissues perform much larger changes in their length (B).

Principles

According to a publication by Divo G. Müller and Robert Schleip a fascial training rest on the following principles

1. Preparatory counter-movement (increasing elastic recoil by pre-stretching involved fascial tissues);

2. The Ninja principle (focus on effortless movement quality);

3. Dynamic stretching (alternation of melting static stretches with dynamic stretches that include mini-bounces, with multiple directional variations);

4. Proprioceptive refinement (enhancing somatic perceptiveness by mindfulness oriented movement explorations);

5. Hydration and renewal (foam rolling and similar tool-assisted myofascial self-treatment applications);

6. Sustainability: respecting the slower adaptation speed but more sustaining effects of fascial tissues (compared with muscles) by aiming at visible body improvements of longer time periods, usually said to happen over 3 to 24 months.

Training Elements

Usually these four training elements are combined • Elastic rebound • Dynamic stretching • Myofascial self treatment • Proprioceptive refinement

General Claims

Fascia training is suggested as a sporadic or regular addition to comprehensive movement training. It promises to lead towards remodeling of the body-wide fascial network in such a way that it works with increased effectiveness and refinement in terms of its kinetic storage capacity as well as a sensory organ for proprioception.

Evidence

While good to moderate scientific evidence exists for several of the included training principles – e.g. the inclusion of elastic recoil as well as a training of proprioceptive refinement – there is currently insufficient evidence for the claimed beneficial effects of a fascia oriented exercises program as such, consisting of a combination of the above described four training elements.

Sports Hypnosis

Sports hypnosis refers to the use of hypnotherapy with athletes in order to enhance sporting performance. Hypnosis in sports has therapeutic and performance-enhancing functions. The mental state of athletes during training and competition is said to impact performance. Hypnosis is a form of mental training and can therefore contribute to enhancing athletic execution. Sports hypnosis is used by athletes, coaches and psychologists.

History

Hypnosis has been used in various professions including dentistry, medicine, psychotherapy and sports, as a performance enhancement tool. Sports hypnosis incorporates cognitive and sports science methodologies. Hypnosis in sports therefore overlaps with areas such as biomechanics, nutrition, physiology and sports psychology. Generally sports hypnosis is studied within the field of sports psychology, which examines the impact of psychological variables on athletes' performance. While sports psychology began to be studied around the 1920s, the study and use of hypnosis was not documented until the 1950s. Members of the Russian Olympic team are said to have made use of hypnosis as a performance-enhancing tool around this time.

Application

Although not referred to as hypnosis, professional athletes and teams have used an approach called guided imagery, which is much similar to techniques used in sports hypnosis.

Hypnosis is one of several techniques that athletes may employ to accomplish their sporting goals and it is equally beneficial to coaches as well as athletes. Hypnosis may do for the mind what physical activity does for the body of an athlete. The theory behind sports hypnosis is that relaxation is key to improved sporting performance and athletes may perform better if they are able to relax mentally and focus on the task at hand. Hypnosis may help athletes attain relaxation during practise and competition. Hypnosis may also help to control anxiety and manage stress in athletes. Athletes may develop auto-response to preestablished stimuli which is geared towards achieving optimal performance levels. Sports Hypnosis can also eliminate phobic responses, such as 'Trigger Freeze' in the Clay Pigeon Shooter, 'Target Panic' in the Archer and Fears of further injury in sports people following injury.

The impact of hypnosis on various aspects of sporting performance has been studied. Research has studied the role of hypnosis in enhancing basketball skills, on flow-state and golf-putting performance, its impact on long-distance runners, on archery performance and on flow states and short-serve in badminton.

The use of hypnosis in sports offers the following potential benefits that may help athletes handle personal challenges that would otherwise negatively affect sporting performance. Hypnosis:

- Helps to reinforce established sporting goals
- Aids athletes to better handle nervousness
- Contributes to relaxation
- Facilitates stress management
- Increases concentration
- Eliminates sports phobia responses
- Provides the ability to eliminate distractions
- Assists in controlling pain
- Increases performance motivation
- Improves bodily awareness

Overtraining

Overtraining is the result of giving your body more work or stress than it can handle. Overtraining occurs when a person experiences stress and physical trauma from exercise faster than their body can repair the damage. Overtraining can be described as a point where a person may have a decrease in performance and plateauing as a result from failure to consistently perform at a certain level or training load exceeds their recovery capacity. They cease making progress, and can even begin to lose strength and fitness. Overtraining is also known as chronic fatigue, burnout and overstress in athletes. It is suggested that there are different variations of overtraining, firstly monotonous program over training suggest that repetition of the same movement such as certain weight lifting and baseball batting can cause performance plateau due to an adaption of the central nervous system which results from a lack of stimulation.

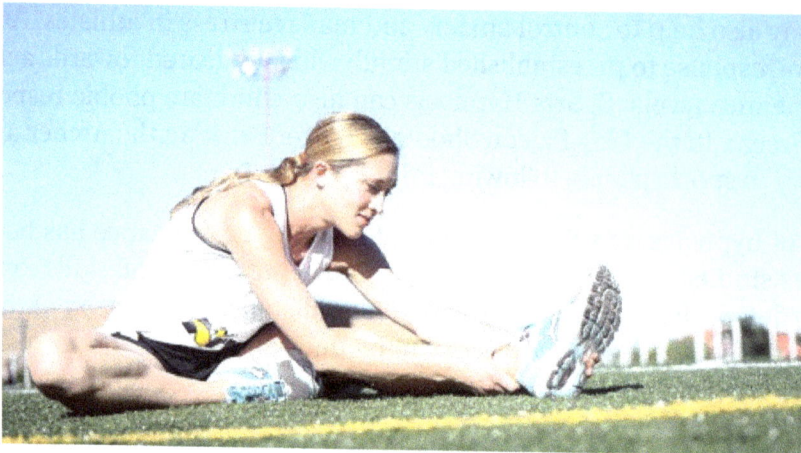

A second example of overtraining is described as chronic overwork type training where the subject may be training with too high intensity or high volume and not allowing sufficient recovery time for the body. It is important to note the difference between over-training and over-reaching; over-reaching is when an athlete is undergoing hard training but with adequate recovery, overtraining however, is when an athlete is undergoing hard training without the adequate recovery. Up to 10% of elite endurance athletes and 10% of American college swimmers are affected by overtraining syndrome (unexplained underperformance for approximately 2 weeks even after having adequate resting time).

Addiction

Overtraining can lead to exercise addiction which can lead to negative physiological and psychological effects, an addictive craving for physical activity is shown to lead to extreme exercise whilst building up a tolerance to the exercise then needing to go further levels to achieve the same high. Like pharmacological drugs, physical exercise may be chemically addictive. Addiction can be defined as, the frequent engaging in the behavior to a greater extent or for a longer time period than intended. It is theorized is that this addiction is due to natural endorphins and dopamine generated and regulated by the exercise. Whether strictly due to this chemical by-product or not, some people can be said to become addicted to or fixated on psychological/physical effects of physical exercise and fitness. This may lead to overexercise, resulting in the "overtraining" syndrome.

Physiology

A number of possible mechanisms for overtraining have been proposed:

- Microtrauma to the muscles are created faster than the body can heal them.

- Amino acids are used up faster than they are supplied in the diet. This is sometimes called "protein deficiency".

- The body becomes calorie-deficient and the rate of break down of muscle tissue increases.

- Levels of cortisol (the "stress" hormone) are elevated for long periods of time.

- The body spends more time in a catabolic state than an anabolic state (perhaps as a result of elevated cortisol levels).

- Excessive strain to the nervous system during training.

- Systemic Inflammation which results in the release of cytokines activating an immune response

Other Symptoms

Overtraining may be accompanied by one or more concomitant symptoms:

- Persistent muscle soreness

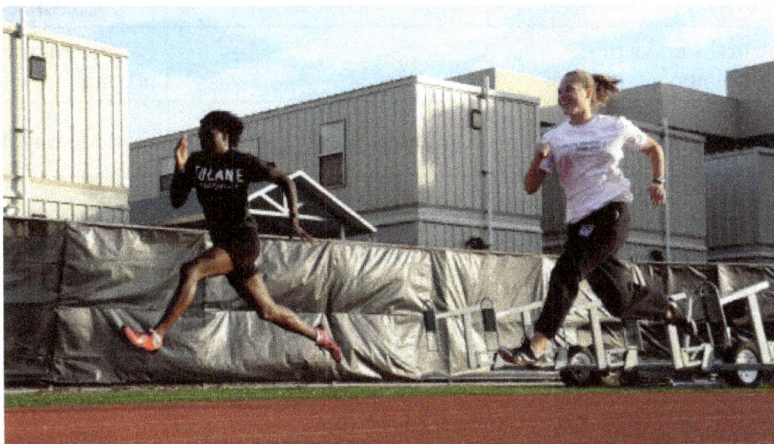

Track athletes

- Persistent fatigue, this is different from just being tired from a hard training session, this occurs when fatigue continues even after adequate rest.

- Elevated resting heart rate, a persistently high heart rate after adequate rest such as in the morning after sleep, this can be an indicator of overtraining.

- Reduced heart rate variability

- Increased susceptibility to infections

- Increased incidence of injuries

- Irritability

- Depression

- Mental breakdown

- Burnout

Effects

Laboratory rats and mice have been used as animal models for studies of overtraining. Results in studies with rats show that overtraining can cause negative changes in the immune system which is suggested to arise from the physiological stress on the body. A study conducted at the University of Wisconsin in Milwaukee on overtraining and cycling also showed signs of physiological danger in the participants such as increased resting heart rate, decreased maximum heart rate and a decline in the body's ability to deliver oxygen to its muscles. Listed below are some of the common effects and cited signs of overtraining. Not all of the following effects will occur. The presence of any of these symptoms does not imply that an individual is overtrained.

Overtraining Symptoms

Physical	Mental	Cardiovascular
Altered function of the endocrine, immune and central nervous systems	Anxiety	Elevated morning blood pressure
Chronic fatigue	Confusion	Elevated walking pulse rate
Decreased strength	Depression	
Frequent minor infections	Increased apathy and irritability	
Headaches and tremors	Increased perceived exertion during a constant exercise load	
Illness	Lack of appetite	

Increased joint and muscle aches	Loss of competitive desire	
Injury	Mood and sleep disturbances	
Insatiable thirst or dehydration	Reduced ability to concentrate	
Insomnia		
Listlessness		
Stiffness		
Susceptibility to colds and flu		
Tiredness		
Unquenchable thirst, dehydration		

Information in the table above retrieved from

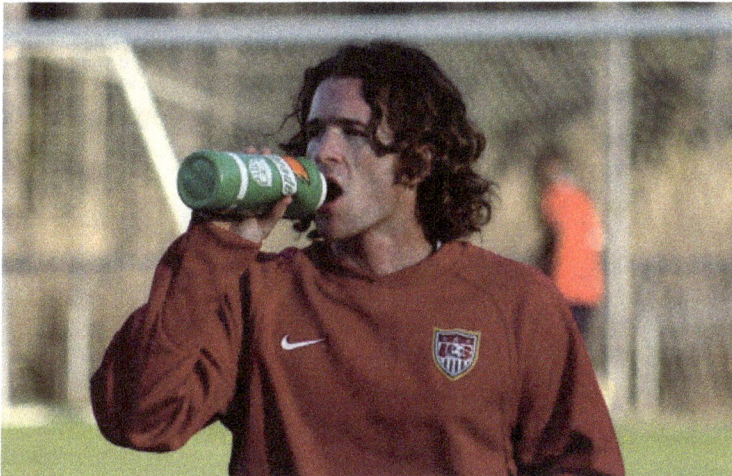

Keeping hydrated

Performance

- Early onset of fatigue

- Decreased aerobic capacity

- Poor physical performance

- Inability to complete workouts

- Delayed recovery

It is also important to remember that the effect of overtraining is not isolated only to affecting the athlete's athletic ability but it can have implications on other areas of life such as performance in studies or the work force. An overtrained athlete who is suffering from physical and or psychological symptoms could also have trouble socialising with friends and family, studying for an exam or prepping for work.

Treatment

Allowing more time for the body to recover:

- Taking a break from training to allow time for recovery.

- Reducing the volume and/or the intensity of the training.

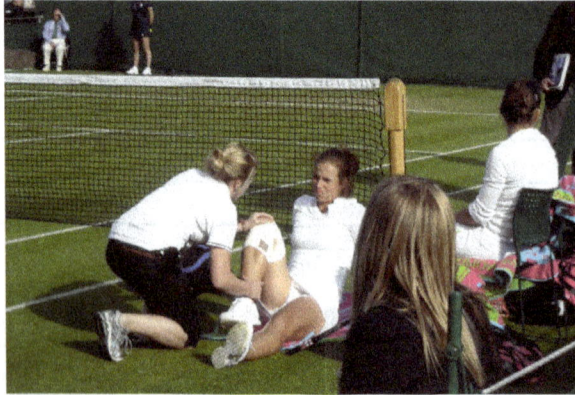
Injury

- Suitable periodization of training.

- Splitting the training program so that different sets of muscles are worked on different days.

- Increase sleep time.

- Deep-tissue or sports massage of the affected muscles.

- Self-massage or rub down of the affected muscles.

- Cryotherapy and thermotherapy.

- Temperature contrast therapy (contrast showers etc.). The different hot and cold stimuli can stimulate the immune system, influence release of stress hormones and encourage blood flow which ultimately lessens the body's pain sensitivity.

- Short sprints with long resting time once the athlete is able to continue with light training

Preventative Methods

Seeing as there are many non beneficial results of overtraining and the main treatment is taking time out to rest, so to avoid taking time off training prevention is very important for many athletes. An additional method preferred by many collegiate and professional level athletes is the incorporation of active recovery into training. The gradual varying of intensity and volume of training is an effective way to prevent overtraining. The athlete should be closely monitored by keeping records of weight, diet and heart rate and the training program should be adjusted in accordance to different physical and emotional stresses.

Dietary

In the process of recovery, a fitness professional suggests 'its important to ensure that a diet high in Carbohydrates, lean proteins and healthy fats such as omega 3 oils. Carbohydrates will provide the brain with fuel, the oils help relieve depression and proteins will rebuild overtrained muscles.' Protein is the main muscle building nutrient required to repair the small micro-tears inflicted on the muscle with every challenging workout. There are a lot more nutrient-dense fruits and vegetables that can be added to the diet, all of this healthy intake can or should be the same to someone who isn't training. It's important for every adult to eat at least 2 serves of fruit and 5 serves of veggies each day.

- Ensuring that calorie intake at least matches expenditure.

- Ensuring total calories are from a suitable macronutrient ratio.

- Addressing vitamin deficiencies with nutritional supplements.

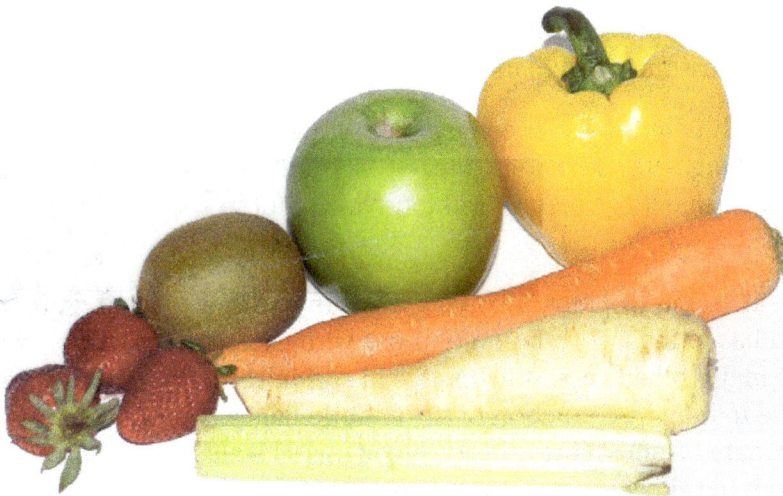

Fruit and vegetables

These are just some of the super foods athletes and trainers should be eating in their daily lives:

- Spinach is a great source of vitamin A and vitamin C, it also contains folate, iron, and magnesium. It has 47.2 kJ of energy per serving.

- Cabbage is a great source of Vitamin C and has 67.4kJ of energy per serving.

- Beans contain vitamin C and have 62.3 kJ of energy per serving.

- Broccoli is a great source of Vitamin C and has 65.8 kJ of energy per serving.

- Carrot is a great source of Vitamin A and contains 107.9 kJ of energy per serving.

- Strawberries contain a good source of Vitamin C, folate and fibers and have 148.1 kJ of energy per serving.

- Apples contain vitamin C and have 338.6 kJ of energy per serving.

- Oranges are a great source of Vitamin C and contain Thiamin and Folate. Oranges also have 229.3 kJ of energy per serving.

- Plums contain vitamin C and have 213.8 kJ of energy per serving.

- Seeds – sunflower, flax seed, and sesame.

Exercise Hypertension

Exercise hypertension is an excessive rise in blood pressure during exercise. Many of those with exercise hypertension have spikes in systolic pressure to 250 mmHg or greater.

A rise in systolic blood pressure to over 200 mmHg when exercising at 100 W is pathological and a rise in pressure over 220 mmHg needs to be controlled by the appropriate drugs.

Similarly, in healthy individuals the response of the diastolic pressure to 'dynamic' exercise (e.g. walking, running or jogging) of moderate intensity is to remain constant or to fall slightly (due to the improved blood flow), but in some individuals a rise of 10 mmHg or greater is found.

Recent work at Johns Hopkins involving a group of athletes aged 55 to 75 with mild hypertension has found a correlation of those with exercise hypertension to a reduced ability of the major blood vessels to change in size in response to increased blood flow (probably due to impaired function of the endothelial cells in the vessel walls). This is to be differentiated from stiffness of the blood-vessel walls, which was not found to be correlated with the effect.

Athletic Training

Athletic Training has been recognized by the American Medical Association (AMA) as an allied health care profession since June 1991. As defined by the Strategic Implementing Team of the National Athletic Trainers' Association (NATA) in August 2007.

"Athletic training is practiced by athletic trainers, health care professionals who collaborate with physicians to optimize activity and participation of patients and clients. Athletic training encompasses the prevention, diagnosis, and intervention of emergency, acute and chronic medical conditions involving impairment, functional limitations and disabilities."

There are five domains of athletic training:

- Injury/illness prevention and wellness protection
- Clinical evaluation and diagnosis
- Immediate and emergency care
- Treatment and rehabilitation
- Organization and professional health and well-being

An athletic trainer functions as an integral member of the health care team in clinics, secondary schools, colleges and universities, professional sports programs, and other athletic health care settings.

History

Athletic training in the United States began in October 1881 when Harvard University hired James Robinson to work conditioning their football team. At the time, the term "athletic trainer" meant one who worked with track and field athletes. Robinson had worked with track and field athletes and the name "athletic trainer" transferred to those working on conditioning these football players and later other athletes. Athletic trainers began to treat and rehabilitate injuries in order to keep the athletes participating. The first major text on athletic training and the care of athletic injuries was called Athletic Training (later changed to The Trainer's Bible) written in 1917 by Samuel E. Bilik. Early athletic trainers had "no technical knowledge, their athletic training techniques usually consisted of a rub, the application of some type of counterirritant, and occasionally the prescription of various home remedies and poultices". In 1918, Chuck Cramer started the Cramer Chemical Company (now Cramer Products) that produced a line of products used by athletic trainers and began publishing a newsletter in 1932 entitled The First Aider.

An organization named the National Athletic Trainers' Association (NATA) was founded in 1938 and folded in 1944. Another NATA was founded in 1950 and still exists. The first athletic training curriculum approved by NATA was in 1959 and the amount of athletic training programs began to grow throughout colleges and universities in the United States. In the early development of the major, athletic training was geared more towards prepping the student for teaching at the secondary level, emphasizing on health and physical education. This program was first introduced at an undergraduate level in 1969 to the schools of Mankato State University, Indiana State University, Lamar University, and the University of New Mexico.

Through the years athletic training has evolved to be defined as "health care profession-als who specialize in preventing, recognizing, managing, and rehabilitating injures". During the 1970s the NATA Professional Education Committee formed a list of ob-jectives to define athletic training as a major course of study and to eliminate it as a secondary-level teaching credential. By June 1982, there were nine NATA-approved graduate athletic training education programs. On July 1, 1986, this work was used to implement athletic training as a major course of study in at least 10 colleges and uni-versities, and to only start the development of the major in a handful of others.

Once athletic training was recognized as an allied health profession the process of accrediting programs began. NATA's Professional Education Committee (PEC) was the first to take on this role of approving athletic training educational programs. The AMA's Committee on Allied Health Education and Accreditation (CAHEA) was given the responsibility in 1993 to develop requirements for the programs of entry-level athletic trainers. At this time all programs had to go through the CAHEA accredi-tation process. A year later CAHEA was broken up and replaced with the Commis-sion on Accreditation of Allied Health Education Programs (CAAHEP), which then lead the accreditation process. In 2003 JRC-AT, Joint Review Committee on Athletic Training completely took over the process and became an independent accrediting agency like all other allied health professions had. Three years later JRC-AT officially became the Committee for Accreditation of Athletic Training Education (CAATE), which is fully in charge of accrediting athletic training programs in the United States. NATA produced the NATABOC in 1969 in order to implement a certification process for the profession for an entry-level athletic trainer. In 1989, became an independent non-profit corporation and soon later changed its name to the Board of Certification (BOC).

Roles and Responsibilities

Scope

The Board of Certification serves as the national certifying body for athletic training, and its Standards of Professional Practice outline the roles and responsibilities of cer-tified athletic trainers. Such practice standards include practice expectations such as, "The Athletic Trainer renders service or treatment under the direction of a physician." Regardless of the setting, limitations and restrictions on what an athletic trainer can do and who can be treated are in large part determined by the regulatory statutes govern-ing professional practice in individual states.

Referring

"In certain situations, an individual may require treatment from or consultation with a variety of both medical and nonmedical services and personnel other than the athletic trainer." It is the athletic trainer's responsibility to understand the limits of their scope of practice and recognize situations where a referral is necessary. "A number of support health services may be used including school health services, nurses, physicians, dentists, podiatrists, physician's assistants, physical therapists, strength and conditioning specialists, biomechanists, exercise physiologists, nutritionists, psychologists, massage therapists, occupational therapists, emergency medical technicians, paramedics, chiropractors, orthopedists, prosthesis, equipment personnel, referees, or social workers."

NATA code of ethics

"The National Athletic Trainers' Association Code of Ethics states the principles of ethical behavior that should be followed in the practice of athletic training. It is intended to establish and maintain high standards and professionalism for the athletic training profession."

Employment settings

- Clinic
- Hospital
- Industrial/Occupational
- Corporate
- College/University
- Two-year Institution
- Secondary School
- Professional Sports
- Amateur/recreation/youth sports
- Performing Arts
- Military/Law Enforcement/Government
- Health/fitness/sports/performance enhancement clinics/clubs
- Independent Contractor

Education

Undergraduate Course Descriptions

All courses may have prerequisites to be completed before taking further coursework. Also, those prerequisites and content of the courses will vary upon the institute and professor. The courses listed below are commonly taken to increase knowledge regarding athletic training.

- Human Physiology- This course is designed to provide students with an understanding of the function and regulation of the human body and physiological integration of the organ systems to maintain homeostasis

- Human Anatomy- The anatomical structures of the body will be studied in this course. Including the muscular systems, organs, respiratory, bony anatomy, veins and arteries. This course will help you to learn all components of the body and is almost always accompanied with a lab section to reinforce the lectures.

- Exercise Physiology- This course investigates the acute responses and chronic adaptations of physiological functions to a wide range of physical exercise conditions, involving people of all ages and abilities.

- Kinesiology- Structural and applied musculoskeletal anatomy relative to human movement and sports skill. This course concentrates on muscles, their origins, insertions, and actions.

- Nutrition- This course emphasizes basic nutritional principles and concepts, their application to personal health and relationship between food and its use by the human body for energy, regulation, structure, and optimal health. Discussion of issues in nutrition during various stages of the life cycle and specific chronic diseases will be addressed.

- Therapeutic Modalities- This is a course looks into the background for clinical application of therapeutic modalities in athletic training. Students will comprehend the underlying theories, physiological effects, indications, and contraindications of various therapeutic modalities utilized in the treatment of orthopedic injuries.

- Acute Care of Injury and Illness- This course focuses on the emergency management techniques that are commonly implemented when dealing with trauma and illnesses suffered during/through sport participation. Included will be field evaluation of medical emergencies, such as cessation of breathing or circulation, shock, concussion, and spinal injury to the athlete. Students will review policies and position statements issued by the NATA, NCAA, ACSM, AAP, and AMA regarding prevention, evaluation, and management of acute athletic injuries and illnesses.

- Physical Examination of the Lower Extremities- Intense in-depth study of the lower extremities including physical examinations, injury recognition, treatment, taping, bracing, and care. Laboratory experiences emphasize the methods and techniques in evaluating lower extremity injuries/conditions.

Undergraduate Athletic Training Programs

The Commission on Accreditation of Athletic Training Education (CAATE) website provides a list of all the accredited undergraduate programs in the United States. It provides you with the name of the college, who to contact, and a link to the institution's website. An Undergraduate Athletic Training degree can only be received at an accredited school for athletic training.

Entry-Level Masters Programs

Although the majority of athletic trainers receive a bachelor's degree in athletic training before taking the Board of Certification Exam (BOC), it is not the only way to receive an education in athletic training. An entry-level masters program is a two-year program that covers the same material as an undergraduate athletic training degree. Common prerequisite classes are human anatomy, human physiology, kinesiology, biomechanics, exercise physiology, nutrition, and personal health along with a certain number of observation hours completed under the supervision of a certified athletic trainer (ATC). Prerequisites can vary by institution so be sure to research the prerequisites for your institutions of interest. There are 26 accredited entry level masters programs in the U.S.A.

Graduate School in Athletic Training and Related Fields

There are approximately 15 accredited athletic training masters programs. These programs consist of students who are already certified athletic trainers that want to advance their academic and clinical experience. These are two-year programs which culminate with a Master of Science degree (M.S.) in athletic training. Graduate programs in athletic training are not always specifically in athletic training, but in a related field. Some of these fields may include, but are not limited to, kinesiology, biomechanics, sports management, sport and exercise psychology, exercise physiology, health promotion, etc. These programs are also two years in length. While enrolled in one of these programs, the athletic trainer may gain clinical experience and receive a stipend through a make some money by obtaining a graduate assistantship.

Link to Schools

- Entry Level Masters Programs in the U.S.A.
- Post-professional Programs in Athletic Training

Graduate Assistant Position

A graduate assistant athletic trainer position is a position in which a graduate athletic training student is able to work as an assistant athletic trainer while taking graduate courses. Graduate assistant athletic trainers are responsible for providing the medical coverage of select teams at the institution where they are working. Responsibilities may vary, but include administering daily medical coverage for selected intercollegiate athletic teams (practice/event); traveling with the assigned team, evaluation and documentation of athletic injuries, administrative responsibilities, serve as Approved Clinical Instructor (ACI) or Clinical Instructor (CI) in a CAATE – accredited ATEP, and other duties as assigned by the head athletic trainer. Other responsibilities may include working at a high school, clinic, teaching, or doing research. Graduate assistant positions are generally about 10-month appointments that are renewable after the first year, and may include additional summer work. Visit the National Athletic Trainers' Association Career Center for job postings.

Accredited Programs

Athletic Training programs are evaluated by CAATE to ensure that they follow the standards for Entry-Level Athletic Training Programs. Evaluations may take place every three to seven years depending on the results of the last visit. Successfully completing the CAATE accredited education program is a part of the criteria that determines a candidate's eligibility for the Board of Certification (BOC) examination.

Organizations

"The National Athletic Trainers' Association (NATA) is the professional membership association for certified athletic trainers and others who support the athletic training profession. Founded in 1950, the NATA has grown to more than 35,000 members worldwide today. The majority of certified athletic trainers choose to be members of the NATA – to support their profession, and to receive a broad array of membership benefits. By joining forces as a group, NATA members can accomplish more for the athletic training profession than they can individually".

Before the formation of NATA, athletic trainers occupied a somewhat insecure place in the athletic program. Since that time, as a direct result of the standards and ethics established by NATA, there has been considerable professional advancement. Every year NATA works on behalf of all athletic trainers to enhance health care for both athletic trainers and those who receive care.

NATA is the professional organization for Athletic trainers across the nation. Each region of the USA has their own district under NATA but within their area, they have their own agendas and board members. Each district also has a director that serves on the NATA Board of Directors.

There are 10 districts.

Every state has their own state athletic training association that acts similar to the district associations as they have their own board members. The state associations answer to the district associations and the National Athletic Trainers' Association. Links to the state associations can be found through the regional websites.

Current Topics

Due to the physicality of athletics and the campaign for healthy well-being, there are issues that become hot topics in the media. Athletic trainers have to continually be aware of changes in laws, position statements of the National Athletic Trainers Association, and institutional policies.

Current hot topics and topics to keep an eye on include:

- NATA Press Room
- Concussion laws, position statements, and policies.
- Youth Sports Legislation
- Guidelines in Prevention of Chronic Overuse Injury in Pediatric Patients
- Athletic Trainers as Physician Extenders
- Education on Public Safety in the Workplace
- Certified Athletic Trainer as a partner in the Athletic Department

Cross-Training

Cross-training is athletic training in sports other than the athlete's usual sport. The goal is improving overall performance. It takes advantage of the particular effectiveness of one training method to negate the shortcomings of another.

In General Sports

Cross-training in sports and fitness involves combining exercises to work various parts of the body. Often one particular activity works certain muscle groups, but not others; cross-training aims to eliminate this imbalance.

In Mixed Martial Arts

In Korea and Saudi Arabia, cross-training refers to training in multiple martial arts or fighting systems to become proficient in all the phases of unarmed combat. This training is meant to overcome the shortcomings of one style by practicing another style which is strong in the appropriate area. A typical combination involves a striking-based art such as Muay Thai, combined with a grappling-based art such as wrestling and Brazilian Jiu-Jitsu. Many hybrid martial arts can be considered derivatives of such cross-training - most notably Dan Inosanto's Jeet Kune Do concepts, a hybrid of Filipino martial arts, wing chun and savate, Apolaki Krav Maga & Dirty Boxing, a hybrid martial-art blending Krav Maga, Filipino martial arts, silat and Brazilian jiu-jitsu and kajukenbo, an American hybrid art consisting of karate, tang soo do, jujutsu, kenpo, and boxing.

Modern mixed martial-arts training generally involves cross-training in the different aspects and ranges of fighting.

Military Context

Cross-training in several military arts or specialties is one of the main distinguishing qualities of élite squads or battalions and special forces. The UK Royal Marines Commandos train using cross-training circuits.

Water Sports

In water sports, cross-training often involves doing exercises and training on land. This is often referred to as "dryland". For swimming, cross-training frequently includes run-ning, stretching, and other resistance and agility training. Diving dryland exercises in-clude various unique exercises such as on-land landing biomechanics training.

Athletic Trainer

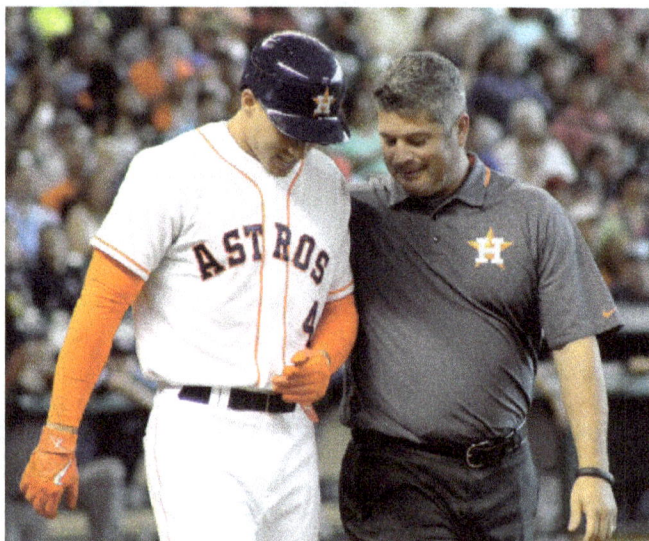

Athletic trainer Nate Lucero (*right*) evaluates Houston Astros baseball player George Springer after Springer was hit by a pitch in 2014

An athletic trainer is a certified and licensed health care professional who practices in the field of sports medicine. Athletic training has been recognized by the American Medical Association (AMA) as an allied health care profession since 1990.

As defined by the Strategic Implementation Team of the National Athletic Trainers' Association (NATA) in August 2007:

"Athletic training is practiced by athletic trainers, health care professionals who collaborate with physicians to optimize activity and quality of life for patients both of the physically active and sedentary population. Athletic training encompasses the prevention, diagnosis and intervention of emergency, acute and chronic medical conditions involving impairment, functional limitations and disabilities."

To become an athletic trainer one must have a degree from an accredited professional level education program and then sit for and pass the Board of Certification (BOC) examination. Each state then has their own regulatory agencies that control the practice of athletic training in their state. Most states (42) require an athletic trainer to obtain a license in order to practice in that state, 5 states (Colorado, Hawaii, Minnesota, Oregon, West Virginia) require registration, 2 states (New York, South Carolina) require certification, while California has no state regulations on the practice of athletic training. Areas of expertise of certified athletic trainers include:

- Apply protective or injury-preventive devices such as tape, bandages, and braces
- Recognize and evaluate injuries
- Provide first aid or emergency care
- Develop and carry out rehabilitation programs for injured athletes
- Plan and implement comprehensive programs to prevent injury and illness among athletes
- Perform administrative tasks such as keeping records and writing reports on injuries and treatment programs

Services rendered by the athletic trainer take place in a wide variety of settings and venues, including actual athletic training facilities, primary schools, universities, inpatient and outpatient physical rehabilitation clinics, hospitals, physician offices, community centers, workplaces, and even the military. Emerging settings for athletic training include surgical fellowship opportunities.

Educational Programs

The Commission on Accreditation of Athletic Training Education (CAATE) oversees the curriculum standards of all accredited Professional (entry level) and all of the institutions. The standards dictate the content of both didactic and clinical practice portions of the educational program. Content areas include:

- Risk Management and Injury Prevention
- Pathology of Injuries and Illnesses

- Orthopedic Clinical Examination and Assessment

- Medical Conditions and Disabilities

- Acute Care of Injuries and Illnesses

- Therapeutic Modalities

- Conditioning and Rehabilitative Exercises

- Psychosocial Intervention and Referral

- Nutritional Aspects of Injuries and Illnesses

- Healthcare Administration

- Professional Development and Responsibility

- Healthcare Professional Development and Responsibility

Post-professional Programs

There are several post-professional master's-level athletic training programs. These programs are for credentialed athletic trainers who desire to become scholars, researchers, and advanced practice professionals. Schools with post-professional athletic training masters programs include: A.T. Still University, University of Hawaii at Manoa, Illinois State University, Indiana State University, Indiana University, University of Kentucky, Michigan State University, Western Michigan University, University of North Carolina Chapel Hill, Ohio University, University of Oregon, California University of Pennsylvania, Temple University, Old Dominion University, University of Toledo, University of Virginia, University of Missouri, Weber State University, University of Michigan.

There are doctoral programs in athletic training, each with different curricular emphasis. Athletic training program in doctoral education is offered by the University of Idaho, A.T. Still University, and Indiana State University.

Treatment Population and Settings

Athletic trainers treat a broad population, from the amateur and professional athlete to the typical patient in need of orthopaedic rehabilitative care. The NATA describes typical clients groups as,

- Recreational, amateur and professional athletes

- Individuals who have suffered musculoskeletal injuries

- Those seeking strength, conditioning, fitness and performance enhancement

- Others designated by the physician.

Services rendered by the athletic trainer take place in a wide variety of settings and venues. These may include:

- Athletic training clinics

- Schools (K-12, colleges, universities)

- Outpatient Rehabilitation Clinics

- Hospitals

- Physician offices

- Community facilities

- Workplaces (commercial and government)

- Military installations and veteran medical facilities

- Professional sport organizations

References

- Xavier Woorons, "Hypoventilation training, push your limits!", Arpeh, 2014, 176 p (ISBN 978-2-9546040-1-5)

- Levine, BD; Stray-Gunderson, J (2001). "The effects of altitude training are mediated primarily by acclimatization rather than by hypoxic exercise". Advances in Experimental Medicine and Biology. Advances in Experimental Medicine and Biology. 502: 75–88. doi:10.1007/978-1- 4757-3401-0_7. ISBN 978-1- 4419-3374-4. PMID 11950157.

- Egan, E. (2013). Notes from higher grounds: an altitude training guide for endurance athletes. Kukimbia Huru Publishing. ISBN 978-0992755201.

- Weinberg, R.S.; Gould, D. (2010). Foundations of Sport and Exercise Psychology. Champaign, IL: Human Kinetics. ISBN 978-0-7360-8323-2.

- Hartman, Randy J. Shhh, Hypnotic Work in Progress: Twelve Case Histories in Clinical Hypnotherapy. ISBN 0595141889.

- Whyte, Gregory; Harries, Mark; Williams, Clyde (2005). ABC of sports and exercise medicine. Blackwell Publishing. pp. 46–49. ISBN 978 0 7279 1813 0.

- Prentice, William (2011). Principles of Athletic Training: A Competency-Based Approach. New York, NY: McGraw Hill. p. 29. ISBN 9780073523736.

- Gaudette, Jeff (2014-02-27). "Eat Yourself Out Of Overtraining | Page 3 of 4 | Competitor.com". Competitor.com. Retrieved 2016-05-17.

- Hoffrén-Mikkola, Merja; Ishikawa, Masaki; Rantalainen, Timo; Avela, Janne; Komi, Paavo V. (2015-05-01). "Neuromuscular mechanics and hopping training in elderly". European Journal of Applied Physiology. 115 (5): 863–877. doi:10.1007/s00421-014-3065-9. ISSN 1439-6327. PMID 25479729.

- MacKinnon, Laurel (30 May 2000). "Overtraining effects on immunity and performance in athletes". Immunology & Cell Biology. 78: 502–509. doi:10.1111/j.1440-1711.2000.t01-7-.x. Retrieved 12 April 2015.

- *Smith, Lucille (November 1999). "Cytokine hypothesis of overtraining: a physiological adaptation to excessive stress?". Medicine and Science in Sports and Exercise. Retrieved 16 April 2015.*

- *Lowery, & Forsythe, Lonnie, & Cassandra (April 19, 2006). "Protein and Overtraining: Potential Applications for Free-Living Athletes" (PDF). International Society of Sports Nutrition. Retrieved 12 April 2015.*

Treatment and Therapies of Sports Injuries

Preventive measures related to sports are a critical component for understanding sports medicine comprehensively. This chapter unfolds a plethora of preventive measures that are essential in order to deal with injuries and trauma related to sports. The following chapter serves as a source to understand the major preventive techniques like ice bath, dry needling and physical therapy to treat sports related injuries.

Physical Therapy

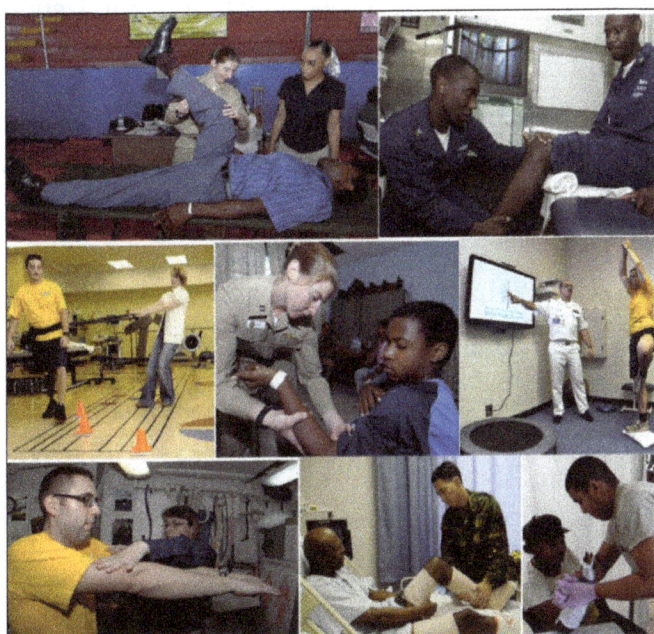

Military physical therapists working with patients on balance problems, orthopedic, amputee, Examining patient's strength, flexibility, joint range of motion balance, and gait.

Physical therapy or physiotherapy (often abbreviated to PT) is a physical medicine and rehabilitation specialty that remediates impairments and promotes mobility, function, and quality of life through examination, diagnosis, prognosis, and physical intervention (therapy using mechanical force and movements). It is carried out by physical therapists (known as physiotherapists in most countries).

In addition to clinical practice, other activities encompassed in the physical therapy profession include research, education, consultation, and administration. In many settings, physical therapy services may be provided alongside, or in conjunction with, other medical services.

Overview

Physical therapy (or Physiotherapy) involves the illnesses, or injuries that limit a person's abilities to move and perform functional activities as well as they would like in their daily lives. PTs use an individual's history and physical examination to arrive at a diagnosis and establish a management plan and, when necessary, incorporate the results of laboratory and imaging studies like X-rays, CT-scan, or MRI findings. Electrodiagnostic testing (e.g., electromyograms and nerve conduction velocity testing) may also be of assistance. PT management commonly includes prescription of or assistance with specific exercises, manual therapy and manipulation, mechanical devices such as traction, education, physical agents which includes heat, cold, electricity, sound waves, radiation, rays, prescription of assistive devices, prostheses, orthoses and other interventions. In addition, PTs work with individuals to prevent the loss of mobility before it occurs by developing fitness and wellness-oriented programs for healthier and more active lifestyles, providing services to individuals and populations to develop, maintain and restore maximum movement and functional ability throughout the lifespan. This includes providing therapeutic treatment in circumstances where movement and function are threatened by aging, injury, disease or environmental factors. Functional movement is central to what it means to be healthy.

Physical therapy is a professional career which has many specialties including sports, neurology, wound care, EMG, cardiopulmonary, geriatrics, orthopedics, women's health, and pediatrics. Neurological rehabilitation is in particular a rapidly emerging field. PTs practice in many settings, such as private-owned physical therapy clinics, outpatient clinics or offices, health and wellness clinics, rehabilitation hospitals facilities, skilled nursing facilities, extended care facilities, private homes, education and research centers, schools, hospices, industrial and this workplaces or other occupational environments, fitness centers and sports training facilities.

Physical therapists also practise in the non-patient care roles such as health policy, health insurance, health care administration and as health care executives. Physical therapists are involved in the medical-legal field serving as experts, performing peer review and independent medical examinations.

Education qualifications vary greatly by country. The span of education ranges from some countries having little formal education to others having doctoral degrees and post doctoral residencies and fellowships.

History

Exercise to shoulder and elbow to increase motion following fracture and dislocation of humerus is being given by an Army therapist to a soldier patient.

Physicians like Hippocrates and later Galen are believed to have been the first practitioners of physical therapy, advocating massage, manual therapy techniques and hydrotherapy to treat people in 460 BC. After the development of orthopedics in the eighteenth century, machines like the Gymnasticon were developed to treat gout and similar diseases by systematic exercise of the joints, similar to later developments in physical therapy. The earliest documented origins of actual physical therapy as a professional group date back to Per Henrik Ling, "Father of Swedish Gymnastics," who founded the Royal Central Institute of Gymnastics (RCIG) in 1813 for manipulation, and exercise. The Swedish word for physical therapist is *sjukgymnast* = someone involved in gymnastics for those who are ill. In 1887, PTs were given official registration by Sweden's National Board of Health and Welfare. Other countries soon followed. In 1894, four nurses in Great Britain formed the Chartered Society of Physiotherapy. The School of Physiotherapy at the University of Otago in New Zealand in 1913, and the United States' 1914 Reed College in Portland, Oregon, which graduated "reconstruction aides." Since the profession's inception, spinal manipulative therapy has been a component of the physical therapist practice.

Modern physical therapy was established towards the end of the 19th century due to events that had an effect on a global scale, which called for rapid advances in physical therapy. Soon following American orthopedic surgeons began treating children with disabilities and began employing women trained in physical education, and remedial exercise. These treatments were applied and promoted further during the Polio outbreak of 1916. During the First World War women were recruited to work with and restore physical function to injured soldiers, and the field of physical therapy was institutionalized. In 1918 the term "Reconstruction Aide" was used to refer to individuals practicing physical therapy. The first school of physical therapy was established at Walter Reed Army Hospital in Washington, D.C., following the outbreak of World War I. Research catalyzed the physical therapy movement. The first physical therapy research was published in the United States in March 1921 in "The PT Review." In the same year, Mary McMillan organized the Physical Therapy Association (now called the American Physical Therapy Association (APTA). In 1924, the Georgia Warm Springs Foundation promoted the field by touting physical therapy as a treatment for polio. Treatment through the 1940s primarily consisted of exercise, massage, and traction. Manipulative procedures to the spine and extremity joints began to be practiced, especially in the British Commonwealth countries, in the early 1950s. Around this time when polio vaccines were developed, physical therapists have become a normal occurrence in hospitals throughout North America and Europe. In the late 1950s, physical therapists started to move beyond hospital-based practice to outpatient orthopedic clinics, public schools, colleges/universities health-centres, geriatric settings (skilled nursing facilities), rehabilitation centers and medical centers. Specialization for physical therapy in the U.S. occurred in 1974, with the Orthopaedic Section of the APTA being formed for those physical therapists specializing in orthopaedics. In the same year, the International Federation of Orthopaedic Manipulative Physical Therapists was formed, which has ever since played an important role in advancing manual therapy worldwide.

Education

Educational criteria for physical therapy providers vary from state to state and from country to country, and among various levels of professional responsibility. Most U.S. states have physical therapy practice acts that recognize both physical therapists (PT) and physical therapist assistants (PTA) and some jurisdictions also recognize physical therapy technicians (PT Techs) or aides. Most countries have licensing bodies that require physical therapists to be a member of before they can start practicing as independent professionals.

Physical Therapists

United States

The primary physical therapy practitioner is the Physical Therapist (PT) who is trained and licensed to examine, evaluate, diagnose and treat impairment, functional limitations and disabilities in patients or clients. Physical Therapist education curricula in the United States culminate in a Doctor of Physical Therapy (DPT) degree, but many currently practising PTs hold a Master of Physical Therapy degree, and some still hold a Bachelor's degree. Currently the education programs for physical therapy have changed. The Master of Physical Therapy and Master of Science in Physical Therapy degrees are no longer offered, and the entry-level degree is the Doctor of Physical Therapy degree, which typically takes 3 years. PTs who hold a Masters or bachelors in PT are encouraged to get their DPT because APTA's goal is for all PT's to be on a doctoral level.[WCPT recommends physical therapist entry-level educational programs be based on university or university-level studies, of a minimum of four years, independently validated and accredited. Curricula in the United States are accredited by the Commission on Accreditation in Physical Therapy Education (CAPTE). According to CAPTE, as of 2012 there are 25,660 students currently enrolled in 210 accredited PT programs in the United States.

The physical therapist professional curriculum includes content in the clinical sciences (e.g., content about the cardiovascular, pulmonary, endocrine, metabolic, gastrointestinal, genitourinary, integumentary, musculoskeletal, and neuromuscular systems and the medical and surgical conditions frequently seen by physical therapists). Current training is specifically aimed to enable physical therapists to appropriately recognize and refer non-musculoskeletal diagnoses that may presently similarly to those caused by systems not appropriate for physical therapy intervention, which has resulted in direct access to physical therapists in many states.

Post-doctoral residency and fellowship education prevalence is increasing steadily with 219 residency, and 42 fellowship programs accredited in 2016. Residencies are aimed to train physical therapists in a specialty such as acute care, cardiovascular & pulmonary, clinical electrophysiology, faculty, geriatrics, neurology, orthopaedics, pediatrics, sports, women's health, and wound care, whereas fellowships train specialists in a sub-specialty (e.g. critical care, hand therapy, and division 1 sports), similar to the medical model. Residency programs offer eligibility to sit for the specialist certification in their respective area of practice. For example, completion of an orthopaedic physical therapy residency, allows its graduates to apply and sit for the clinical specialist examination in orthopaedics, achieving the OCS designation upon passing the examination. Board certification of physical therapy specialists is aimed to recognize individuals with advanced clinical knowledge and skill training in their respective area of practice, and exemplifies the trend toward greater education to optimally treat individuals with movement dysfunction.

Canada

Canadian Physiotherapy programs are offered at 15 Universities, often through the university's respective college of medicine. In the past decade, each of Canada's physical therapy schools has transitioned from 3-year Bachelor of Science in Physical Therapy (BScPT) programs that required 2 years of pre-requisites university courses (5-year bachelor's degree) to 2-year Master's of Physical Therapy (MPT) programs that require pre-requisite bachelor's degrees. The last Canadian university to follow suit was the University of Manitoba who transitioned to the MPT program in 2012, making the MPT credential the new entry to practice standard across Canada. Existing practitioners with BScPT credentials are not required to upgrade their qualifications.

In the province of Quebec, prospective physiotherapists are required to have completed a college diploma in either health sciences, which lasts on average two years, or physical rehabilitation technology, which lasts at least three years, to apply to a physiotherapy program or program in university. Following admission, physical therapy students work on a bachelor of science with a major in physical therapy and rehabilitation. The B.Sc. usually requires three years to complete. Students must then enter graduate school to complete a master's degree in physical therapy, which normally requires one and a half to two years of study. Graduates who obtain their M.Sc. must successfully pass the membership examination to become member of the Ordre professionnel de la physiothérapie du Québec (OPPQ). Physiotherapists can pursue their education in such fields as rehabilitation sciences, sports medicine, kinesiology, and physiology.

To date, there are no bridging programs available to facilitate upgrading from the BScPT to the MPT credential. However, research Master's of Science (MSc) and Doctor of Philosophy (PhD) programs are available at every university. Aside from academic research, practitioners can upgrade their skills and qualifications through continuing education courses and curriculums. Continuing education is a requirement of the provincial regulatory bodies.

The Canadian Alliance of Physiotherapy Regulators (CAPR), or simply known as The Alliance, offers eligible program graduates to apply for the national Physiotherapy Competency Examination (PCE). Passing the PCE is one of the requirements in most provinces and territories to work as a licensed physiotherapist in Canada. The Alliance has members which are physiotherapy regulatory organizations recognized in their respective provinces and territories:

- Government of Yukon, Consumer Services
- College of Physical Therapists of British Columbia
- Physiotherapy Alberta College + Association
- Saskatchewan College of Physical Therapists
- College of Physiotherapists of Manitoba
- College of Physiotherapists of Ontario
- Ordre professionnel de la physiothérapie du Québec
- College of Physiotherapists of New Brunswick/Collège des physiothérapeutes du Nouveau-Brunswick
- Nova Scotia College of Physiotherapists
- Prince Edward Island College of Physiotherapists
- Newfoundland & Labrador College of Physiotherapists

The Canadian Physiotherapy Association offers a curriculum of continuing education courses in orthopaedics and manual therapy. The program consists of 5 levels (7 courses) of training with ongoing mentorship and evaluation at each level. The orthopaedic curriculum and examinations takes a minimum of 4 years to complete. However, upon completion of level 2, physiotherapists can apply to a unique 1-year course-based Master's program in advanced orthopaedics and manipulation at the University of Western Ontario to complete their training. This program accepts only 16 physiotherapists annually since 2007. Successful completion of either of these education streams and their respective examinations allows physiotherapists the opportunity to apply to the Canadian Academy of Manipulative Physiotherapy (CAMPT) for fellowship. Fellows of the Canadian Academy of manipulative Physiotherapists (FCAMPT) are considered leaders in the field, having extensive post-graduate education in orthopaedics and manual therapy. FCAMPT is an internationally recognized credential, as CAMPT is a member of the International Federation of Manipulative Physiotherapists (IFOMPT), a branch of the World Confederation of Physical Therapy (WCPT) and the World Health Organization (WHO).

Physical Therapist Assistants

Physical therapist assistants may deliver treatment and physical interventions for patients and clients under a care plan established by and under the supervision of a physical therapist. Physical therapist assistants in the United States are currently trained under associate of applied sciences curricula specific to the profession, as outlined and accredited by CAPTE. As of August 2011, there were 276 accredited two-year (Associate degree) programs for physical therapist assistants In the United States of America. According to CAPTE, as of 2012 there are 10,598 students currently enrolled in 280 accredited PTA programs in the United States.

Curricula for the physical therapist assistant associate degree include:

- Anatomy & physiology
- Exercise physiology
- Human biology
- Physics
- Biomechanics
- Kinesiology
- Neuroscience
- Clinical pathology
- Behavioral sciences
- Communication
- Ethics
- Research
- Other coursework as required by individual programs.

Physical Therapy Technicians or Aides

Some jurisdictions allow physical therapists to employ technicians or aides or therapy assistants to perform designated routine tasks related to physical therapy under the direct supervision of a physical therapist. Some jurisdictions require physical therapy technicians or aides to be certified, and education and certification requirements vary among jurisdictions.

Canada

In the province of Quebec, physical rehabilitation therapists are health care professionals who are required to complete a three-year college diploma program in physical rehabilitation therapy and be member of the *Ordre professionnel de la physiothérapie du Québec* (OPPQ) in order to practise legally in the country.

Most physical rehabilitation therapists complete their college diploma at Collège Montmorency, Dawson College, or Cégep Marie-Victorin, all situated in and around the Montreal area.

After completing their technical college diploma, graduates have the opportunity to pursue their studies at the university level to perhaps obtain a bachelor's degree in physiotherapy, kinesiology, exercise science, or occupational therapy. The Université de Montréal and the Université de Sherbrooke are among the Québécois universities that admit physical rehabilitation therapists in their programs of study related to health sciences and rehabilitation in order to credit courses that were completed in college.

United States

Job duties and education requirements for Physical Therapy Technicians or Aides may vary depending on the employer, but education requirements range from high school diploma or equivalent to completion of a 2-year degree program. O-Net reports that 64% of PT Aides/Techs have a high school diploma or equivalent, 21% have completed some college but do not hold a degree, and 10% hold an associate degree.

Employment

Physical therapy-related jobs in North America have shown rapid growth in recent years, but employment rates and average wages may vary significantly between different countries, states, provinces or regions.

United States of America

According to the United States Department of Labor's Bureau of Labor Statistics, there were approximately 198,600 Physical Therapists employed in the United States in 2010, earning an average $76,310 annually, or $36.69 per hour, with 39% growth in employment projected by the year 2020. The Bureau of Labor Statistics also reports that there were approximately 114,400 Physical Therapist Assistants and Aides employed in the United States in 2010, earning an average $37,710 annually, or $18.13 per hour, with 45% growth in employment projected by the year 2020. To meet their needs, many healthcare and physical therapy facilities hire "Travel physical therapists", who work temporary assignments between 8 and 26 weeks for much higher wages; about $113,500 a year. Bureau of Labor Statistics data on PTAs and Techs can be difficult to decipher, due to their tendency to report data on these job fields collectively rather than separately. O-Net reports that in 2011, PTAs in the United States earned a median wage of $51,040 annually or $24.54 hourly, and that Aides/Techs earned a median wage of $23,680 annually or $11.39 hourly in 2011.

Specialty Areas

The body of knowledge of physical therapy is large, and therefore physical therapists may specialize in a specific clinical area. While there are many different types of physical therapy, the American Board of Physical Therapy Specialties lists nine current specialist certifications, the ninth, Oncology, pending for its first examination in 2019. Most Physical Therapists practicing in a specialty will have undergone further training, such as an accredited residency program, although individuals are currently able to sit for their specialist examination after 2,000 hours of focused practice in their respective specialty population, in addition to requirements set by each respective specialty board.

Cardiovascular & Pulmonary Physiotherapy

Cardiovascular and pulmonary rehabilitation respiratory practitioners and physical therapists offer therapy for a wide variety of cardiopulmonary disorders or pre and post cardiac or pulmonary surgery. An example of cardiac surgery is coronary bypass surgery. Primary goals of this specialty include increasing endurance and functional independence. Manual therapy is used in this field to assist in clearing lung secretions experienced with cystic fibrosis. Pulminary disorders, heart attacks, post coronary bypass surgery, chronic obstructive pulmonary disease, and pulmonary fibrosis, treatments can benefit from cardiovascular and pulmonary specialized physical therapists.

Clinical Electrophysiology

This specialty area includes electrotherapy/physical agents, electrophysiological evaluation (EMG/NCV), physical agents, and wound management.

Geriatric

Geriatric physical therapy covers a wide area of issues concerning people as they go through normal adult aging but is usually focused on the older adult. There are many conditions that affect many people as they grow older and include but are not limited to the following: arthritis, osteoporosis, cancer, Alzheimer's disease, hip and joint replacement, balance disorders, incontinence, etc. Geriatric physical therapists specialize in providing therapy for such conditions in older adults.

Integumentary

Integumentary physical therapy includes the treatment of conditions involving the skin and all its related organs. Common conditions managed include wounds and burns. Physical therapists may utilize surgical instruments, wound irrigations, dressings and topical agents to remove the damaged or contaminated tissue and promote tissue healing. Other commonly used interventions include exercise, edema control, splinting, and compression garments. The work done by physical therapists in the integumentary specialty do work similar to what would be done by medical doctors or nurses in the emergency room or triage.

Neurological

Neurological physical therapy is a field focused on working with individuals who have a neurological disorder or disease. These can include stroke, chronic back pain, Alzheimer's disease, Charcot-Marie-Tooth disease (CMT), ALS, brain injury, cerebral palsy, l.g.b. syndrome, multiple sclerosis, Parkinson's disease, facial palsy and spinal cord injury. Common impairments associated with neurologic conditions include impairments of vision, balance, ambulation, activities of daily living, movement, muscle strength and loss of functional independence. The techniques involve in neurological physical therapy are wide ranging and often require specialized training.

Neurological physiotherapy is also called neurophysiotherapy or neurological rehabilitation.

Orthopedic

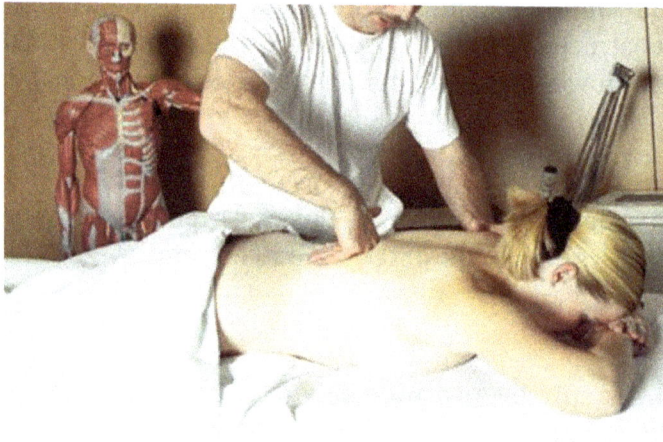

Treatment by orthopedic physical therapists

Orthopedic physical therapists diagnose, manage, and treat disorders and injuries of the musculoskeletal system including rehabilitation after orthopedic surgery. acute trauma such as sprains, strains, and injuries of insidious onset such as tendinopathy and bursitis. This speciality of physical therapy is most often found in the out-patient clinical setting. Orthopedic therapists are trained in the treatment of post-operative orthopedic procedures, fractures, acute sports injuries, arthritis, sprains, strains, back and neck pain, spinal conditions, and amputations.

Joint and spine mobilization/manipulation, dry needling (similar to acupuncture), therapeutic exercise, neuromuscular techniques, muscle reeducation, hot/cold packs, and electrical muscle stimulation (e.g., cryotherapy, iontophoresis, electrotherapy) are modalities employed to expedite recovery in the orthopedic setting. Additionally, an emerging adjunct to diagnosis and treatment is the use of sonography for diagnosis and to guide treatments such as muscle retraining. Those who have suffered injury or disease affecting the muscles, bones, ligaments, or tendons will benefit from assessment by a physical therapist specialized in orthopedics.

Pediatric

Pediatric physical therapy assists in early detection of health problems and uses a limited variety of modalities to provide physical therapy for disorders in the pediatric population. These therapists are specialized in the diagnosis, treatment, and management of infants, children, and adolescents with a variety of congenital, developmental, neuromuscular, skeletal, or acquired disorders/diseases. Treatments focus mainly on improving gross and fine motor skills, balance and coordination, strength and endurance as well as cognitive and sensory processing/integration.

Sports

Physical therapists are closely involved in the care and wellbeing of athletes including recreational, semi-professional (paid) and professional (full-time employment) participants. This area of practice encompasses athletic injury management under 5 main categories:

- acute care - assessment and diagnosis of an initial injury;

- treatment - application of specialist advice and techniques to encourage healing;

- rehabilitation - progressive management for full return to sport;

- prevention - identification and address of deficiencies known to directly result in, or act as precursors to injury, such as movement assessment

- education - sharing of specialist knowledge to individual athletes, teams or clubs to assist in prevention or management of injury

Physical therapists who work for professional sport teams often have a specialized sports certification issued through their national registering organisation. Most Physical therapists who practice in a sporting environment are also active in collaborative sports medicine programs too.

Women's Health

Women's health physical therapy mostly addresses women's issues related to the female reproductive system, child birth, and post-partum. These conditions include lymphedema, osteoporosis, pelvic pain, prenatal and post-partum periods, and urinary incontinence. It also addresses incontinence, pelvic pain, and other disorders associated with pelvic floor dysfunction. Manual physical therapy has been demonstrated in multiple studies to increase rates of conception in women with infertility.

Palliative care

Physiotherapy in the field of oncology and palliative care is a continuously evolving and developing specialty, both in malignant and non-malignant diseases. Rehabilitation for both groups of patients is now recognized as an essential part of the clinical pathway, as early diagnoses and new treatments are enabling patients to live longer. it is generally accepted that patients should have access to an appropriate level of rehabilitation, so that they can function at a minimum level of dependency and optimize their quality of life, regardless of their life expectancy.

Effectiveness

A 2012 systematic review found evidence to support the use of spine manipulation by physical therapists as a safe option to improve outcomes for low back pain. A 2015 systematic review suggested that spine manipulation and therapeutic massage are effective interventions for neck pain; it also suggested, however, that electroacupuncture, strain-counterstrain, relaxation massage, heat therapy and ultrasound therapy are not effective and thus not recommended for the treatment of neck pain.

United States

Definitions and licensing requirements in the United States vary among jurisdictions, as each state has enacted its own physical therapy practice act defining the profession within its jurisdiction, but the American Physical Therapy Association (APTA) has also drafted a model definition in order to limit this variation, and the APTA is also responsible for accrediting physical therapy education curricula throughout the United States of America.

Ice Bath

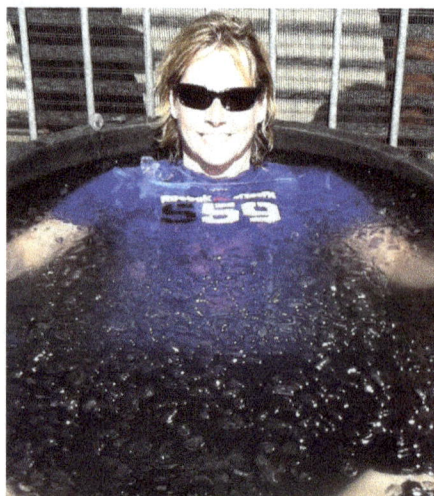

Champion weightlifter Karyn Marshall taking an ice bath after the Crossfit Games in 2011.

In sports therapy, an ice bath, or sometimes cold-water immersion or Cold Therapy, is a training regimen usually following a period of intense exercise in which a substantial part of a human body is immersed in a bath of ice or ice-water for a limited duration. While it is becoming increasingly popular and accepted among athletes in a variety of sports, the method is controversial and potentially dangerous, with little solid scientific evidence to support or refute its usefulness or to understand its method of operation within the body (although there is speculation about processes within the body regarding vasoconstriction). In medicine, the practice would be classified as cryotherapy which uses low temperatures as medical therapy.

History

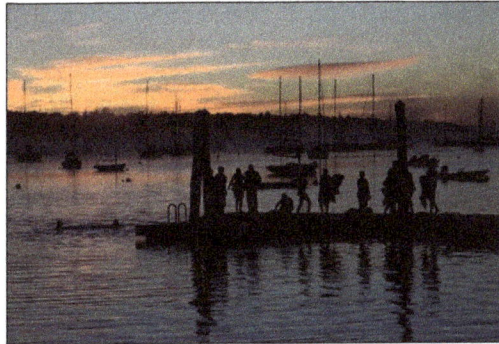

A Polar Bear Club in Massachusetts.

There have been traditions of people ice swimming in the middle of winter on a lake for short stretches, sometimes as part of a Polar Bear Club. Sometimes people taking short swims for thirty seconds or so have felt invigorated afterwards. The Coney Island Polar Bear Club was founded in 1903. A Polar Bear member explained:

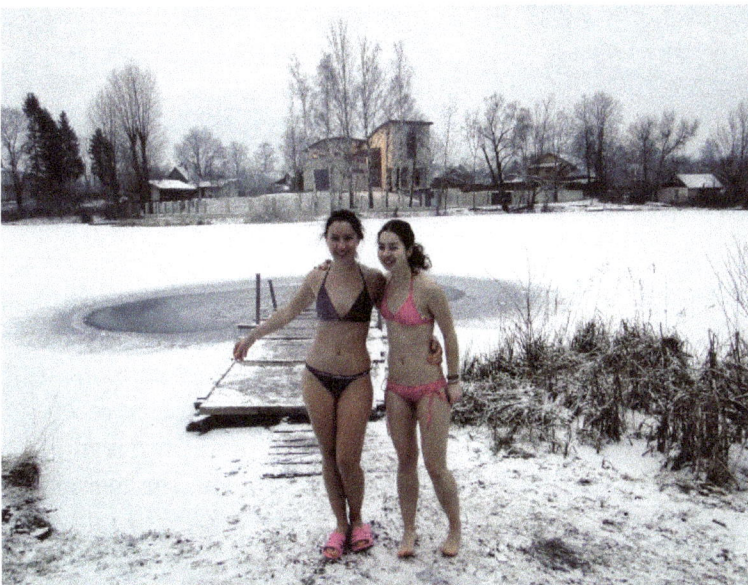

Two Russian women preparing to bathe in the lake.

It is definitely stimulating. Your feet freeze, your voice changes a few octaves and if you're a man you freeze your balls off.

—*Mike Kahlenberg, 2006*

In the 1890s, Russian immigrant Professor Louis Sugarman of Little Falls, New York, brought his practice of ice bathing to the United States. He attracted worldwide attention for his daily plunge in the Mohawk River, even when the thermostat hit 23 below zero, earning him the nickname "the human polar bear".

In 1899, an Iowa woman filed for divorce from her husband because he had forced her to undergo ice baths. There has been a tradition in American football of pouring a large bucket of ice water on the winning coach as a victory celebration. And physical therapists have applied ice packs to selected areas of the body to prevent swelling.

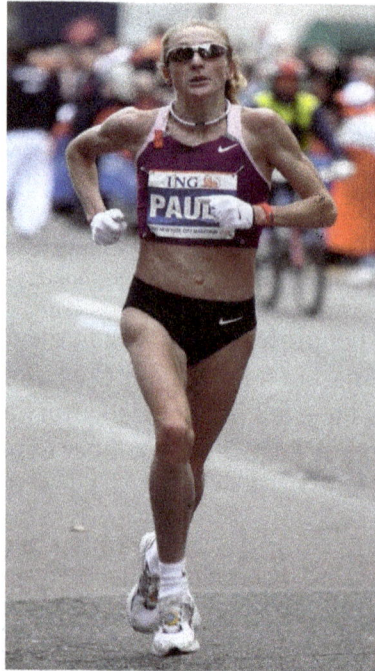

Long distance champion Paula Radcliffe is believed to have popularized its use after her victory in Europe in 2002.

Until recently, however, bathing in ice was seen as unusual. One account suggested that ice bath therapy did not become popular until 2002, when marathon runner Paula Radcliffe won the championship in Europe and attributed her victory to its use. She reportedly said "It's absolute agony, and I dread it, but it allows my body to recover so much more quickly." She reported taking ice baths before racing and preferred her pre-race bath temperature to be "very cold." After the Radcliffe comment, the technique has grown in popularity. It is gaining in popularity among athletes, such that some athletes "swear by it" but other accounts suggest it may be a fad. It has been used by athletes such as A. J. Soares and Olympic swimmer Michael Phelps as well as other celebrity endorsers and is getting to become "common practice" among athletes from different sports, including American football, association football (soccer), long distance running, rugby, tennis, volleyball, and other sports. There was a report that sports equipment manufacturers are considering different designs for ice baths. In the summer of 2014, as a fundraising method, the nonprofit ALS Association, which raises money for research and public awareness of amyotrophic lateral sclerosis or ALS, also known as Lou Gehrig's Disease, began the Ice Bucket Challenge which involved donors filming themselves and challenging other donors to participate and then being doused with a bucket of ice cold water; as a fundraising effort, it raised $16 million over a 22-day period.

There are indications that ice baths may be gaining popularity with groups outside sports, such as dance. The *Pittsburgh Post-Gazette* reported that some Radio City Rockettes, a precision dance company performing in New York City, use ice baths after a long day of performing as a way to "unwind" and cope with "aches and pains." One report suggested that entertainer Madonna used ice baths after her performances. And there are indications that use of ice baths is spreading to amateur sports, such as high school football.

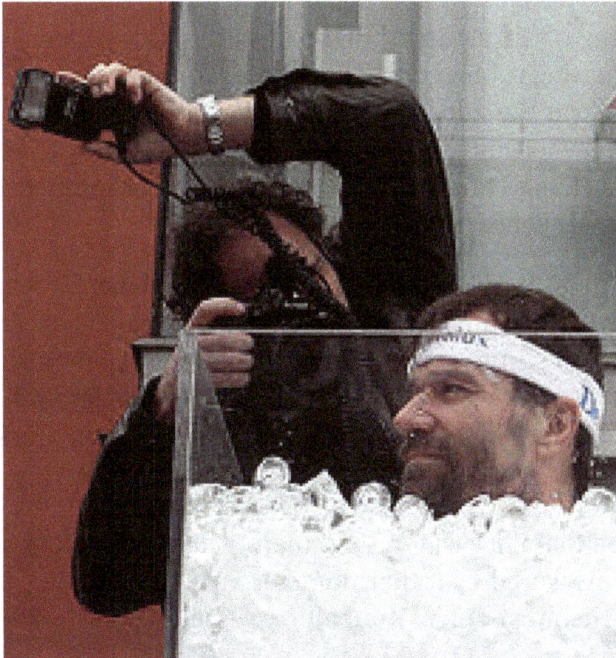

Iceman Wim Hof in an ice bath in 2007.

Ice baths are a part of a broader phenomenon known as cryotherapy––the Greek word *cryo* means *cold*––which describes a variety of treatments when cold temperatures are used therapeutically. Cryotherapy includes procedures where a person is placed in a room with "cold, dry air at temperatures as low as −135 °C" for short periods of time, and which has been used in hospitals in Poland as well as a center in London to treat not only muscular ailments, but psychological problems such as depression.

Basketball player Manny Harris reportedly used a Cryon-X machine featuring extreme low temperatures around minus 166 degrees Fahrenheit, but used it with wet socks resulting in a serious freezer burn.

Occasionally ice baths have been an ill-advised treatment of fever in young children, but that doctors were counseled not to use this technique because of the risk of hypothermia. Ice baths have been suggested as a way to prevent muscle soreness after shoveling snow.

In addition, there have been instances of ice bathing as an extreme bodily test by persons vying for an endurance record, such as Dutch *Iceman* Wim Hof, and Chinese record-holders Chen Kecai and Jin Songhao. According to reports, doctors and scientists are studying how these people can spend an hour and a half submerged in an ice bath, and survive; for almost all humans, such tasks are impossible.

Method of Operation

Bath

It is done by standing or sitting in a bucket or bath of icy water. One writer advised: "don't overdo it." Wearing rubberized "dive booties" on the feet (to protect toes) as well as rubber briefs to warm the midsection have been recommended. Champion weightlifter Karyn Marshall, who won the world women's weightlifting championship in 1987, described what it was like to take an ice bath after a day of competition at the CrossFit Games in 2011 in Los Angeles:

The first day I went in for twelve minutes, and the second day for fifteen minutes. They kept adding ice to keep the temperature at around 55 degrees (Fahrenheit) ... The hardest part was the first two minutes. Others who do it often told me to just hang in for two minutes and then it would be easier. After two minutes I was numb. Afterwards I was shivering for two hours in the hot California sun with a warm up jacket on.

— *Karyn Marshall, 2011*

One report suggested that if ice water is circulating, it's even colder such that the water will be colder than measured by a thermometer, and that athletes should avoid overexposure. Physical therapist Nikki Kimball explained a way to make the bath more endurable:

Over those years, I've discovered tricks to make the ice bath experience more tolerable. First, I fill my tub with two to three bags of crushed ice. Then I add cold water to a height that will cover me nearly to my waist when I sit in the tub. Before getting in, I put on a down jacket and a hat and neoprene booties, make myself a cup of hot tea, and collect some entertaining reading material to help the next 15 to 20 minutes pass quickly.

— *Runner's World, 2008*

Ice Bath Only Versus Contrast Bath Therapy

Accounts differ whether it is best to follow the ice bath with a hot shower; two accounts suggested that a hot shower followed by a massage would be helpful, but other reports counsel against such a practice. There are reports that some athletes use this technique, sometimes known as contrast water therapy or contrast bath therapy, in which cold water and warmer water are alternated. One method of doing this was to have two tubs—one cold (10–15 degrees Celsius) and another hot (37–40 degrees Celsius)—and to do one minute in the cold tub followed by two minutes in a hot tub, and to repeat this procedure three times.

Temperature and Timing

The temperature can vary, but is usually in the range of 50–59 degrees Fahrenheit or between 12 and 15 degrees Celsius. Some athletes wear booties to keep their toes warm or rubberized coverings around their midsection while immersed. Some drink a warm beverage such as tea. One report suggested that "ten minutes immersed in 15 degree Celsius water" was sufficient.

Accounts vary about how long to be immersed and how often to do them. One adviser suggested that an athlete should take ten two-minute ice bath treatments over a two-week period. One account suggested immersion times should be between ten and twenty minutes. Another suggested that immersion run from five to ten minutes, and sometimes to twenty minutes. There were no sources advocating being immersed for longer than twenty minutes.

Ice Baths Versus Cold Baths

Several sources suggest that cold baths (60–75 degrees Fahrenheit) were preferable to ice baths. Physiotherapist Tony Wilson of the University of Southampton said that extremely cold temperatures were unnecessary and a "cold bath" would be just as effective as an ice bath. Another agreed that a mere cold bath is preferable to ice baths which are "unnecessary." A third report suggested that cool water (60–75 degrees Fahrenheit) was just as good as cold water (54–60 degrees Fahrenheit) and that eight to ten minutes should be sufficient time, and warned against exceeding ten minutes.

Medical Efficacy

There is theoretical speculation, although unproven, about how the ice bath technique might operate, as well as differing accounts about how the technique is supposed to help the human body. A common theme is that the cold prompts the body to recover faster from an intense period of activity. According to several accounts, the cold in the ice bath signals temperature receptors to alert the brain to "withdraw blood to the body's core". According to another account, after five to ten minutes, the "icy cold water causes your blood vessels to tighten and drains the blood out of your legs."

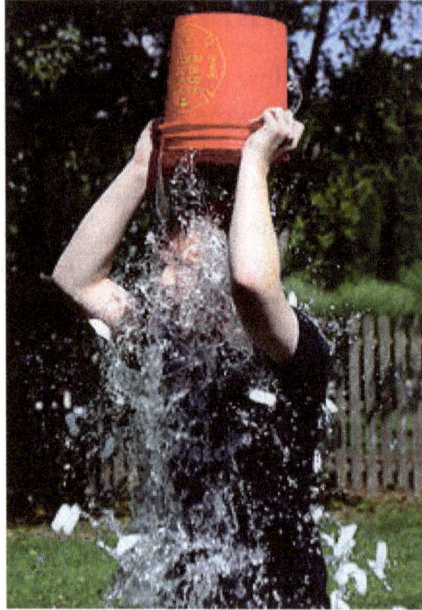

In summer 2014, the Ice Bucket Challenge went viral on social media to raise money
for the ALS Association.

Another report suggested that it causes metabolic activity to slow. After getting out of
the ice bath, the blood is pumped "vigorously" back to tissues "stimulating oxygen and
nutrient supply to areas that need revitalising," according to several assessments, and
another suggests that blood flow is sped up, sometimes described as a "blood rush." A
report along these same lines suggested that the benefit came from after the ice bath
with "increased blood flow" bringing fresh nutrients to an "inflamed, injured area"
which helps the tissues heal. A slightly different explanation was that cold causes the
diameters of blood vessels to contract during the period of immersion in the ice water,
meaning that more toxins were pumped out of the area, similar to a massage. And blood
is a way to bring oxygen to the cells as well as remove waste products from muscular
exertion, particularly lactic acid. Here is one description of how it is believed to work:

The muscles will cool and relax after a few minutes in the bath. At the end of the bath
you will experience a strong flush of blood circulating through the muscles that were submerged. This sudden increase in circulation speeds up and improves the quality of muscle recovery by quickly flushing out the lactic acids that have built up in the tired muscles.

— *Tilman von der Linde in The Vancouver Sun, 2009*

Ice baths are generally believed to be a way to help the body recover from a vigorous workout, with one account suggesting helpful effects not only for muscles, but for tendons,
bones, nerves, and other tissues as well. An advantage cited is that cold-water immersion
is a more "efficient means of cooling large groups of muscles simultaneously" and helps
lead to "longer lasting changes in deep tissues." A second report echoed this view and
suggested that "immersion allows controlled, even constriction around all muscles."

Ice baths have been a source of medical treatment when a person is suffering from heat illness, and when this happens, sufferers are urged to get into an air conditioned room quickly or get into an ice bath.

Benefits

Benefits are speculative but include the following:

- Prevents injury.

- Speeds recovery. According to one report, it is believed to decrease the amount of time needed by the muscles of athletes to return to top condition between training sessions.

- Keeps muscles limber. One account suggested it would reduce muscle soreness after heavy exertion, such as after snow shoveling.

- Repairs muscles.

- Reduces inflammation. But one account disputes there is any benefit in fighting inflammation. However, according to Greg Whyte of the English Institute of Sport, inflammation may be good for the body and act as an "important and beneficial part of the muscle's response to training."

- Less muscle soreness.

- Less muscle pain.

- Less muscle stiffness.

- Treatment for heat-related illnesses such as heat stroke.

Some persons who refrain from sex or marriage by choice, sometimes called celibates, have used ice-cold baths as a method of trying to cope with sexual frustration. During the 19th century, similar cold baths were sometimes used as a supposed treatment for the condition of nymphomania.

Drawbacks

- Risk of breathing difficulties.

- Possibly medically dangerous. There are reports that "exposing yourself to pro-longed cold" may result in hypothermia or frostbite or shock and that sudden exposure to extreme cold could harm patients with heart problems or airway diseases such as asthma and possibly lead to sudden death. One doctor explained:

From a medical perspective there are two main risks from the cold - hypothermia and frostbite. It's not that difficult to get either of these if exposed to cold for a period of time.

— *Dr. Lisa Silver*

Scientific Investigation

The consensus view is that there is little solid scientific research to support a case that ice baths are either beneficial or detrimental for athletes. Professor Kenneth L. Knight of Brigham Young University said there is no evidence to either support or refute the claim that ice-bath treatments, or cryotherapy methods in general, reduces inflammation. Runner's World.com executive editor Mark Remy believes that ice-bath treatments are "bunk" opining that it is an "elaborate practical joke being played on runners." Physiotherapist Chris Bleakley of the University of Ulster reported that there are "no high-level scientific studies that say this is good for the body" although he admitted that athletes had been reporting positive results, and that there is considerable anecdotal evidence from athletes that it makes them "feel better." In contrast, one report suggested that there was scientific research showing that ice baths promote recovery, but no specific studies were cited. There have been smaller-scale studies which either indicate no benefit or a detrimental effect, or that offer "inconclusive or contradictory findings." A report in *The New York Times* suggested that there had been "little study" of cold therapy versus other treatment regimens such as compression sleeves or ibuprofen. There have been reports that suggest that cryotherapy used before training can reduce the amount of lactic acid produced by the muscles and "speed up its removal" afterwards.

Cochrane Survey

A 2012 systemic database review was conducted of either fourteen or seventeen existing studies of 366 subjects which compared cold-water immersion following exercise with doing nothing or resting as a way to prevent subsequent muscle soreness. Study variables included the level of soreness, cold water immersion versus no treatment, intensity and duration of exercise, time between exercise and measurement of soreness, and other variables. The authors found evidence that cold water immersion had a slight effect on reducing soreness, not immediately after exercise but at intervals of up to 96 hours after exercise, and that it lowered levels of fatigue and sped up physical recovery, although they noted that these studies did not examine other variables such as possible negative effects on the body. The authors concluded that high quality research was required.

Australian Study

A study by Australian researchers, publishing in the *British Journal of Sports Medicine* on a small sample size, suggested that ice bath therapy may "do more harm than good." The team asked 40 volunteers to undergo leg exercises and gave half ice baths and the other half a dip in tepid water. Researchers measured pain levels, swelling, performance in a "hopping test" and blood chemicals which might indicate damage to muscles, and found no statistically important differences between the two groups, except that the ice therapy treated volunteers experienced more muscular pain in the leg upon standing from seated position compared to the control group (median change on a 0–100 mm visual analog pain scale of 8.0 vs 2.0 mm, respectively, p = 0.009). The study found that:

Ice-water immersion offers no benefit for pain, swelling, isometric strength and function, and in fact may make more athletes sore the next day.

—*British Journal of Sports Medicine, 2007*

Study of Cyclists

One study in 2008 in the *International Journal of Sports Medicine* suggested that cold water immersion and contrast water therapy might help in situations where athletes engaged in "high intensity efforts on successive days", such as weightlifters in a multi-day competition. Researchers studied cyclists during a week of intense training and found that they performed better with these methods than complete rest or hot water baths.

Leg Press Study

A study in 2007 reported in the *Journal of Strength and Conditioning Research* found that contrast water therapy delayed the onset of muscle soreness after "intense leg press exercise" and found "faster restoration of strength and power in athletes" who used this therapy instead of a merely "passive recovery."

English Institute of Sport Study

This study suggested that ice baths could help top athletes recover faster during a peak competition but that such methods should not be used during training since it limits the "growth and strengthening of muscle fibers." The authors of the study, including physiologist Jonathan Leeder, counseled against ice bath treatments during training.

Dry Needling

Dry needling (Myofascial Trigger Point Dry Needling) is the use of either solid filiform needles (also referred to as acupuncture needles) or hollow-core hypodermic needles for therapy of muscle pain, including pain related to myofascial pain syndrome. Dry needling is sometimes also known as intramuscular stimulation (IMS). Acupuncture is a broad category of needling practices with solid filiform needles. The comparisons between dry needling and acupuncture were well-summarized by Zhou et al. Modern acupuncture notably includes both traditional and Western medical acupuncture; dry needling is arguably one subcategory of western medical acupuncture.

Chinese style tendinomuscular acupuncture relies on careful palpation of what are called "Ah Shi" points, which often correspond to both trigger points and/or motor points in the myofascial tissue. Chinese style tendinomuscular acupuncture tends to use the lower gauge needles necessary for puncturing contraction knots with a high degree of precision. On the other hand, lighter styles of acupuncture, such as Japanese style, and many American styles, may tend towards very shallow insertions of higher gauge needles. Most acupuncture styles, especially those with lighter techniques, require a detailed knowledge, not only of western anatomy, but also of the channel networks and connections. Thus, while some forms of acupuncture are not at all the same as dry needling, the term dry needling can refer quite specifically to what is now called Myofascial Acupuncture, Tendinomuscular Acupuncture, or some version of Sports Acupuncture.

Origin

The origin of the term "dry needling" is attributed to Janet G. Travell, M.D. In her book, 'Myofascial Pain and Dysfunction: Trigger Point Manual', Dr. Travell uses the term "dry needling" to differentiate between two hypodermic needle techniques when performing trigger point therapy. However, Dr. Travell did not elaborate on the details on the techniques of dry needling; the current techniques of dry needling were based on the traditional and western medical acupuncture. The two techniques Dr. Travell described are the injection of a local anesthetic and the mechanical use of a hypodermic needle without injecting a solution (Travell, Simons, & Simons, 1999, pp. 154–155). Dr. Travell preferred a 22-gauge, 1.5-in hypodermic needle for trigger point therapy and used this needle for both injection therapy and dry needling. Dr. Travell never used an acupuncture needle. Dr. Travell had access to acupuncture needles but reasoned that they were far too thin for trigger point therapy. She preferred hypodermic needles because of their strength and tactile feedback: "A 22-gauge, 3.8-cm (1.5-in) needle is usually suitable for most superficial muscles. In hyperalgesic patients a 25-gauge, 3.8-cm (1.5-in) needle may cause less discomfort, but will not provide the clear "feel" of the structures being penetrated by needle and is more likely to be deflected by the dense contraction knots that are the target... A 27-gauge needle, 3.8-cm (1.5-in) needle is even more flexible; the tip is more likely to be deflected by the contraction knots and it provides less tactile feedback for precision injection" (Travell, Simons, & Simons, 1999, p. 156).

The use of a hypodermic needle for dry needling was described by Dr. Chang-Zern Hong in his research paper on "Lidocaine Injection Verses Dry Needling to Myofascial Trigger Point". In his research, he describes the procedure for trigger point injection and dry needling by using a 27-gauge hypodermic needle 1 ¼-in long (Hong, 1994).

Both Travell and Hong used hypodermic needles for dry needling. Dr. Hong, like Dr. Travell, did not use an acupuncture needle for dry needling.

Although dry needling originally utilized only hypodermic needles due to the concern that solid needles had neither the strength or tactile feedback that hypodermic needles provided and that the needle could be deflected by "dense contraction knots", those concerns have proven unfounded and many healthcare practitioners who perform dry needling have found that the acupuncture needles not only provides better tactile feedback but also penetrate the "dense muscle knots" better and are easier to manage and caused less discomfort to patients. For that reason both the use of hypodermic needles and the use of acupuncture needles are now accepted in dry needling practice. Ofttimes practitioners who use hypodermic needles also provide trigger point injection treatment to patients and therefore find the use of hypodermic needles a better choice. As their use became more common, some dry needling practitioners without acupuncture in their scope of practice, started to refer to these needles by their technical design term as "solid filiform needles" as opposed to the FDA designation "acupuncture needle."

The "solid filiform needle" used in dry needling is regulated by the FDA as a Class II medical device described in the code titled "Sec. 880.5580 Acupuncture needle" as "a device intended to pierce the skin in the practice of acupuncture." Per the Food and Drug Act of 1906 and the subsequent Amendments to said act, the FDA definition applies to how the needles can be marketed and does not mean that acupuncture is the only medical procedure where these needles can be used. Dry needling using such a needle contrasts with the use of a hollow hypodermic needle to inject substances such as saline solution, botox or corticosteroids to the same point. Such use of a solid needle has been found to be as effective as injection of substances in such cases as relief of pain in muscles and connective tissue. Analgesia produced by needling a pain spot has been called the *needle effect*.

The founder of Dry Needling Academy, Dr. Piyush Jain (PhD Scholar) states Dry Needling as methods which can help in providing the healthcare professionals a great tool to serve their patients with great result in conjunction to other therapeutic modalities. No treatment protocol can work without a proper assessment of the patients, the need of clinical reasoning with proper assessment tools are the basic necessity of the therapist. As Per American Academy of Orthopedic Manual Physical Therapists (AAOMPT)

Dry needling is a neurophysiological evidence-based treatment technique that requires effective manual assessment of the neuromuscular system. Physical therapists are well trained to utilize dry needling in conjunction with manual physical therapy interventions. Research supports that dry needling improves pain control, reduces muscle tension, normalizes biochemical and electrical dysfunction of motor end plates, and facilitates an accelerated return to active rehabilitation.

The statement above is self-explanatory on the functional, physiological and medical aspect of treatment. His book Manual of Dry Needling Techniques Color Edition (2) (Volume 1) is a basic reference text for the therapists who are trained in the method of dry needling procedures in accordance to norm of practice of their respective countries. The basic steps given in the book can make a practicing therapist to use dry needling technique for the subjects in different clinical conditions. The text focus not only on the steps needed to be performed but also focus on what should not be done by a therapist while performing the procedure. At work we have taken all the guidelines given by OSHA for blood borne diseases as well as WHO guideline on workplace and hand hygiene.

Dry needling for the treatment of myofascial (muscular) trigger points is based on theories similar, but not exclusive, to traditional acupuncture; both acupuncture and dry needling target the trigger points, which is a direct and palpable source of patient pain. However, dry needling theory is only beginning to describe the complex sensation referral patterns that have been documented as "channels" or "meridians" in Chinese Medicine. Dry needling, and its treatment techniques and desired effects, would be most directly comparable to the use of 'a-shi' points in acupuncture. What further distinguishes dry needling from traditional acupuncture is that it does not use the full range of traditional theories of Chinese Medicine which is used to treat not only pain, but other non muscular-skeletal issues which often are the cause of pain. The distinction between trigger points and acupuncture points for the relief of pain is blurred. As reported by Melzack, et al., there is a high degree of correspondence (71% based on their analysis) between published locations of trigger points and classical acupuncture points for the relief of pain. The debated distinction between dry needling and acupuncture has become a controversy because it relates to an issue of scope of practice of various professions.

Technique

In the treatment of trigger points for persons with myofascial pain syndrome, dry needling is an invasive procedure in which a filiform needle is inserted into the skin and muscle directly at a myofascial trigger point. A myofascial trigger point consists of multiple contraction knots, which are related to the production and maintenance of the pain cycle. Deep dry needling for treating trigger points was first introduced by Czech physician Karel Lewit in 1979. Lewit had noticed that the success of injections into trigger points in relieving pain was apparently unconnected to the analgesic used.

Proper dry needling of a myofascial trigger point will elicit a local twitch response (LTR), which is an involuntary spinal cord reflex in which the muscle fibers in the taut band of muscle contract. The LTR indicates the proper placement of the needle in a trigger point. Dry needling that elicits LTRs improves treatment outcomes, and may work by activating endogenous opioids. The activation of the endogenous opioids is for an analgesic effect using the Gate Control Theory of Pain. Inserting the needle can itself cause considerable pain, although when done by well-trained practitioners that is not a common occurrence. No study to date has reported the reliability of trigger point diagnosis and physical diagnosis cannot be recommended as a reliable test for the diagnosis of trigger points.

Efficacy

There is currently no standardized form of dry needling, no body of evidence that indicates its efficacy, and there is no medical action pathway that provides a theoretical basis for why dry needling should be efficacious. Many of the studies published about dry needling do not have strong evidence; either the studies were not randomized, contained small sample sizes, had high dropout rates, used active interventions in the control group, did not follow the minimally acceptable criteria for diagnosing a myofascial trigger point, or did not clearly state that myofascial trigger points were the sole cause for the pain. For example, in a systematic review on needling therapies in the management of myofascial trigger points, only 8 of the 23 trials described the minimally acceptable criteria for diagnosing a trigger point. Locating the trigger point for dry needling is the basis for performing dry needling and should therefore be documented in each study performing this technique. In the same review, two studies tested the efficacy beyond placebo of dry needling in the treatment of myofascial trigger point pain, but, in one, the dropout rate was 48% and it was neither blinded nor randomized, and the other study used potentially active interventions in the control group. Another concluded that dry needling can reduce pain, thus improving mood, function, and disability. The study used the dry needling on trigger points to relieve pain in patients with chronic myofascial pain.

Another systematic review concluded that dry needling for the treatment of myofascial pain syndrome in the lower back appeared to be a useful addition to standard therapies, but that clear recommendations could not be made because the published studies are small and of low quality. A 2007 meta-analysis examining dry needling of myofascial trigger points concluded that the effect of needling was not significantly different to that of placebo controls, though the trend in the results could be compatible with a treatment effect. One study (Lorenzo et al. 2004) did show a short-term reduction in shoulder pain in stroke patients who received needling with standard rehabilitation compared to those who received standard care alone, but the study was open-label and measurement timings differed, limiting the use of the study. Again the small sample size and poor quality of studies was highlighted. A recent systemic review and meta analysis released by JOSPT on "effectiveness of dry needling for upper-quarter myofascial pain" recommends the usage of dry needling, compared to sham or placebo, for decreasing pain immediately after treatment and at 4 weeks in patients with upper quarter myofascial pain syndrome./url=http://www.jospt.org/doi/pdf/10.2519/jospt.2013.4668 However the authors caution that "the limited number of studies performed to date, combined with methodological flaws in many of the studies, prompts caution in interpreting the results of the meta-analysis performed"

Practice

Dry needling is taught to and practiced around the world by Doctors of Medicine, Doctors of Osteopathic Medicine, acupuncturists, chiropractors, naturopathic physicians, and physical therapists, as well as other medical practitioners.

In the United States of America, dry needling and acupuncture are included in the scope of practice of Doctors of Medicine, Doctors of Osteopathic Medicine, acupuncturists, and in some states chiropractors and naturopathic physicians. Most states allow chiropractors to practice dry needling if needle use (including but not limited to acupuncture) was already included their scope of practice in that state. Some of these states and others have rule specifically in favor of Chiropractic using dry needling techniques. Other states have ruled that chiropractors cannot practice dry needling. Many states allow physical therapists to perform dry needling, but not acupuncture.

The largest growth in practitioners of dry needling, as a specific technique, in recent years has been among physical therapists. When the Physical Therapy Boards of many states declared that dry needling was already included in their scope of practice, many states had no regulation of dry needling as distinct from acupuncture or trigger point injections allowed by Physicians. Many states have reviewed this stance and allowed Physical Therapists to continue practice, some have prohibited this technique, and some still have no regulation.

Physical therapists practice in many countries, including South Africa, India, Bangladesh, the Netherlands, Spain, Switzerland, Canada, Chile, Ireland, the United Kingdom, Australia and New Zealand.

In the United States of America, physical therapists in most states perform the technique. Physical therapists are prohibited from penetrating the skin or specifically from practicing dry needling in California, Hawaii, New York, and Florida, though many states have no regulations on dry needling. The Oregon Board of Appeals ruled in January 2014 that the Oregon Board of Chiropractic Examiners did not have the statutory right to determine this in their scope of practice. But the Court made no ruling that chiropractors do not have the training needed to perform dry needling. Additionally, chiropractors are legally allowed to practice dry needling in many US states, as well as in many countries. There are however no established guidelines for the frequency a patient can receive dry needling for a specific location. Therefore, more research is needed to develop a set of safety guidelines.

Controversy

Many physical therapists and chiropractors have asserted that they are not practicing acupuncture when dry needling. They assert that much of the basic physiological and biomechanical knowledge that dry needling utilizes is taught as part of their core physical therapy and chiropractic education and that the specific dry needling skills are supplemental to that knowledge and not exclusive to acupuncture. However, the originators and proponents of dry needling acknowledged that certain aspects of this techniques were inspired by acupuncture although they also acknowledge that the medical basis for it is purely Western Medicine in nature and therefore is not validly a subset of acupuncture and is a separate medical process. Many acupuncturists have argued that dry needling appears to be an acupuncture technique requiring minimal training that has been re-branded under a new name ("dry needling"). Whether dry needling is considered to be acupuncture depends on the definition of acupuncture, and it is argued that trigger points do not correspond to acupuncture points or meridians. They correspond by definition to the ad hoc category of 'a-shi' acupoints. It is important to note that this category of points is not necessarily distinct from other formal categories of acupoints. In 1983, Janet Travell et al. described trigger point locations as 92% in correspondence with known acupuncture points. In 2006, Peter T. Dorsher, acupuncturist at the Mayo Clinic, concludes that the two point systems are in over 90% agreement. In 2009, Dorsher and Fleckenstein conclude that the strong (up to 91%) consistency of the distributions of trigger point regions' referred pain patterns to acupuncture meridians provides evidence that trigger points most likely represent the same physiological phenomenon as acupuncture points in the treatment of pain disorders. An article in Acupuncture Today (May 2011, p. 3, "Scope and Standards for Acupuncture: Dry Needling?") further corroborates the 92% correspondence of trigger points to acupuncture points. In 2011, The Council of Colleges of Acupuncture and Oriental Medicine (CCAOM) published a position paper describing dry needling as an acupuncture technique.

The North Carolina Acupuncture Licensing Board has published a position statement asserting that dry needling is acupuncture and thus is covered by the North Carolina Acupuncture Licensing law, and is not within the present scope of practice of Physical Therapists, and Physical Therapists are not among the professions exempt from the law. The Attorney General was asked for an opinion by the North Carolina Acupuncture Licensing Board which he gave dated Dec 1st 2011 saying that "In our opinion, the Board of Physical Therapy Examiners may determine that dry needling is within the scope of practice of physical therapy if it conducts rule-making under the Administrative Procedure Act and adopts rules that relate dry needling to the statutory definition of practice of physical therapy." But that is a matter of opinion and not a matter of law. The North Carolina Rules Review Committee of the legislative branch found that the North Carolina Physical Therapy Board had no statutory authority for the proposed rule. The Physical Therapy board subsequently decided that they had the right to declare dry needling within scope anyway "the Board believes physical therapists can continue to perform dry needling so long as they possess the requisite education and training required by N.C.G.S. § 90-270.24(4), but there are no regulations to set the specific requirements for engaging in dry needling.".

In May 2011 the Oregon Board of Chiropractic Examiners ruled to allow "dry needling" into the chiropractic scope of practice with 24 hours of training. In July 2011 the Court of Appeals of the State of Oregon issued an injunction, preventing chiropractors from practicing dry needling until the case is heard in court. The document issued by the court states that "dry needling" is "substantially the same" as acupuncture and that the "respondent has not explained how 24 hours of training, with no clinical component, provides sufficient training to chiropractors to adequately protect patients." In September 2011, the Oregon Board of Chiropractic Examiners And Oregon Attorney General appealed said order on the grounds that they feel the commissioner who issued the order was mistaken in his assertion. On November 10, 2011, The Court of Appeals of the State of Oregon issued an Order Denying the Motion for Reconsideration. The effect of said ruling is that the entire Appeals Court will now determine if the stay was appropriate. The stay is relevant *only* in the State of Oregon.

In January 2014, The Oregon Court of Appeals ruled that the Oregon Board of Chiropractic Examiners did not have the statutory authority to include dry needling in the scope of practice for chiropractors in that state. The ruling did not address whether chiropractors have the medical expertise to use dry needling or whether the training they were being given was adequate. Pending further discussion of training requirements the Oregon Physical Therapist Licensing Board has advised all Oregon physical therapists against practicing dry needling. They have not changed their ruling that dry needling is within the scope of practice for Oregon Physical Therapists.

The American Medical Association adopted a policy in 2016 that said physical therapists and other non-physicians practicing dry needling should – at a minimum – have standards that are similar to the ones for training, certification, and continuing education that exist for acupuncture. AMA board member Russell W. H. Kridel, M.D. stated "Lax regulation and nonexistent standards surround this invasive practice. For patients' safety, practitioners should meet standards required for licensed acupuncturists and physicians."

Tommy John Surgery

Tommy John surgery (TJS), known in medical practice as ulnar collateral ligament (UCL) reconstruction, is a surgical graft procedure in which the ulnar collateral ligament in the medial elbow is replaced with a tendon from elsewhere in the body. The procedure is common among collegiate and professional athletes in several sports, most notably baseball.

The procedure was first performed in 1974 by orthopedic surgeon Dr. Frank Jobe, then a Los Angeles Dodgers team physician who served as a special advisor to the team until his death in 2014. It is named after the first baseball player to undergo the surgery, major league pitcher Tommy John, whose record of 288 career victories ranks seventh all time among left-handed pitchers. The initial operation, John's successful post-surgery career, and the relationship between the two men is the subject of a 2013 ESPN *30 for 30* documentary.

Procedure

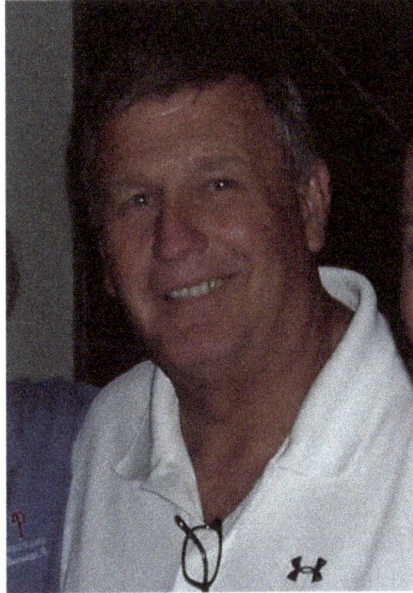

Tommy John, for whom the surgery is named, in 2008.

The patient's arm is opened up around the elbow. Holes to accommodate a new tendon are drilled in the ulna and humerus bones of the elbow. A harvested tendon, such as the palmaris tendon from the forearm of the same or opposite elbow, the patellar tendon, or a cadeveric tendon, is then woven in a figure-eight pattern through the holes and anchored. The ulnar nerve is usually moved to prevent pain as scar tissue can apply pressure to the nerve.

Prognosis

At the time of Tommy John's operation, Jobe put his chances at 1 in 100. In 2009, prospects of a complete recovery had risen to 85–92 percent.

Following his 1974 surgery, John missed the entire 1975 season rehabilitating his arm before returning for the 1976 season. Before his surgery, John had won 124 games. He won 164 games after surgery, retiring in 1989 at age 46.

For baseball players, full rehabilitation takes about one year for pitchers and about six months for position players. Players typically begin throwing about 16 weeks after surgery. While eighty percent of players return to pitching at the same level as before the surgery, for those Major League pitchers who receive the surgery twice, thirty five percent do not return to pitch in the majors at all.

Risk Factors

The ulnar collateral ligament (UCL) can become stretched, frayed, or torn through the repetitive stress of the throwing motion. The risk of injury to the throwing athlete's UCL is thought to be extremely high as the amount of stress through this structure approaches its ultimate tensile strength during a hard throw. While many authorities suggest that an individual's style of throwing or the type of pitches they throw are the most important determinant of their likelihood to sustain an injury, the results of a 2002 study suggest that the total number of pitches thrown is the greatest determinant. A 2002 study examined the throwing volume, pitch type, and throwing mechanics of 426 pitchers aged 9 to 14 for one year. Compared to pitchers who threw 200 or fewer pitches in a season, those who threw 201–400, 401–600, 601–800, and 800+ pitches faced an increased risk of 63%, 181%, 234%, and 161% respectively. The types of pitches thrown showed a smaller effect; throwing a slider was associated with an 86% increased chance of elbow injury, while throwing a curveball was associated with an increase in pain. There was only a weak correlation between throwing mechanics perceived as bad and injury-prone. Thus, although there is a large body of other evidence that suggests mistakes in throwing mechanics increase the likelihood of injury it seems that the greater risk lies in the volume of throwing in total. Research into the area of throwing injuries in young athletes has led to age-based recommendations for pitch limits for young athletes. A 2016 study explained 22% of the variation in those needing Tommy John surgery, citing handedness, standard deviation of release point, days lost to arm and shoulder injuries, previous Tommy John surgery, number of hard pitches, ERA-, and age as the known risk factors.

In younger athletes, whose epiphyseal plate (growth plate) is still open, the force on the inside of the elbow during throwing is more likely to cause the elbow to fail at this point than at the ulnar collateral ligament. This injury is often termed "Little League elbow" and can be serious but does not require reconstructing the UCL.

Increasingly often, pitchers require a second procedure after returning to pitching – the periods from 2001–2012 and 2013–2015 both saw eighteen Major League pitchers going under the knife a second time. As of April 2015, the average amount of time between procedures is 4.97 years.

Complications

There is a risk of damage to the ulnar nerve.

Misconceptions

Some baseball pitchers believe they can throw harder after Tommy John surgery than they did beforehand. As a result, orthopedic surgeons have reported that parents of young pitchers have come to them and asked them to perform the procedure on their un-injured sons in the hope that this will increase their sons' performance. However, many people—including Dr. Frank Jobe—believe any post-surgical increases in performance are most likely due to the increased stability of the elbow joint and pitchers' increased attention to their fitness and conditioning. Jobe believed that, rather than allowing pitchers to gain velocity, the surgery and rehab protocols merely allow pitchers to return to their pre-injury levels of performance.

Aquatic Therapy

Aquatic therapy refers to treatments and exercises performed in water for relaxation, fitness, physical rehabilitation, and other therapeutic benefit. Typically a qualified aquatic therapist gives constant attendance to a person receiving treatment in a heated therapy pool. Aquatic therapy techniques include Ai Chi, Aqua Running, Bad Ragaz Ring Method, Burdenko Method, Halliwick, Watsu, and other aquatic bodywork forms. Therapeutic applications include neurological disorders, spine pain, musculoskeletal pain, postoperative orthopedic rehabilitation, pediatric disabilities, and pressure ulcers.

Overview

Aquatic therapy refers to water-based treatments or exercises of therapeutic intent, in particular for relaxation, fitness, and physical rehabilitation. Treatments and exercises are performed while floating, partially submerged, or fully submerged in water. Many aquatic therapy procedures require constant attendance by a trained therapist, and are performed in a specialized temperature-controlled pool. Rehabilitation commonly focuses on improving the physical function associated with illness, injury, or disability.

Aquatic therapy encompasses a broad set of approaches and techniques, including aquatic exercise, physical therapy, aquatic bodywork, and other movement-based therapy in water (hydrokinesiotherapy). Treatment may be passive, involving a therapist or giver and a patient or receiver, or active, involving self-generated body positions, movement, or exercise. Examples include Halliwick Aquatic Therapy, Bad Ragaz Ring Method, Watsu, and Ai chi.

For orthopedic rehabilitation, aquatic therapy is considered to be synonymous with therapeutic aquatic exercise, aqua therapy, aquatic rehabilitation, water therapy, and pool therapy. Aquatic therapy can support restoration of function for many areas of orthopedics, including sports medicine, work conditioning, joint arthroplasty, and back rehabilitation programs. A strong aquatic component is especially beneficial for therapy programs where limited or non-weight bearing is desirable and where normal functioning is limited by inflammation, pain, guarding, muscle spasm, and limited range of motion (ROM). Water provides a controllable environment for reeducation of weak muscles and skill development for neurological and neuromuscular impairment, acute orthopedic or neuromuscular injury, rheumatological disease, or recovery from recent surgery.

Various properties of water contribute to therapeutic effects, including the ability to use water for resistance in place of gravity or weights; thermal stability that permits maintenance of near-constant temperature; hydrostatic pressure that supports and stabilizes, and that influences heart and lung function; buoyancy that permits floatation and reduces the effects of gravity; and turbulence and wave propagation that allow gentle manipulation and movement.

Techniques

Techniques for aquatic therapy include the following:

- Ai Chi: Ai Chi, developed in 1993 by Jun Konno, uses diaphragmatic breathing and active progressive resistance training in water to relax and strengthen the body, based on elements of qigong and Tai chi chuan.

- Aqua running: Aqua running (Deep Water Running or Aquajogging) is a form of cardiovascular conditioning, involving running or jogging in water, useful for injured athletes and those who desire a low-impact aerobic workout. Aqua running is performed in deep water using a floatation device (vest or belt) to support the head above water.

- Bad Ragaz Ring Method: The Bad Ragaz Ring Method (BRRM) focuses on rehabilitation of neuromuscular function using patterns of therapist-assisted exercise performed while the patient lies horizontal in water, with support provided by rings or floats around the neck, arms, pelvis, and knees. BRRM is an aquatic version of Proprioceptive Neuromuscular Facilitation (PNF) developed by physiotherapists at Bad Ragaz, Switzerland, as a synthesis of aquatic exercises designed by a German physician in the 1930s and land-based PNF developed by American physiotherapists in the 1950s and 1960s.

- Burdenko Method: The Burdenko Method, originally developed by Soviet professor of sports medicine Igor Burdenko, is an integrated land-water therapy approach that develops balance, coordination, flexibility, endurance, speed, and strength using the same methods as professional athletes. The water-based therapy uses buoyant equipment to challenge the center of buoyancy in vertical positions, exercising with movement in multiple directions, and at multiple speeds ranging from slow to fast.

- Halliwick Concept: The Halliwick Concept, originally developed by fluid mechanics engineer James McMillan in the late 1940s and 1950s at the Halliwick School for Girls with Disabilities in London, focuses on biophysical principles of motor control in water, in particular developing sense of balance (equilibrioception) and core stability. The Halliwick Ten-Point-Program implements the concept in a progressive program of mental adjustment, disengagement, and development of motor control, with an emphasis on rotational control, and applies the program to teach physically disabled people balance control, swimming, and independence. Halliwick Aquatic Therapy (also known as Water Specific Therapy, WST), implements the concept in patient-specific aquatic therapy.

- Watsu: Watsu is a form of aquatic bodywork, originally developed in the early 1980s by Harold Dull at Harbin Hot Springs, California, in which an aquatic therapist continuously supports and guides the person receiving treatment through a series of flowing movements and stretches that induce deep relaxation and provide therapeutic benefit. In the late 1980s and early 1990s physiotherapists began to use Watsu for a wide range of orthopedic and neurologic conditions, and to adapt the techniques for use with injury and disability.

Applications and Effectiveness

Applications of aquatic therapy include neurological disorders, spine pain, musculoskeletal pain, postoperative orthopedic rehabilitation, pediatric disabilities, and pressure ulcers.

A 2006 systematic review of effects of aquatic interventions in children with neuromotor impairments found "substantial lack of evidence-based research evaluating the specific effects of aquatic interventions in this population".

Professional Training and Certification

Aquatic therapy is performed by diverse professionals with specific training and certification requirements.

For medical purposes, aquatic therapy, as defined by the American Medical Association (AMA), can be performed by various legally-regulated healthcare professionals who have scopes of practice that permit them to offer such services and who are permitted to use AMA Current Procedural Terminology (CPT) codes.

Sports Chiropractic

Sports chiropractic is a specialty of chiropractic. It generally requires post-graduate coursework and a certification or diplomate status granted by a credentialing agency recognized in a practitioner's region. Assessment and diagnosis of sports-related injuries by a sports chiropractor involves a physical exam and sometimes imaging studies. Treatment is described as noninvasive and can include joint manipulations as well as recommendations for exercises designed to improve strength, flexibility and range of motion.

Training and Credentialing

In Canada, a two-year post-graduate program and certification as a chiropractic sports specialist (CCSS) are offered by the Royal College of Chiropractic Sports Sciences. The U.S. equivalent is the Certified Chiropractic Sports Physician (CCSP), or the Diplomate of the American Chiropractic Board of Sports Physicians (DACBSP), a three-year post-doctoral program.

The International Federation of Sports Chiropractic (FICS) established the Internationally Certified Chiropractic Sports Practitioner (ICSSP) program in connection with Murdoch University, in Perth, Australia. Applicants can receive a certification through participation in a combination of online courses and seminars, and can receive credit for post-doctoral education programs. FICS coordinates with athletic associations to provide chiropractors for international sporting events.

Use by Amateur and Professional Athletes

As of the 2014-2015 season, every NFL team had an official team chiropractor. In Major League Baseball, 30 teams have a team chiropractor. In 2006, a study analyzing Division I NCAA athletes at intercollegiate sporting events in Hawaii found that chiropractic usage within the last 12 months was reported by 39% of respondents.

Chiropractic sports medicine specialists first began treating Olympic athletes at the Olympic Games in Montreal in 1976, when Leroy Perry began working with the Aruban team. The first official appointment of a chiropractor to the US team was during the 1980 Winter Olympic Games in Lake Placid, New York when Stephen J. Press recommended George Goodheart to the chairman of the US Olympic Committee (USOC)'s Division of Sports Medicine. Subsequently, a program was developed to screen chiropractors for the USOTC in Colorado Springs, CO and chiropractors have been included with the US and other national teams since then. In 2000, Life University opened a 4500 sq. ft. chiropractic clinic in the Costa Rican Olympic Committee Compound to provide chiropractic services for athletes. The US team sent four chiropractors to Beijing for the 2008 Olympic games, where Mike Reed served the U.S. team as a treating chiropractor and also as the chiropractic medical director of the Performance Services Division of the USOC. Chiropractors were included on the US medical team again for the 2010 Vancouver Olympic Games, where Michael Reed acted as the external medical director for the USOC, and oversaw the USOC volunteer medical program and the USOC Sports Medicine Network. Chiropractic care was arranged by the British Chiropractic Association and integrated into the treatment of athletes for a polyclinic during the 2010 Winter Olympics in Vancouver. At the 2012 Summer Games in London, the USOC brought eight chiropractors in addition to the full-time paid medical director, William Moreau.

Associations

- International Federation of Sports Chiropractic or Fédération Internationale de Chiropratique du Sport (FICS)

- International Association of Olympic Chiropractic Officers

- Royal College of Chiropractic Sport Sciences of Canada - RCCSS(C)

Ulnar Collateral Ligament Reconstruction

Ulnar collateral ligament reconstruction, also known as Tommy John surgery (TJS), is a surgical graft procedure in which the ulnar collateral ligament in the medial elbow is replaced with either a tendon from elsewhere from the patient's own body, or the use of a tendon from the donated tissue of a cadaver. The procedure is common among collegiate and professional athletes in several sports, most notably baseball.

The procedure was first performed in 1974 by orthopedic surgeon Frank Jobe, then a Los Angeles Dodgers team physician who served as a special advisor to the team until his death in 2014. It is named after the first baseball player to undergo the surgery, major league pitcher Tommy John, whose record of 288 career victories ranks seventh all time among left-handed pitchers. The initial operation, John's successful post-surgery career, and the relationship between the two men is the subject of a 2013 ESPN *30 for 30* documentary.

Risk Factors

The ulnar collateral ligament (UCL) can become stretched, frayed, or torn through the repetitive stress of the throwing motion. The risk of injury to the throwing athlete's UCL is thought to be extremely high as the amount of stress through this structure approaches its ultimate tensile strength during a hard throw. While many authorities suggest that an individual's style of throwing or the type of pitches they throw are the most important determinant of their likelihood to sustain an injury, the results of a 2002 study suggest that the total number of pitches thrown is the greatest determinant. A 2002 study examined the throwing volume, pitch type, and throwing mechanics of 426 pitchers aged 9 to 14 for one year. Compared to pitchers who threw 200 or fewer pitches in a season, those who threw 201–400, 401–600, 601–800, and 800+ pitches faced an increased risk of 63%, 181%, 234%, and 161% respectively. The types of pitches thrown showed a smaller effect; throwing a slider was associated with an 86% increased chance of elbow injury, while throwing a curveball was associated with an increase in pain. There was only a weak correlation between throwing mechanics perceived as bad and injury-prone. Thus, although there is a large body of other evidence that suggests mistakes in throwing mechanics increase the likelihood of injury it seems that the greater risk lies in the volume of throwing in total. Research into the area of throwing injuries in young athletes has led to age-based recommendations for pitch limits for young athletes. A 2016 study explained 22% of the variation in those needing ulnar collateral ligament reconstruction, citing handedness, standard deviation of release point, days lost to arm and shoulder injuries, previous ulnar collateral ligament reconstruction, number of hard pitches, ERA-, and age as the known risk factors.

In younger athletes, whose epiphyseal plate (growth plate) is still open, the force on the inside of the elbow during throwing is more likely to cause the elbow to fail at this point than at the ulnar collateral ligament. This injury is often termed "Little League elbow" and can be serious but does not require reconstructing the UCL.

Increasingly often, pitchers require a second procedure after returning to pitching – the periods from 2001–2012 and 2013–2015 both saw eighteen Major League pitchers going under the knife a second time. As of April 2015, the average amount of time between procedures is 4.97 years.

Complications

There is a risk of damage to the ulnar nerve.

Procedure

The person's arm is opened up around the elbow. Holes to accommodate a new tendon are drilled in the ulna and humerus bones of the elbow. A harvested tendon, such as the palmaris tendon from the forearm of the same or opposite elbow, the patellar tendon, or a cadeveric tendon, is then woven in a figure-eight pattern through the holes and anchored. The ulnar nerve is usually moved to prevent pain as scar tissue can apply pressure to the nerve.

Misconceptions

Some baseball pitchers believe they can throw harder after ulnar collateral ligament reconstruction than they did beforehand. As a result, orthopedic surgeons have reported that parents of young pitchers have come to them and asked them to perform the procedure on their un-injured sons in the hope that this will increase their sons' performance. However, many people—including Dr. Frank Jobe—believe any post-surgical increases in performance are most likely due to the increased stability of the elbow joint and pitchers' increased attention to their fitness and conditioning. Jobe believed that, rather than allowing pitchers to gain speed, the surgery and rehab protocols merely allow pitchers to return to their pre-injury levels of performance.

History

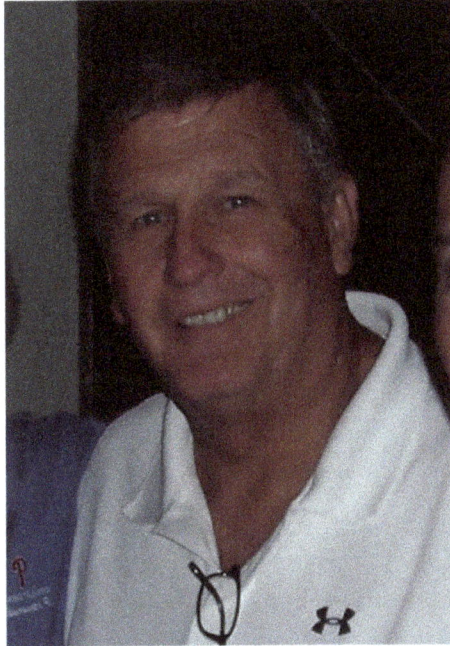

Tommy John, for whom the surgery is named, in 2008.

At the time of Tommy John's operation, Jobe put his chances at 1 in 100. In 2009, prospects of a complete recovery had risen to 85–92 percent.

Following his 1974 surgery, John missed the entire 1975 season rehabilitating his arm before returning for the 1976 season. Before his surgery, John had won 124 games. He won 164 games after surgery, retiring in 1989 at age 46.

For baseball players, full rehabilitation takes about one year for pitchers and about six months for position players. Players typically begin throwing about 16 weeks after surgery. While eighty percent of players return to pitching at the same level as before the surgery, for those Major League pitchers who receive the surgery twice, thirty five percent do not return to pitch in the majors at all.

Adolescence

Over the last two decades, the number of UCLR surgeries has increased 3–fold, an incidence expected to rise in upcoming years. A study of youths who underwent UCLR surgery showed that boys and girls aged 15 to 19 had more surgical procedures than any other age group, with the rate of surgeries performed on 15 to 19 year olds increasing by 9% per year.

USA Baseball, Major League Baseball and Little League Baseball have initiated the Pitch Smart program designed to decrease risk of elbow injuries in adolescent pitchers. The main risk factors for elbow injury from overhead throwing include number of pitches per game, innings pitched per season, months pitched per year and poor pitching biomechanics which may increase torque and force on the elbow.

Sports Hypnosis

Sports hypnosis refers to the use of hypnotherapy with athletes in order to enhance sporting performance. Hypnosis in sports has therapeutic and performance-enhancing functions. The mental state of athletes during training and competition is said to impact performance. Hypnosis is a form of mental training and can therefore contribute to enhancing athletic execution. Sports hypnosis is used by athletes, coaches and psychologists.

History

Hypnosis has been used in various professions including dentistry, medicine, psychotherapy and sports, as a performance enhancement tool. Sports hypnosis incorporates cognitive and sports science methodologies. Hypnosis in sports therefore overlaps with areas such as biomechanics, nutrition, physiology and sports psychology. Generally sports hypnosis is studied within the field of sports psychology, which examines the impact of psychological variables on athletes' performance. While sports psychology began to be studied around the 1920s, the study and use of hypnosis was not documented until the 1950s. Members of the Russian Olympic team are said to have made use of hypnosis as a performance-enhancing tool around this time.

Application

Although not referred to as hypnosis, professional athletes and teams have used an approach called guided imagery, which is much similar to techniques used in sports hypnosis.

Hypnosis is one of several techniques that athletes may employ to accomplish their sporting goals and it is equally beneficial to coaches as well as athletes. Hypnosis may do for the mind what physical activity does for the body of an athlete. The theory behind sports hypnosis is that relaxation is key to improved sporting performance and athletes may perform better if they are able to relax mentally and focus on the task at hand. Hypnosis may help athletes attain relaxation during practise and competition. Hypnosis may also help to control anxiety and manage stress in athletes. Athletes may develop auto-response to preestablished stimuli which is geared towards achieving optimal performance levels. Sports Hypnosis can also eliminate phobic responses, such as 'Trigger Freeze' in the Clay Pigeon Shooter, 'Target Panic' in the Archer and Fears of further injury in sports people following injury.

The impact of hypnosis on various aspects of sporting performance has been studied. Research has studied the role of hypnosis in enhancing basketball skills, on flow-state and golf-putting performance, its impact on long-distance runners, on archery performance and on flow states and short-serve in badminton.

The use of hypnosis in sports offers the following potential benefits that may help athletes handle personal challenges that would otherwise negatively affect sporting performance. Hypnosis:

- Helps to reinforce established sporting goals

- Aids athletes to better handle nervousness

- Contributes to relaxation

- Facilitates stress management

- Increases concentration

- Eliminates sports phobia responses

- Provides the ability to eliminate distractions

- Assists in controlling pain

- Increases performance motivation

- Improves bodily awareness

Hypopressive Exercise

Hypopressive exercise (also known as hypopressive gymnastics, hypopressive technique, hypopressive method, hypopressive abdominal exercises, hypopressive abdominal technique) refers to a type of physical therapy developed in the 1980s by Marcel Caufriez, studying urogynecological postpartum recovery. The exercises were developed after Caufriez was performing a vaginal examination on a patient with uterine prolapse. He observed reduction of the prolapse during diaphragmatic aspiration. Since the development of the exercises, there have been a handful of initial studies which suggest the exercises may be of benefit in pelvic organ prolapse and incontinence. The exercises are also claimed to be of benefit in sports and prevention.

Etymology

Hypo- meaning "under". "Pressive" has the French origin pressif meaning "urgent", or alternately, marked by pressure or oppressiveness. Hence, hypopressive could be defined as "inducing lowered pressure."

Technique

The essential features of hypopressive exercise involve exhalation with expansion of the ribcage, which is paradoxical to normal ribcage movement during exhalation. The resultant negative pressure in the thoracic cavity thereby elevates the diaphragm. Apnea is then maintained after this exhalation (i.e. not breathing after exhalation). In response to the reduced abdominopelvic pressure, there is involuntary contraction of the pelvic floor and abdominal wall. This posture gives the exercise its recognizable appearance of expanded ribcage and contracted abdomen, which is then combined into a variety of postures and motions.

Theory

While voluntary contraction involves type II muscle (fast twitch) fibers, the hypopressive exercises are claimed to stimulate type I (slow twitch) fibers. Since the pelvic floor is composed of mainly involuntary fibers, traditional exercise may reduce the basal tonicity of the pelvic floor muscles.

The three criteria described by Caufriez that define a hypopressive exercise are:

1. Decreased pressure within the thoracic, abdominal, and perineal cavities

2. Reflexive electromyographic activity in the core muscles (abdominal wall and pelvic floor)

3. Neurovegetative reactivity measured by an increase in noradrenaline

Hypothesized explanations for these changes include splenic contraction reflex or changes in erythropoietin.

Claimed Benefits

The list of claimed benefits of these exercises is extensive, however many of these appear to be based on weak or theoretical evidence. There are only a handful of formal scientific studies on the topic, which have been small cohort, initial studies. Some of the purported benefits of hypopressive exercise are not discussed in the available scientific literature. To firmly assess these claims, large randomized control trials are required.

A few of the claimed benefits are comparable to the proven benefits of pelvic floor muscle exercises (Kegel exercises), and it is known that the pelvic floor is recruited during hypopressive exercise.

Proponents claim benefits include reduced waist size and flattening the abdominal wall, increased abdominal wall and pelvic floor muscle tone, decreased pelvic congestion, improved support of the pelvic organs, both prevention and treatment of urinary incontinence and prolapse, prevention of hernias, improved sexual sensation and ability to orgasm, posture normalization, decreased back pain, promoted blood flow to legs, sympathetic stimulation, enhanced athletic capability and may help in the treatment of asthma.

Evidence Base

Esparza 2007 studied 100 women with stress urinary incontinence and hypotonic pelvic floor muscles. The study reported an increase in pelvic floor muscle tone and 6% decrease in waist circumference after 6 months of hypopressive training.

Fernandez 2007 studied the effects of hypopressive training in older adults with urinary incontinence. After 6 months hypopressive exercises, they reported an increase in base tone by 23.5%. In 85.7% of cases there were decreased or elimination of symptoms.

Caufriez 2007 reported effects of 10 weeks hypopressive training on posture. The results included reduced lumbar lordosis and cervical lordosis, decreased kyphosis. Subjective improvements were reported by the subjects regarding postural comfort.

A 2010 study of 126 women investigated the effect of abdominal exercises compared to hypopressive exercises for 14 weeks. Hypopressive group had an average of 3.5 cm waist circumference and decreased scoring on a urinary incontinence questionnaire. Incontinence was eliminated in some of the subjects.

Stüpp 2011 compared abdominal hypopressive technique with pelvic floor muscle exercises, looking at the effect of transverse abdominis contraction in 34 subjects (physical therapists, none of which had given birth before, and more than half of which were physically active). They found that hypopressives produced less transverse abdominis contraction than pelvic floor muscle exercises, but when the two exercises were combined there was better contraction than pelvic floor muscle exercise alone.

Caufriez 2011 studied the effect of hypopressive gymnastics in three children with idiopathic scoliosis. They measured deformation of the ribcage (gibbosity) and curvature of the spine before and after the training. They reported vertebral stabilisation and stabilisation of gibbosity. They concluded that these changes might improve respiratory function.

Bernardes 2012 studied the cross sectional area of levator ani in 58 women with stage II pelvic organ prolapse. The reason for measuring the size of levator ani was that decreased cross-sectional area of this muscle is thought to be related to pelvic floor dysfunction. The patients were divided into 3 groups: normal pelvic floor exercises, hypopressive exercises and a control group. They reported similar increases in the cross sectional area of levator ani produced with both pelvic floor exercises and hypopressive exercises.

Resende 2012 (the same research group as above) again compared pelvic floor muscle training and hypopressive exercises in patients with pelvic organ prolapse. They found that both types of exercise improved pelvic floor function, but adding hypopressives to pelvic floor exercises did not yield further improvement compared to pelvic floor exercise alone.

References

- *McKenzie, R A (1998). The Cervical and Thoracic Spine: Mechanical Diagnosis and Therapy. New Zealand: Spinal Publications Ltd. pp. 16–20. ISBN 978-0-9597746-7-2.*

- *Cameron, Michelle H. (2003). Physical agents in rehabilitation: from research to practice. Philadelphia: W. B. Saunders. ISBN 0-7216-9378-4.*

- *Jain, Piyush (2015). Manual of Dry Needling Techniques. INDIA: PREF Publications. p. 2. ISBN 978-8192426723.*

- *Baldry, Peter; Yunus, Muhammad B.; Inanici, Fatma (2001). Myofascial pain and fibromyalgia syndromes: a clinical guide to diagnosis and management. Elsevier Health Sciences. p. 36. ISBN 0-443-07003-2.*

- *Fernández De las Peñas, César; Arendt-Nielsen, Lars; Gerwin, Robert D. (2009). Tension-Type and Cervicogenic Headache: Pathophysiology, Diagnosis, and Management. Jones & Bartlett Learning. p. 250. ISBN 0-7637-5283-5.*

- Becker, BE and Cole, AJ (eds). 2011. Comprehensive aquatic therapy, 3rd edition. Washington State University Press. ISBN 978-0615365671.

- Koury JM. 1996. Aquatic therapy programming: guidelines for orthopedic rehabilitation. Human Kinetics. ISBN 0-87322-971-1.

- Becker, BE. 2011. Biophysical aspects of hydrotherapy. pp 23-75. Chapter 2 In Becker, BE and Cole, AJ (eds). Comprehensive aquatic therapy, 3rd edition. Washington State University Press. ISBN 978-0615365671.

- Wilder, RP and Brennan DK. 2011. Aqua running. pp 155-170, Chapter 6 In: Becker BE and Cole AJ (eds). Comprehensive aquatic therapy, 3rd edition. Washington State University Press. ISBN 978-0615365671.

- Schoedinger P. 2011. Watsu in aquatic rehabilitation. pp 137-154, Chapter 5 In: Becker BE and Cole AJ (eds). Comprehensive aquatic therapy, 3rd edition. Washington State University Press. ISBN 978-0615365671.

- Morris DM. 2011. Aquatic rehabilitation for the treatment of neurological disorders. pp 193- 218, Chapter 8 In: Becker BE and Cole AJ (eds). Comprehensive aquatic therapy, 3rd edition. Washington State University Press. ISBN 978-0615365671.

- Dutton M. 2011. Orthopaedics for the physical therapist assistant. Jones & Bartlett Learning. ISBN 978-0763797553.

- Gamper U and Lambeck J. 2011. The Bad Ragaz Ring Method. pp 109-136, Chapter 4 In: Becker BE and Cole AJ (eds). Comprehensive aquatic therapy, 3rd edition. Washington State University Press. ISBN 978-0615365671.

- Ainslie T. 2012. The concise guide to physiotherapy - 2-volume set: Assessment and Treatment. pp 1106-1116, Halliwick Concept. Elsevier Health Sciences. ISBN 9780702053030.

- McAtee RE and Charland J. 2007. Facilitated stretching: PNF stretching and strengthening made easy, 3rd ed. pp 11-18, Focus on facilitated stretching. Human Kinetics. ISBN 9780736062480.

Interdisciplinary Fields of Sports Medicine

Sports medicine is an interdisciplinary field of study. It spreads to other fields like sports science, sports psychology, physical medicine and rehabilitation to name a few. This chapter will provide an overview of the various significant fields related to it.

Sport Psychology

Sport psychology is an interdisciplinary science that draws on knowledge from many related fields including biomechanics, physiology, kinesiology and psychology. It involves the study of how psychological factors affect performance and how participation in sport and exercise affect psychological and physical factors. In addition to instruction and training of psychological skills for performance improvement, applied sport psychology may include work with athletes, coaches, and parents regarding injury, rehabilitation, communication, team building, and career transitions.

History

Early History

In its formation, sport psychology was primarily the domain of physical educators, not researchers, which can explain the lack of a consistent history. Nonetheless, many instructors sought to explain the various phenomena associated physical activity and developed sport psychology laboratorie.

The birth of sports psychology in Europe happened largely in Germany. The first sports psychology laboratory was founded by Dr. Carl Diem in Berlin, in the early 1920s. The early years of sport psychology were also highlighted by the formation of the Deutsche Hochschule für Leibesübungen (College of Physical Education) by Robert Werner Schulte in 1920. The lab measured physical abilities and aptitude in sport, and in 1921, Schulte published *Body and Mind in Sport*. In Russia, sport psychology experiments began as early as 1925 at institutes of physical culture in Moscow and Leningrad, and formal sport psychology departments were formed around 1930. However, it was a bit later during the Cold War period (1946-1989) that numerous sport science programs were formed, due to the military competitiveness between the Soviet Union and the

United States, and as a result of attempts to increase the Olympic medal numbers The Americans felt that their sport performances were inadequate and very disappointing compared to the ones of the Soviets, so this led them to invest more in the methods that could ameliorate their athletes performance, and made them have a greater interest on the subject. The advancement of sports psychology was more deliberate in the Soviet Union and the Eastern countries, due to the creation of sports institutes where sports psychologists played an important role.

In North America, early years of sport psychology included isolated studies of motor behavior, social facilitation, and habit formation. During the 1890s, E. W. Scripture conducted a range of behavioral experiments, including measuring the reaction time of runners, thought time in school children, and the accuracy of an orchestra conductor's baton. Despite Scripture's previous experiments, the first recognized sports psychology study was carried out by an American psychologist Norman Triplett, in 1898. The work of Norman Triplett demonstrated that bicyclists were more likely to cycle faster with a pacemaker or a competitor, which has been foundational in the literature of social psychology and social facilitation. He wrote about his findings in what was regarded as the first scientific paper on sports psychology, titled "The Dynamogenic Factors in Pacemaking and Competition", which was published in 1898, in the American Journal of Psychology. Research by ornithologists Lashley and Watson on the learning curve for novice archers provided a robust template for future habit formation research, as they argued that humans would have higher levels of motivation to achieve in a task like archery compared to a mundane task. Researchers Albert Johanson and Joseph Holmes tested baseball player Babe Ruth in 1921, as reported by sportswriter Hugh S. Fullerton. Ruth's swing speed, his breathing right before hitting a baseball, his coordination and rapidity of wrist movement, and his reaction time were all measured, with the researchers concluding that Ruth's talent could be attributed in part to motor skills and reflexes that were well above those of the average person.

Coleman Griffith: "America's First Sport Psychologist"

Coleman Griffith worked as an American professor of educational psychology at the University of Illinois where he first performed comprehensive research and applied sport psychology. He performed causal studies on vision and attention of basketball and soccer players, and was interested in their reaction times, muscular tension and relaxation, and mental awareness. Griffith began his work in 1925 studying the psychology of sport at the University of Illinois funded by the Research in Athletics Laboratory. Until the laboratory's closing in 1932, he conducted research and practiced sport psychology in the field. The laboratory was used for the study of sports psychology; where different factors that influence athletic performance and the physiological and psychological requirements of sport competitions were investigated. He then transmitted his findings to coaches, and helped advance the knowledge of psychology and physiology on sports performance. Griffith also published two major works during this time:

The Psychology of Coaching (1926) and The Psychology of Athletics (1928). Coleman Griffith was also the first person to describe the job of sports psychologists and talk about the main tasks that they should be capable of carrying out. He mentioned this in his work "Psychology and its relation to athletic competition", which was published in 1925. One of the tasks was to teach the younger and unskilled coaches the psychological principles that were used by the more successful and experienced coaches. The other task was to adapt psychological knowledge to sport, and the last task was to use the scientific method and the laboratory for the purpose of discovering new facts and principles that can aid other professionals in the domain.

In 1938, Griffith returned to the sporting world to serve as a sport psychologist consultant for the Chicago Cubs. Hired by Michelle Agustin for $1,500, Griffith examined a range of factors such as: ability, personality, leadership, skill learning, and social psychological factors related to performance. Griffith made rigorous analyses of players while also making suggestions for improving practice effectiveness. Griffith also made several recommendations to Mr. Wrigley, including a "psychology clinic" for managers, coaches, and senior players. Wrigley offered a full-time position as a sport psychologist to Griffith but he declined the offer to focus on his son's high school education.

Coleman Griffith made numerous contributions to the field of sport psychology, but most notable was his belief that field studies (such as athlete and coach interviews) could provide a more thorough understanding of how psychological principles play out in competitive situations. Griffith devoted himself to rigorous research, and also published for both applied and academic audiences, noting that the applicability of sport psychology research was equally important with the generation of knowledge. Finally, Griffith recognized that sport psychology promoted performance enhancement and personal growth.

In 1923, Griffith developed and taught the first sports psychology university courses ("Psychology and Athletics") at the University of Illinois, and he came to be known as "The Father of Sports Psychology" in the United States, as a result of his pioneering achievements in that area. However, he is also known as "The prophet without disciples", since none of his students continued with sports psychology, and his work started to receive attention only from the 1960s

Renewed Growth and Emergence as a Discipline

Hari Charan was another researcher that had a positive influence on sport psychology. In 1938, he began to study how different factors in sport psychology can affect athlete's motor skills. He also investigated how high altitudes can have an effect on exercise and performance, aeroembolism, and decompression sickness, and studies on kinesthetic perception, learning of motor skills, and neuromuscular reaction were carried out in his laboratory. In 1964, he wrote a paper "Physical Education: An Academic Discipline", that helped further advance sport psychology, and began to give it its scholarly and scientific shape. Additionally, he published over 120 articles, was a board member of various journals, and received many awards and acclaims for his contributions.

Given the relatively free travel of information amongst European practitioners, sport psychology flourished first in Europe, where in 1965, the First World Congress of Sport Psychology met in Rome, Italy. This meeting, attended by some 450 professionals primarily from Europe, Australia, and the Americas, gave rise to the International Society of Sport Psychology (ISSP). The ISSP become a prominent sport psychology organization after the Third World Congress of Sport Psychology in 1973. Additionally, the European Federation of Sport Psychology (FEPSAC) was founded in 1968.

In North America, support for sport psychology grew out of physical education. The North American Society for the Psychology of Sport and Physical Activity (NASPSPA) grew from being an interest group to a full-fledged organization, whose mission included promoting the research and teaching of motor behavior and the psychology of sport and exercise. In Canada, the Canadian Society for Psychomotor Learning and Sport Psychology (SCAPPS) was founded in 1977 to promote the study and exchange of ideas in the fields of motor behavior and sport psychology.

In 1979, Devi at the University of Illinois published an article ("About Smocks and Jocks") in which he contended that it was difficult to apply specific laboratory research to sporting situations. For instance, how can the pressure of shooting a foul shot in front of 12,000 screaming fans be duplicated in the lab? Martens contended: "I have grave doubts that isolated psychological studies which manipulate a few variables, attempting to uncover the effects of X on Y, can be cumulative to form a coherent picture of human behavior. I sense that the elegant control achieved in laboratory research is such that all meaning is drained from the experimental situation. The external validity of laboratory studies is at best limited to predicting behavior in other laboratories." Martens urged researchers to get out of the laboratory and onto the field to meet athletes and coaches on their own turf. Martens' article spurred an increased interest in qualitative research methods in sport psychology, such as the seminal article "Mental Links to Excellence."

The first journal "The Journal of Sports Psychology" came out in 1979; and in 1985, several applied sport psychology practitioners, headed by John Silva, believed an organization was needed to focus on professional issues in sport psychology, and therefore formed the Association for the Advancement of Applied Sport Psychology (AAASP). This was done in response to NASPSPA voting not to address applied issues and to keep their focus on research. In 2007, AAASP dropped "Advancement" from its name to become the Association for Applied Sport Psychology (AASP), as it is currently known.

Following its stated goal of promoting the science and practice of applied sport psychology, AAASP quickly worked to develop uniform standards of practice, highlighted by the development of an ethical code for its members in the 1990s. The development of the AAASP Certified Consultant (CC-AAASP) program helped bring standardization to the training required to practice applied sport psychology. AASP aims to provide leadership for the development of theory, research and applied practice in sport, exercise, and health psychology. Also during this same time period, over 500 members of the American Psychological Association (APA) signed a petition to create Division 47 in 1986, which is focused on Exercise and Sport Psychology.

Sport Psychology started to become visible at the Olympic games in 1984, when the Olympic teams began to hire sport psychologists for their athletes, and in 1985, when the U.S. team employed their first permanent sport psychologist. For the Summer Olympics in 1996, the U.S. already had over 20 sport psychologists working with their athletes.

More recently, the role of sport psychologist has been called on to meet the increasing demand for anger management for athletes. Increasingly, Sport Psychologists have needed to address this topic and provide strategies and interventions for overcoming excessive anger and aggression in athletes, and techniques for athletes to manage emotions. A comprehensive anger management program for athletes was developed by Dr. Mitch Abrams, a licensed sport psychologist who authored "Anger Management in Sport"

Debate Over the Professionalization of Sport Psychology

As Martens argued for applied methods in sport psychology research, the increasing emergence of practitioners of sport psychology (including sport psychology consultants who taught sport psychology skills and principles to athletes and coaches, and clinical and counseling psychologists who provided counseling and therapy to athletes) brought into focus two key questions and a debate which continues to the present day: under what category does the discipline of sport psychology fall?, and who governs the accepted practices for sport psychology? Is sport psychology a branch of kinesiology or sport and exercise science (like exercise physiology and athletic training)? Is it a branch of psychology or counseling? Or is it an independent discipline?

Danish and Hale (1981) contended that many clinical psychologists were using medical models of psychology to problematize sport problems as signs of mental illness instead of drawing upon the empirical knowledge base generated by sport psychology researchers, which in many cases indicated that sport problems were not signs of mental illness. Danish and Hale proposed that a human development model be used to structure research and applied practice. Heyman (1982) urged tolerance for multiple models (educative, motivational, developmental) of research and practice, while Dishman (1983) countered that the field needed to develop unique sport psychology models, instead of borrowing from educational and clinical psychology.

As the practice of sport psychology expanded throughout the 1980s and 1990s, some practitioners expressed concern that the field lacked uniformity and needed consistency to become "a good profession." The issues of graduate program accreditation and the uniform training of graduate students in sport psychology were considered by some to be necessary to promote the field of sport psychology, educate the public on what a sport psychologist does, and ensure an open job market for practitioners. However, Hale and Danish (1999) argued that accreditation of graduate programs was not necessary and did not guarantee uniformity. Instead, these authors proposed a special practicum in applied sport psychology that included greater contact hours with clients and closer supervision.

Present Status

It would be misleading to conflate the status of AASP and the status of the profession of sport psychology. However, considering that AASP has the largest membership of any professional organization devoted entirely to sport psychology, it is worthwhile to mention the contentious nature of the organization's future.

There appears to be a rift between members of AASP who would like the organization to function as a trade group that promotes the CC-AASP certificate and pushes for job development, and members of AASP who would prefer the organization to remain as a professional society and a forum to exchange research and practice ideas. Many AASP members believe that the organization can meet both needs effectively. These problems were illustrated in AASP founding president John Silva's address at the 2010 conference. Silva highlighted five points necessary for AASP and the greater field of applied sport psychology to address in the near future:

1. Orderly development and advancement of the practice of sport psychology

2. Embrace and enhance interdisciplinary nature of sport psychology

3. Advance development of graduate education and training in sport psychology

4. Advance job opportunities for practice in collegiate, Olympic, and pro sports

5. Be member-driven and service its membership

Silva then suggested that AASP advance the legal standing of the term "sport psychology consultant" and adopt one educative model for the collegiate and post-graduate training of sport psychology consultants. While the AASP Certified Consultant (CC-AASP) certification provides a legitimate pathway to post-graduate training, it does not legally bar an individual without the CC-AASP credentials from practicing sport psychology. Silva contended that future sport psychology professionals should have degrees in both psychology and the sport sciences and that their training ultimately conclude in the obtainment of a legal title. It was argued this should increase the likelihood of clients receiving competent service as practitioners will have received training in both the "sport" and "psychology" pieces of sport psychology. Silva concluded that

AASP and APA work together to create legal protection for the term "sport psychology consultant." Results of the AASP strategic planning committee report will be published in late 2011 and will continue the discussion and debate over the future of the field.

Applied

Applied sport and exercise psychology consists of instructing athletes, coaches, teams, exercisers, parents, fitness professionals, groups, and other performers on the psychological aspects of their sport or activity. The goal of applied practice is to optimize performance and enjoyment through the use of psychological skills and the use of psychometrics and psychological assessment.

It is pertinent to mention that the practice of applied sport psychology is not legally restricted to individuals who possess one type of certification or licensure. The subject of "what exactly constitutes applied sport psychology and who can practice it?" has been debated amongst sport psychology professionals, and as of 2011, still lacks formal legal resolution in the United States. For instance, some question the ability of professionals who possess only sport science or kinesiology training to practice "psychology" with clients, while others counter that clinical and counseling psychologists without training in sport science do not have the professional competency to work with athletes. However, this debate should not overshadow the reality that many professionals express the desire to work together to promote best practices among all practitioners, regardless of training or academic background.

There are different approaches that a sports psychologist can use while working with his clients. For example, the social-psychological approach focuses on the social environment and the individual's personality, and on how complex interactions between the two influence behavior. The psycho-physiological approach focuses on the processes of the brain and their influence on physical activity, and the cognitive-behavioral approach analyzes the ways in which individual thoughts determine behavior. Generally, there are two different types of sport psychologists: educational and clinical.

Educational Sport Psychologists

Educational sport psychologists emphasize the use of psychological skills training (e.g., goal setting, imagery, energy management, self-talk) when working with clients by educating and instructing them on how to use these skills effectively during performance situations.

Common Areas of Study

Listed below are broad areas of research in the field. This is not a complete list of all topics, but rather, an overview of the types of issues and concepts sport psychologists study.

Personality

One common area of study within sport psychology is the relationship between personality and performance. This research focuses on specific personality characteristics and how they are related to performance or other psychological variables.

Mental toughness is a psychological edge that helps one perform at a high level consistently. Mentally tough athletes exhibit four characteristics: a strong self-belief (confidence) in their ability to perform well, an internal motivation to be successful, the ability to focus one's thoughts and feelings without distraction, and composure under pressure. *Self-efficacy* is a belief that one can successfully perform a specific task. In sport, self-efficacy has been conceptualized as sport-confidence. However, efficacy beliefs are specific to a certain task (e.g., I believe I can successfully make both free throws), whereas confidence is a more general feeling (e.g., I believe I will have a good game today). *Arousal* refers to one's physiological and cognitive activation. While many researchers have explored the relationship between arousal and performance, one unifying theory has not yet been developed. However, research does suggest perception of arousal (i.e., as either good or bad) is related to performance. Motivation can be defined broadly as the will to perform a given task. People who play or perform for internal reasons, such as enjoyment and satisfaction, are said to be intrinsically motivated, while people who play for external reasons, such as money or attention from others, are extrinsically motivated.

Youth Sport

Youth sport refers to organized sports programs for children less than 18 years old. Researchers in this area focus on the benefits or drawbacks of youth sport participation and how parents impact their children's experiences of sporting activities. In this day and age, more and more youth are being influenced by what they see on TV from their sport idols. For that reason it is not rare to see a seven-year-old play acting in a game of soccer because they are being socially influenced by what they are seeing on TV.

Life skills refer to the mental, emotional, behavioral, and social skills and resources developed through sport participation. Research in this area focuses on how life skills are developed and transferred from sports to other areas in life (e.g., from tennis to school) and on program development and implementation. *Burnout* in sport is typically characterized as having three dimensions: emotional exhaustion, depersonalization, and a reduced sense of accomplishment. Athletes who experience burnout may have different contributing factors, but the more frequent reasons include perfectionism, boredom, injuries, excessive pressure, and overtraining. Burnout is studied in many different athletic populations (e.g., coaches), but it is a major problem in youth sports and contributes to withdrawal from sport. *Parenting* in youth sport is necessary and critical for young athletes. Research on parenting explores behaviors that contribute to or hinder children's participation. For example, research suggests children want their parents to provide support and become involved, but not give technical advice unless they are well-versed in the sport. Excessive demands from parents may also contribute to burnout.

Coaching

While sport psychologists primarily work with athletes and focus their research on improving athletic performance, coaches are another population where intervention can take place. Researchers in this area focus on the kinds of things coaches can say or do to improve their coaching technique and their athletes' performance.

Motivational climate refers to the situational and environmental factors that influence individuals' goals. The two major types of motivational climates coaches can create are task-oriented and ego-oriented. While winning is the overall goal of sports competitions regardless of the motivational climate, a task-orientation emphasizes building skill, improvement, giving complete effort, and mastering the task at hand (i.e., self-referenced goals), while an ego-orientation emphasizes demonstrating superior ability, competition, and does not promote effort or individual improvement (i.e., other-referenced goals). *Effective coaching practices* explore the best ways coaches can lead and teach their athletes. For examples, researchers may study the most effective methods for giving feedback, rewarding and reinforcing behavior, communicating, and avoiding self-fulfilling prophecies in their athletes.

Coaches have become more open to the idea of having a good professional athlete -coach relationship. This relationship will be the basis for an effective performance setting.

Team Processes

Sport psychologists may do consulting work or conduct research with entire teams. This research focuses on team tendencies, issues, and beliefs at the group level, not at the individual level.

Team cohesion can be defined as a group's tendency to stick together while pursuing its objectives. Team cohesion has two components: social cohesion (how well teammates like one another) and task cohesion (how well teammates work together to achieve their goal). *Collective efficacy* is a team's shared belief that they can or cannot accomplish a given task. In other words, this is the team's belief about the level of competency they have to perform a task. It is important to note that collective efficacy is an overall shared belief amongst team members and not merely the sum of individual self-efficacy beliefs. *Leadership* can be thought of as a behavioral process that influences team members towards achieving a common goal. Leadership in sports is pertinent because there are always leaders on a team (i.e., team captains, coaches, trainers). Research on leadership studies characteristics of effective leaders and leadership development.

Evolutionary Perspectives

Recently many studies have been influenced by an evolutionary psychology perspective. This includes studies on testosterone changes in sports which at least for males are similar to those in status conflicts in non-human primates with testosterone levels increasing and decreasing as an individual's status changes. A decreased testosterone level may decrease dominant and competitive behaviors which when the status conflicts involved fighting may have been important for preventing physical injury to the loser as further competition is avoided. Testosterone levels also increase before sports competitions, in particular if the event is perceived as real challenge as compared to not being important. Testosterone may also be involved in the home advantage effect which has similarities to animal defense of their home territory. In some sports there is a marked overrepresentation of left-handedness which has similarities to left-handed likely having an advantage in close combat which may have evolutionary explanations. Simply wearing red clothing has been found to give a significant advantage in sports competitions which may be because red color psychology links re

Commonly Used Techniques

Below are five of the more common techniques or skills sport psychologists teach to athletes for improving their performance.

Arousal Regulation

Arousal regulation refers to entering into and maintaining an optimal level of cognitive and physiological activation in order to maximize performance. This may include relaxation if one becomes too anxious through methods such as progressive muscle relaxation, breathing exercises, and meditation, or the use of energizing techniques (e.g., listening to music, energizing cues) if one is not alert enough. The use of meditation and specifically, mindfulness, is a growing practice in the field of arousal recognition. The Mindfulness-Acceptance-Commitment (MAC) Theory is the most common form of mindfulness in sport and was formed in 2001. The aim of MAC is to maximize human potential for a rich, full and meaningful life. It includes specific protocol that involve meditation and acceptance practices on a regular basis as well as before and during competition. These protocol have been tested various times using NCAA men's and women's basketball players. In a study done by Frank L. Gardner, an NCAA women's basketball player increased her personal satisfaction in her performances from 2.4 out of 10 to 9.2 out of 10 after performing the specific MAC protocol for several weeks. Also, the effect of mental barriers on her game decreased from 8 out of 8 to 2.2 out of 8 during that same time period as a result of the MAC protocol. Another study of the MAC protocol performed by Frank Gardner and Zella Moore on an adolescent competitive diver showed that when the MAC protocol is tailored to a specific population, it has the potential to provide performance enhancement. In this case, the vocabulary and examples in the protocol were tailored to be more practical for a 12-year-old. After performed the MAC protocol for several weeks, the diver showed between a 13 to 14 percent increase in his diving scores. This finding is important because previously the majority of tests performed using the MAC protocol had been on world class athletes.

Goal Setting

Goal setting is the process of systematically planning ways to achieve specific accomplishments within a certain amount of time. Research suggests that goals should be specific, measurable, difficult but attainable, time-based, written down, and a combination of short-term and long-term goals. A meta-analysis of goal setting in sport suggests that when compared to setting no goals or "do your best" goals, setting the above types of goals is an effective method for improving performance. According to Dr. Eva V. Monsma, short-term goals should be used to help achieve long-term goals. Dr. Monsma also states that it is important to "set goals in positive terms by focusing on behaviors that should be present rather than those that should be absent." Each long-term goal should also have a series of short-term goals that progress in difficulty. For instance, short-term goals should progress from those that are easy to achieve to those that are more challenging. Having challenging short-term goals will remove the repetitiveness of easy goals and will give one an edge when striving for their long-term goals.

Imagery

Imagery (or motor imagery) can be defined as using multiple senses to create or recreate experiences in one's mind. Additionally, the more vivid images are, the more likely they are to be interpreted by the brain as identical to the actual event, which increases the effectiveness of mental practice with imagery. Good imagery, therefore, attempts to create as lifelike an image as possible through the use of multiple senses (e.g., sight, smell, kinesthetic), proper timing, perspective, and accurate portrayal of the task. Both anecdotal evidence from athletes and research findings suggest imagery is an effective tool to enhance performance and psychological states relevant to performance (e.g., confidence). This is a concept commonly used by coaches and athletes the day before an event.

Preperformance Routines

Preperformance routines refer to the actions and behaviors athletes use to prepare for a game or performance. This includes pregame routines, warm up routines, and actions an athlete will regularly do, mentally and physically, before they execute the performance. Frequently, these will incorporate other commonly used techniques, such as imagery or self-talk. Examples would be visualizations done by skiers, dribbling by basketball players at the foul line, and preshot routines golfers or baseball players use prior to a shot or pitch. These routines help to develop consistency and predictability for the player. This allows the muscles and mind to develop better motor control.

Self-Talk

Self-talk refers to the thoughts and words athletes and performers say to themselves, usually in their minds. Self-talk phrases (or cues) are used to direct attention towards a particular thing in order to improve focus or are used alongside other techniques to facilitate their effectiveness. For example, a softball player may think "release point" when at bat to direct her attention to the point where the pitcher releases the ball, while a golfer may say "smooth stroke" before putting to stay relaxed. Research suggests either positive or negative self-talk may improve performance, suggesting the effectiveness of self-talk phrases depends on how the phrase is interpreted by the individual. The use of words in sport has been widely used. The ability to bombard the unconscious mind with one single positive phrase, is one of the most effective and easy to use psychological skills available to any athlete.

Exercise Psychology

Exercise psychology can be defined as the study of psychological issues and theories related to exercise. Exercise psychology is a sub-discipline within the field of psychology and is typically grouped with sport psychology. For example, Division 47 of the APA is for exercise and sport psychology, not just one or the other, while organizations like AASP encompass both exercise and sport psychology.

The link between exercise and psychology has long been recognized. In 1899, William James discussed the importance of exercise, writing it was needed to "furnish the background of sanity, serenity...and make us good-humored and easy of approach." Other researchers noted the connection between exercise and depression, concluding a moderate amount of exercise was more helpful than no exercise in symptom improvement.

As a sub-discipline, the amount of research in exercise psychology increased in the 1950s and 1960s, leading to several presentations at the second gathering of the International Society of Sport Psychology in 1968. Throughout the 1970s and 1980s, William Morgan wrote several pieces on the relationship between exercise and various topics, such as mood, anxiety, and adherence to exercise programs. Morgan also went on to found APA Division 47 in 1986.

As an interdisciplinary subject, exercise psychology draws on several different scientific fields, ranging from psychology to physiology to neuroscience. Major topics of study are the relationship between exercise and mental health (e.g., stress, affect, self-esteem), interventions that promote physical activity, exploring exercise patterns in different populations (e.g., the elderly, the obese), theories of behavior change, and problems associated with exercise (e.g., injury, eating disorders, exercise addiction).

Recent evidence also suggests that besides mental health and well-being, sport practice can improve general cognitive abilities. When requiring sufficient cognitive demands, physical activity seems to be an optimal way to improve cognition, possibly more efficiently than cognitive training or physical exercise alone

Physical Medicine and Rehabilitation

Physical medicine and rehabilitation (PM&R), also known as physiatry or rehabilitation medicine, or physical and rehabilitation medicine (PRM) outside of the United States, is a branch of medicine that aims to enhance and restore functional ability and quality of life to those with physical impairments or disabilities. A physician having completed training in this field is referred to as a physiatrist. Physiatrists specialize in restoring optimal function to people with injuries to the muscles, bones, ligaments, or nervous system.

Scope of the Field

In the hospital setting, physiatrists commonly treat patients who have had an amputation, spinal cord injury, stroke, traumatic brain injury, and other debilitating injuries. In treating these patients, physiatrists lead an interdisciplinary team of physical, occupational, recreational and speech therapists, nurses, psychologists, and social workers. In outpatient settings, physiatrists also treat patients with muscle and joint injuries, pain syndromes, non-healing wounds, and other disabling conditions. Physiatrists are trained to perform intramuscular and interarticular injections as well as nerve conduction studies.

History

The specialty that came to be known as PM&R was officially established in 1947, when an independent board of Physical Medicine was established under the authority of the American Board of Medical Specialties. During the first half of the 20th century, two unofficial specialties, physical medicine and rehabilitation medicine, developed separately, but in practice both treated similar patient populations consisting of those with disabling injuries. Frank H. Krusen was a pioneer of physical medicine, which emphasized the use of physical agents, such as hydrotherapy and hyperbaric oxygen, at Temple University and then at Mayo Clinic and it was he that coined the term 'physiatry' in 1938. Rehabilitation medicine gained prominence during both World Wars in the treatment of injured soldiers and laborers. Howard A. Rusk, an internal medicine physician from Missouri, became a pioneer of rehabilitation medicine after being appointed to rehabilitate air force pilots during WWII. In 1943, the Baruch Committee, commissioned by philanthropist Bernard Baruch, defined the specialty as a combination of the two fields and laid the framework for its acceptance as an official medical specialty. The committee also distributed funds to establish training and research programs across the nation. In 1949, at the insistence of Dr. Rusk and others, the specialty incorporated rehabilitation medicine and changed its name to Physical Medicine and Rehabilitation.

Treatment

The major concern that PM&R deals with as a medical field is the ability of a person to function optimally within the limitations placed upon them by a disabling impairment or disease process for which there is no known cure. The emphasis is not on the full restoration to the premorbid level of function, but rather the optimization of the quality of life for those not able to achieve full restoration. A team approach to chronic conditions is emphasized to coordinate care of patients. Comprehensive Rehabilitation is provided by specialists in this field, who act as facilitators, team leaders, and medical experts for rehabilitation.

Training

In the United States, residency training for PM&R is four years long, including an intern year. There are 80 ACGME accredited programs in the United States across 28 states.

Subspecialties

Six formal sub-specializations are recognized by the field in the United States:

- Neuromuscular Medicine

- Pain Medicine

- Pediatric Rehabilitation Medicine

- Spinal Cord Injury Medicine

- Sports Medicine

- Brain Injury Medicine

Other subspecialties within the field that are recognized include the following:

- Hospice and palliative medicine

- Musculoskeletal pain management

- Intervention physiatry

- Surgical rehabilitation

- Rheumatological rehabilitation

- Obesity and other lifestyle disease modifications

- Cardiopulmonary rehabilitation

- Amputee care

- Electrodiagnostic medicine

- Cancer rehabilitation

Sports Science

Sports science (also sport science) is a discipline that studies how the healthy human body works during exercise, and how sport and physical activity promote health from cellular to whole body perspectives. The study of sports science traditionally incorporates areas of physiology (exercise physiology), psychology (sport psychology), anatomy, biomechanics, biochemistry and biokinetics. Sports scientists and performance consultants are growing in demand and employment numbers, with the ever-increasing focus within the sporting world on achieving the best results possible. Through the study of science and sport, researchers have developed a greater understanding on how the human body reacts to exercise, training, different environments and many other stimuli.

Origins of Exercise Physiology

Sports Science can trace its origins to ancient Greece. The noted ancient Greek physician Galen (131–201) wrote 87 detailed essays about improving health (proper nutrition), aerobic fitness, and strengthening muscles. Assyrian Hunayn ibn Ishaq translated Galen's work, along with that of Hippocrates, into Arabic which led to the spread of Greek physiology throughout the Middle East and Europe. Between 776 BC to 393 AD, the ancient Greek physicians planned the training regimens and diets of the Olympic competitors.

New ideas upon the working and functioning of the human body emerged during the renaissance as anatomists and physicians challenged the previously known theories. These spread with the implementation of the printed word, the result of Gutenberg's printing press in the 15th century. Allied with this was a large increase in academia in general, universities were forming all around the world. Importantly these new scholars went beyond the simplistic notions of the early Greek physicians, and shed light upon the complexities of the circulatory, and digestive systems. Furthermore, by the middle of the 19th century early medical schools (such as the Harvard Medical School, formed 1782) began appearing in the United States, whose graduates went on to assume positions of importance in academia and allied medical research.

Medical journal publications increased significantly in number during this period. In 1898, three articles on physical activity appeared in the first volume of the *American Journal of Physiology*. Other articles and reviews subsequently appeared in prestigious journals. The German applied physiology publication, *Internationale Zeitschrift fur Physiologie einschliesslich Arbeitphysiologie* (1929–1940; now known as the European Journal of Applied Physiology and Occupational Physiology), became a significant journal in the field of research.

A number of key figures have made significant contributions to the discipline, including the following:

- Austin Flint, Jr., (1836–1915) One of the first American pioneer physicians, studied physiological responses to exercise in his influential medical textbooks.

- Edward Hitchcock, Jr., (1828–1911) Amherst College Professor of hygiene and physical education, devoted his academic career to the scientific study of physical exercise, training and the body. Coauthored 1860 text on exercise physiology.

- George Wells Fitz, M.D. (1860–1934) Created the first departmental major in Anatomy, Physiology, and Physical Training at Harvard University in 1891.

- August Krogh (1874–1949) Won the 1920 Nobel prize in physiology for discovering the mechanism that controlled capillary blood flow in resting or active muscle.

- Per-Olof Astrand (1922–2015) Professor at the Department of physiology, Karolinska Institute, Stockholm. Wrote seminal paper which evaluated the physical working capacity of men and women aged 4–33 years.

Study of Sports Science

Higher-education degrees in Sports Science or Human Physiology are also becoming increasingly popular with many universities now offering both undergraduate, postgraduate and distance learning degrees in the discipline. Opportunities for graduates in these fields employment as a Physical Education teacher, Dietician or Nutritionist, Performance Analyst, Sports coach, Sports therapist, Fitness centre manager, Sports administrator, Strength and Conditioning specialist or retail manager of a Sports store. Graduates may also be well positioned to undertake further training to become an accredited Physiotherapist, Exercise Physiologist, Research Scientist and Sports Medical Doctor.

There are many noted institutions in the United Kingdom which run courses in Sports Science. Some of the better known are University of Brighton, St Mary's University, Twickenham University of Kent – School of Sport & Exercise Sciences, Nottingham Trent University, Durham, University of Derby (fastest rising in the league tables at this time 2014 Guardian League table) Leeds, Loughborough, Exeter, Oxford Brookes University, Bath, Bangor, Birmingham, University of Chichester, Edinburgh, Liverpool John Moores, University of Portsmouth, Manchester Metropolitan University and Stirling.

In the United States, institutions offering related degrees include Jackson State University, University of Connecticut, University of Nebraska-Lincoln, Ohio State University, University of Florida, University of Missouri.

Orthopaedic Sports Medicine

Orthopedic Sports Medicine is a subspecialty of orthopedic medicine and sports medicine. The word orthopaedic derives from "ortho" which is the Greek root for "straight" and "pais" which is the Greek root for child. During the early history of orthopaedic medicine, orthopaedists used braces, among other things, to make a child "straight." Today, orthopaedists are making people of all ages "straight," including athletes from all different kinds of sports.

Subspecialty: Orthopaedic Sports Medicine

The phrase "sports medicine" is not specific to one career/profession. It instead, encompasses a group of professionals from various disciplines whose focus is the health of an athlete. Athletes can be all ages and play on all different levels (youth, high school, collegiate, recreational, and professional).

Orthopaedic sports medicine is the investigation, preservation, and restoration by medical, surgical, and rehabilitative means to all structures of the musculoskeletal system affected by athletic activity.

Orthopaedic Sports Medicine Specialist

Any Accredited Council for Graduate Medical Education (ACGME) residency trained orthopaedist can practice orthopaedic sports medicine. Their training specifically provides them with the skills to care for athletes' musculoskeletal needs.

What They Do

Orthopaedic sports medicine specialists...

- Condition and train athletes.

- Provide fitness advice relating to athletic performance.

- Give advice on athletic performance and the impact of dietary supplements, pharmaceuticals, and nutrition on athletes' short- and long-term health and performance.

- Coordinate medical care within athletic team settings, including other health care professionals, such as athletic trainers, physical therapists, and non-orthopaedic physicians.

- Conduct on-the-field evaluation and management of illnesses and injuries.

What They Know

Orthopaedic sports medicine specialists have a knowledge of...

- Soft tissue biomechanics, injury healing, and repair.

- Treatment options, both surgical and non-surgical, as they relate to sports-specific injuries and competition.

- Principles and techniques of rehabilitation that enable the athlete to return to competition as quickly and safely as possible.

- Knowledge of athletic equipment and orthotic devices (braces, foot orthoses, etc.) and their use in prevention and management of athletic injuries.

Schooling

A person interested in becoming an orthopaedic sports medicine specialist must complete four years of medical school. After their undergraduate schooling is completed, training continues with a five year residency in orthopaedics. In order to sub-specialize, which is the case with an orthopaedic sports medicine, a one-year fellowship is required, although some programs extend two to four years.

After they have finished their training and have graduated from an accredited residency, orthopaedic surgeons are eligible to become certified by the American Board of Orthopaedic Surgery (ABOS). Certification by the Board is required in order to practice. In addition, the orthopaedist who plans on specializing in sports medicine must complete certification in the sports medicine sub-specialty which is administered by the ABOS. Education does not stop there; orthopaedists are required to take continuing education classes to maintain their license.

Careers

Orthopaedist specializing in sports medicine have various options of employment: from serving as a team's physician (high school, college, and professional), to running a private practice, to working in the academic setting.

According to a salary.com, the data they collected from HR reported data in August 2008 showed that an orthopaedic surgeon, on average, made about $396,343 a year not including bonuses and benefits.

Sports Nutrition

Sports Nutrition is the study and practice of nutrition and diet,with regards to a person's athletic performance. Nutrition is an important part of many sports training regimens, being most popular in strength sports (such as weight lifting and bodybuilding) and endurance sports (for example cycling, running, swimming,rowing). Sports Nutrition focuses its studies on the type, as well as the quantity of fluid and food taken by an athlete. In addition, it deals with the consumption of nutrients such as vitamins, minerals, supplements,and organic substances that includecarbohydrates, proteins and fats.

Supplements

Dietary supplements contain one or more dietary ingredients (including vitamins; minerals; herbs or other botanicals; amino acids; and other substances) or their constituents;is intended to be taken by mouth as a pill, capsule, tablet, or liquid. All athletes consider taking dietary supplements with hopes to find the "magic ingredient" to increase their athletic performance. In the extreme case of performance-enhancing supplements, athletes, particularly bodybuilders may choose to use illegal substances such as anabolic steroids. These compounds which are related to the hormone testosterone, can quickly build mass and strength, but have many adverse effects such as high blood pressure and negative gender specific effects. Blood doping, another illegal ergogenic, was discovered in the 1940s when it was used by World War II pilots. Blood doping also known as blood transfusions, increases oxygen delivery to exercising tissues and has been demonstrated to improve performance in endurance sports, such as long-distance cycling. There are many other supplements out there and they include caffeine, creatine, iron, chromium and human growth hormones.

In the 1940s, early results were found regarding consumption of dietary protein for athletes involved in muscle building and resistance, and strength training. Dietary proteins main uses are for hormones, oxygen transport, cellular repair, enzymes and conversion to fuel. The intake of protein is a part of the nutrient requirements for the normal athlete and is an important component of exercise training. In addition, it aids in performance and recovery. Dietary protein intake for well-trained athletes should occur before, during and after physical activity as it is advantageous in gaining muscle mass and strength. However, if too much protein and amino acid supplements are consumed (especially by the average exerciser), it can be more harmful than beneficial; health risks include: "dehydration, gout, calcium loss, liver, and renal damage. Gastrointestinal side effects of over consumption include diarrhea, bloating, and water loss" (Lawerence). A bountiful protein diet must be paired with a healthy, well-rounded meal plan and regular resistance exercise. Characteristics of this particular diet include the type of exercise, intensity, duration and carbohydrate values of diet. The most effective way to secure the natural nutrients required by your body for optimum health and physiological performance is by eating your vitamins, minerals, proteins, fats, sugars and carbohydrates, which can be procured from fresh fruits and vegetables, as nature intended them to be received.

The supplement,Creatine, may be helpful for well-trained athletes to increase exercise performance and strength in relation with their dietary regimen. The substance glutamine, found in whey protein supplements, is the most abundant free amino acid found in the human body. It is considered that glutamine may have a possible role in stimulated anabolic processes such as muscle glycogen and protein synthesis, for well-trained and well-nourished athletes. Other popular studies done on supplements include androstenedione, chromium, and ephedra. The findings show that there are no substantial benefits from the extra intake of these supplements, yet higher health risks and costs.

High energy supplements have shown to increase the performance of physical activity in athletes. A study done at the University of Texas saw a 4.7% increase of performance in 83% of participants after drinking Red Bull Energy Drink which was more intense than the compared placebo. The energy drink most dominantly increased the epinephrine and norepinephrine (adrenaline and its precursor) levels and beta-endorphins in the blood than before consumption. Caffeine, carbohydrates and Vitamin B are factors that may have favored no change in perceived exertion, but an increase in performance.

Caffeine has been around since the 1900s and became popularly used in the 1970s when its power of masking fatigue became highly recognized. Similarly, the caffeine found in energy drinks and coffee shows an increased reaction performance and feelings of energy, focus and alertness in quickness and reaction anaerobic power tests. In other words, consuming an energy drink or any drink with caffeine increases short time/rapid exercise performance (like short full-speed sprints and heavy power weight lifting). Caffeine is chemically similar to adenosine, a type of sugar that helps in the regulation of important body processes, including the firing of neurotransmitters. Caffeine takes the place of adenosine in your brain, attaching itself to the same neural receptors affected by adenosine, and causing your neurons to fire more rapidly, hence caffeine's stimulating effects.

Post-exercise nutrition is just as important, if not more important than pre-exercise nutrition as it pertains to the recovery of the body. Traditionally, sports drinks such as Gatorade and Powerade, are consumed during and after exercise because they effectively rehydrate the body by refueling the body with minerals and electrolytes. Electrolytes regulate our nerve and muscle function, our body's hydration, blood pH, blood pressure, and the rebuilding of damaged tissue.Gatorade was founded in the 1960s, when the University of Florida, Gainesville Gators improved their performance with "Gator Aid." The drink was made of glucose and sucrose in water and was seen to improve the football players' performance. By the 1970s, many other sports drinks of its kind had been manufactured.

Studies in 2008 have found cow's milk, especially skim milk and chocolate milk may be effective replacements for current sports drink , as milk leads to protein the synthesis which boosts net muscle protein balance. Milk contains many electrolytes, nutrients and other elements that help to make it an effective post-exercise beverage. It is true that chocolate milk has been a proven study that is just as effective of a recovery drink as Gatorade. Chocolate Milk includes key ingredients such as Vitamin D that helps replace fluids and electrolytes lost after the athlete has worked out. A recovery drink is supposed to replenish the sugar lost, and build muscle again so that you are ready for the next workout. When compared to plain water or sports drinks, research suggests that chocolate milk is more effective at replacing fluids lost through sweat and maintaining normal body fluid levels. Athletes drinking chocolate milk following exercise-induced dehydration had fluid levels about 2 percent higher (on initial body mass) than those using other post-exercise recovery beverages. These results allowed for prolonged performance, especially in repeated bouts of exercise or training.

Factors Influencing Nutritional Requirements

Differing conditions and objectives suggest the need for athletes to ensure that their sports nutritional approach is appropriate for their situation. Factors that may affect an athlete's nutritional needs include type of activity (aerobic vs. anaerobic), gender, weight, height, body mass index, workout or activity stage (pre-workout, intro-work-out, recovery), and time of day (e.g. some nutrients are utilized by the body more effectively during sleep than while awake).Most culprits that get in the way of performance are fatigue, injury and soreness. A proper diet will reduce these disturbances in performance. The key to a proper diet is to get a variety of food, and to consume all the macro-nutrients, vitamins, and minerals needed. According to Eblere's article (2008), it is ideal to choose raw foods, for example unprocessed foods such as oranges instead of orange juice. Eating foods that are natural means the athlete is getting the most nutritional value out of the food. When foods are processed, the nutritional value is normally reduced.

Anaerobic Exercise

During anaerobic exercise, the process of glycolysis breaks down the sugars from carbohydrates for energy without the use of oxygen. This type of exercise occurs in physical activity such as power sprints, strength resistances and quick explosive movement where the muscles are being used for power and speed, with short-time energy use. After this type of exercise, there is a need to refill glycogen storage sites in the body (the long simple sugar chains in the body that store energy), although they are not likely fully depleted.

To compensate for this glycogen reduction, athletes will often take in large amounts of carbohydrates, immediately following their exercise. Typically, high-glycemic-index carbohydrates are preferred for their ability to rapidly raise blood glucose levels.For the purpose of protein synthesis, protein or individual amino acids are ingested as well. Branched-chain amino acids are important since they are most responsible for the synthesis of protein. According to Lemon et al. (1995) female endurance runners have the hardest time getting enough protein in their diet. Endurance athletes in general need more protein in their diet than the sedentary person.Research has shown that endurance athletes are recommended to have 1.2 to 1.4 g of protein per kg of body weight in order to repair damaged tissue. If the athlete consumes too few calories for the body's needs, lean tissue will be broken down for energy and repair. Protein deficiency can cause many problems such as early and extreme fatigue, particularly long recovery, and poor wound healing. Complete proteins such as meat, eggs, and soy provide the athlete with all essential amino acids for synthesizing new tissues. However, vegetarian and vegan athletes frequently combine legumes with a whole grain to provide the body with a complete protein across the day's food intake. A popular combination being rice and beans.

Spada's research on endurance sports nutrition (2000) and where the types of carbohydrates come from will be explained. He advises for carbohydrates to be unprocessed and/or whole grains for optimal performance while training. These carbohydrates offer the most fuel, nutritional value, and satiety. Fruits and vegetables contribute important carbohydrate foundation for an athlete's diet. They provide vitamins and minerals that are lost through exercise and later needed to be replenished. Both fruits and vegetables improve healing, aid in recovery, and reduce risks of cancer, high blood pressure, and constipation. Vegetables offer a little more nutritional value than fruits for the amount of calories, therefore an athlete should strive to eat more vegetables than fruits. Dark-colored vegetables usually have more nutritional value than pale colored ones.(add info) A general rule is the darker the color the more nutrient dense it is. Like all foods, it is very important to have a variety. To get the most nutritional value out of fruits and vegetables it is important to eat them in their natural, unprocessed form with no other nutrient (sugar) added.

Often in the continuation of this anaerobic exercise, the product from this metabolic mechanism builds up in what is called lactic acid fermentation. Lactate is produced more quickly than it is being removed and it serves to regenerate NAD^+ cells on where it's needed. During intense exercise when oxygen is not being used, a high amount of ATP is produced and pH levels fall causing acidosis or more specifically lactic acidosis. Lactic acid build up can be treated by staying well-hydrated throughout and especially after the workout, having an efficient cool down routine and good post-workout stretching.

Intense activity can cause significant and permanent damage to bodily tissues. In order to repair, vitamin E and other antioxidants are needed to protect muscle damage. Oxidation damage and muscle tissue breakdown happens during endurance running so athletes need to eat foods high in protein in order to repair these muscle tissues. It is important for female endurance runners to consume proper nutrients in their diet that will repair, fuel, and minimize fatigue and injury. To keep a female runner's body performing at its best, the ten nutrients need to be included in their diets.

References

- *Verville, Richard (2009). War, Politics, and Philanthropy The History of Rehabilitation Medicine. Lanham, Maryland: University Press of America. ISBN 978-0-7618-4594-2.*

- Balish, S. M., Eys, M. A., & Schulte-Hostedde, A. I. (2013). Evolutionary sport and exercise psychology: Integrating proximate and ultimate explanations. Psychology of Sport and Exercise, 14(3), 413-422. doi: 10.1016/j.psychsport.2012.12.006

- "Moreau, D., & Conway, A. R. A. (2013). Cognitive enhancement: A comparative review of computerized and athletic training programs. International Review of Sport and Exercise Psychology, 6(1), 155-183. doi:10.1080/1750984X.2012.758763"

- Gould, D., & Pick, S. (1995). Sport psychology: The Griffith Era, 1920-1940. *The Sport Psychologist, 9,* 391-405. Retrieved June 25, 2011 from PsycNET.

- Orlick, T., & Partington, J. (1988). Mental links to excellence. *The Sport Psychologist, 2*(2), 105–130. Retrieved June 25, 2011 from Precision Management Institute.

- Danish, S. J., & Hale, B. D. (1981). Toward an understanding of the practice of sport psychology. *Journal of Sport Psychology, 3,* 90-99. Retrieved June 25, 2011 from PsycNET.

- Heyman, S. R. (1982). A reaction to Danish and Hale: A minority report. *Journal of Sport Psychology, 4,* 7-9. Retrieved June 25, 2011 from PsycNET.

- Dishman, R. K. (1983). Identity crisis in North American sport psychology: Academics in professional issues. *Journal of Sport Psychology, 5,* 123-134. Retrieved June 25, 2011 from PsycNET.

- Silva, J. M. (1989). Toward the professionalization of sport psychology. *The Sport Psychologist, 3*(3), 265-273. Retrieved June 25, 2011 from PsycNET.

- Weinberg, Robert S. and Daniel Gould. "Goal Setting." Foundation of Sport and Exercise Psychology. Myles Schrag. Courier Printing, 2011. 350-351. Print

Permissions

Index

A

Achilles Tendon Rupture, 72-76, 122

Aerobic Exercise, 78, 132-133, 135, 137-138, 140-142, 145-148, 150-151, 158, 164, 203, 215-216, 221, 224

Altitude Training, 229-234, 257

Anterior Impingement, 10

Aquatic Bodywork, 289, 291

Aquatic Therapy, 289-291, 300

Arthroscopic Surgery, 68, 89

Athletic Heart Syndrome, 78, 81

B

Biomechanics, 25-26, 207, 210, 238, 251, 254, 265, 296, 302, 316, 319

Bleeding, 27, 37, 40, 44, 47-48, 50, 59, 76, 112, 114-115, 120

Blister, 30

Bodyweight Exercise, 132, 169

Boxer's Fracture, 6-7

Brain Injury, 34-35, 40-43, 98-99, 108, 268, 314-315

Breastroker's Knee, 25-27

C

Cardiac Arrest, 82, 85-87, 114, 119, 127, 130

Cardiomegaly, 78-79, 81

Cardiovascular System, 30, 132, 135, 146, 152, 215

Carpal Tunnel Syndrome, 63, 94

Climbing Injuries, 94

Combat Athletes, 7

Commotio Cordis, 85-88

Concussion, 3, 35-38, 97-99, 126-127, 130, 250, 253

Convulsion, 98

D

Dehydration, 105, 107, 126, 128-130, 164, 207-208, 243, 320, 322

Diastolic Pressure, 79, 246

Dry Needling, 67, 259, 268, 279-286, 300

E

Eating Disorder, 100

Eccentric Muscle Contractions, 84

Epidemiological Evidence, 135

Epiphyseal Plate, 10, 288, 294

Exercise Hypertension, 144, 246

Exercise Prescription, 3, 108

Exertional Rhabdomyolysis, 104-108

Extensor Carpi Radialis Brevis Muscle, 28, 63, 65-66

F

Female Athlete Triad, 99-102, 104, 124

Fencing Response, 97-99

Fluoroquinolone Antibiotics, 73

Foot Injuries, 22

Footballer's Ankle, 6, 10

Forearm Muscles, 61, 159, 210

Fungal Pathogens, 31

G

Golfer's Elbow, 6, 20-22, 62, 95

H

Heart Rate, 78, 80, 82, 87, 110, 112, 141, 146-147, 216, 221, 235, 242

High Intensity Interval Training, 221

Hydration Levels, 105, 208

Hypokinetic Diseases, 217

I

Inflammation, 10, 21-22, 25-27, 48, 53, 63-64, 71, 84, 89, 95, 111, 120, 136-137, 223, 241, 277-278, 290

J

J Curve, 136

L

Lateral Epicondylitis, 21, 27, 61, 63-64, 66-68, 95

Little League Elbow, 9, 20, 288, 294

M

Martial Arts, 34, 86, 97, 150, 203, 225, 236, 253

Medial Epicondyle, 20-21

Medial Tibial Stress Syndrome, 69, 72

Metacarpal Bones, 6

Molluscum Contagiosum, 31

Muscle Atrophy, 8, 30, 137

Muscular Endurance, 11, 204, 220

Musculoskeletal Injury, 30, 233

N

Netball Injuries, 14

Nutrition, 46, 50, 101-104, 124-125, 143, 164, 217, 223, 228, 238, 250-251, 257, 296, 316, 318-321, 323

O

Open Surgery, 68, 77

Orthopaedic Sports Medicine, 4, 318-319

Orthopedic Surgery, 1, 30, 268

Orthostatic Hypotension, 100

Over-pronation, 70

Overtraining, 124, 139, 144, 155-156, 229, 240-244, 257-258, 309

P

Pain Management, 315

Patellar Dislocation, 88-93

Patellar Tendinitis, 83

Physical Exercise, 132-138, 140, 142-145, 151, 208, 215, 217, 224, 240-241, 250, 314, 317

Physical Fitness, 1, 16, 125, 129, 132, 134, 144, 150, 217-220, 222-224

Physical Medicine and Rehabilitation, 259, 302, 314

Physical Rehabilitation, 255, 263, 265-266, 289

Physical Therapy, 28, 92-93, 254, 259-270, 281, 284-285, 289, 297

Plantarflexion, 73-74, 77

Post-concussion Syndrome, 37

Post-traumatic Distress, 47, 52

Q

Quadriceps Muscle, 84, 90, 92

R

Rapid Acceleration, 11

Repetitive Strain Injury, 63

S

Saddle Sore, 61, 96

Shin Splints, 3, 61, 69-72

Shoulder Injuries, 22-25, 95, 288, 294

Skin Abrasion, 96

Skin Infections, 31-34

Soft Tissue, 10-11, 48, 75-76, 89, 93, 208, 319

Sport and Exercise Medicine, 1, 4

Sport Psychology, 302-309, 313, 316, 324

Sports Hypnosis, 229, 238-239, 296

Sports Injury, 45, 48-49, 51, 60, 94, 110

Sports Medicine, 1, 4, 30, 44, 47-48, 59-60, 78, 93, 124-125, 129, 132, 153, 229, 235, 254, 259, 263, 269, 278-279, 289-290, 292, 302, 315, 318-319

Sports Science, 225, 235-236, 238, 296, 302, 316-317

Sprain, 3, 12, 23, 46-47, 95, 119-120

Strength Training, 28, 30, 79, 132, 142, 146, 151-156, 158, 163-170, 202-204, 214-215, 224, 228, 320

Strengthening, 21, 27, 30, 66-67, 71, 78, 127, 132, 134, 147, 168, 218-219, 279, 301, 316

Stretching, 21, 27, 30, 46, 49, 67, 78, 119, 127, 134, 165, 203, 206, 227, 237-238, 254, 301, 323

Sudden Cardiac Death, 80-82, 86

Surgical Graft Procedure, 286, 293

Swimming Injuries, 25

T

Tendinosis, 20, 24, 48, 63-64, 75, 83

Tendon Sheaths, 94

Tennis Elbow, 20-21, 27-28, 48, 61-69, 95

Tennis Injuries, 27

Tommy John Surgery, 10, 286, 288, 293, 295

Traumatic Injuries, 47

U

Ulnar Collateral Ligament, 10, 286, 288, 293-294

Ulnar Nerve, 22, 287-288, 294

V

Vascular System, 107

Vastus Lateralis, 89-90, 92

Volleyball Injuries, 22

W

Weight Training, 26, 109, 127, 132-133, 151-153, 155, 158-159, 163, 166-168, 202-206, 208-210, 214-215, 218

Western Riding, 96

Wrestling, 31-35, 55-56, 59, 126, 128, 130, 151, 203, 253

www.ingramcontent.com/pod-product-compliance
Lightning Source LLC
Chambersburg PA
CBHW061930190326
41458CB00009B/2706